MAKING
YOUR
BAD BACK
BETTER

with

THE O'CONNOR TECHNIQUE (TM)
HOW YOU CAN BECOME YOUR OWN CHIROPRACTOR

Copyright © 1997
Revised 1999

by

William T. O'Connor, Jr., M.D.

MAKING YOUR BAD BACK BETTER
WITH THE O'CONNOR TECHNIQUE (TM)
HOW YOU CAN BECOME YOUR OWN CHIROPRACTOR
by
William Thomas O'Connor, Jr., M.D.
Copyright © 1997
Revised 1999

PUBLISHED BY

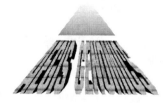

AEGIS GENOMICS
P.O. BOX 808
VACAVILLE, CA. 95696

LIBRARY OF CONGRESS CATALOGUING DATA
O'Connor, William T.
Making your bad back better with the O'Connor technique / by William T. O'Connor, Jr.
1. Backache–Exercise Therapy   2. Backache–Diagnosis   3. Backache–Prevention   4. Intervertebral disk–Diseases
Library of Congress Catalogue Number 98-146084
Call Number: RD771.B217O26 1997   Dewey Number: 617.5/64 21

ISBN 0-9664991-1-5 $37.95
                                                                                                                Softcover
Printed in the United States of America

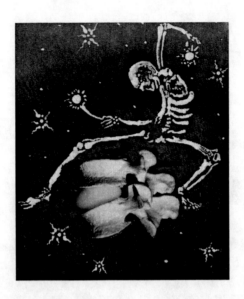

Special thanks to:
Kate Fortin, my wife, for her editorial expertise and support, as well as Ann Fortin (proofreading), David Best (photography), Mindy (modeling), and Gary Rains (printing) for their generous assistance.

Cover: Illustration from a 15th Century Turkish translation of the 12th Century Persian Manuscript: *Imperial Surgery*.

WARNING–DISCLAIMER

THIS BOOK CONTAINS INFORMATION AND INSTRUCTIONS INTENDED TO ALLEVIATE SPINAL PAIN ORIGINATING IN THE INTERVERTEBRAL DISCS. JUDICIOUS AND REASONABLE CARE WAS TAKEN, IN GOOD FAITH, TO INSURE THAT NOTHING INTRINSICALLY DANGEROUS WAS ADVOCATED AND THAT THE TECHNIQUES DISCUSSED WERE BOTH SAFE AND EFFECTIVE. SINCE *THE O'CONNOR TECHNIQUE (TM)* IS A SELF-ADMINISTERED METHOD, THE PERFORMER CREATES, PRECIPITATES, AND HAS THE FULL AND ULTIMATE RESPONSIBILITY FOR ITS EFFECT AND CONSEQUENCES. IT IS IMPOSSIBLE FOR THE AUTHOR, PUBLISHER, OR ANYONE CONNECTED WITH THE DISTRIBUTION OF THIS BOOK TO INDIVIDUALLY DIAGNOSE, OR EXCLUDE AS A DIAGNOSIS, ANY AND ALL DANGEROUS CONDITIONS THAT MAY RESULT IN AN ALLEGATION OF PERSONAL INJURY OR HARM AND/OR PREDICT EVERY POSSIBLE RAMIFICATION FROM PRACTICING THIS METHOD; THEREFORE, <u>BEFORE READING OR PRACTICING THE TECHNIQUES IN THIS BOOK, THE READER OF THIS BOOK OR PRACTITIONER OF THIS TECHNIQUE MUST AGREE TO ASSUME ANY AND ALL LIABILITY FOR ANY POTENTIAL, REAL OR IMAGINED HARM OR RESULTANT DAMAGES BROUGHT ON BY ACTING UPON THE INFORMATION.</u>

NOTHING IN THIS BOOK IS INTENDED TO SUBSTITUTE FOR OR SUPPLANT AN ACCURATE DIAGNOSIS OR PROPER TREATMENT BY A QUALIFIED MEDICAL PRACTITIONER. NOTHING SAID IN THIS BOOK SHOULD BE INTERPRETED TO DISSUADE THE READER FROM SEEKING APPROPRIATE MEDICAL CARE ELSEWHERE FOR THEIR OWN INDIVIDUAL PROBLEM. DUE TO THE COMPLEXITY OF THE HUMAN CONDITION, THE READER IS ENCOURAGED TO SEEK QUALIFIED MEDICAL ADVICE PRIOR TO INITIATING OR ACTING UPON ANY COMPONENT OF THE METHODOLOGY DESCRIBED IN THIS BOOK TO INSURE THAT TO DO SO WOULD BE WITHOUT RISK OF FURTHER DAMAGE OR HARM. TO FURTHER UNDERSTAND THE BULK OF CONSIDERATIONS ATTENDANT WITH PRACTICING *THE O'CONNOR TECHNIQUE (TM)* THE READER IS INSTRUCTED TO READ THE INTRODUCTION AND ALL ELEMENTS PERTINENT TO THE READER'S PROBLEM IN THEIR ENTIRETY PRIOR TO ATTEMPTING ANY PHYSICAL ACTIONS. <u>IF YOU DO NOT CHOOSE TO BE BOUND BY THE ABOVE UNDERSTANDING, RETURN THIS BOOK FOR A FULL REFUND.</u>

TABLE OF CONTENTS

INTRODUCTION

THE MAGIC REVEALED

THE O'CONNOR TECHNIQUE (TM) IS BASED UPON THE UNDERSTANDING THAT THE OVERWHELMING MAJORITY OF BACK PAIN ORIGINATES FROM SPINAL MECHANICAL PROBLEMS IN WHICH DISC MATERIAL HAS BEEN PHYSICALLY DISPLACED. *THE O'CONNOR TECHNIQUE (TM)* DESCRIBES A METHOD IN WHICH BACK PAIN SUFFERERS THEMSELVES CAN IDENTIFY THE NATURE OF THE PROBLEM, RELOCATE THE DISPLACED DISC MATERIAL, AND PREVENT IT FROM DISLOCATING AGAIN.

IN ORTHOPEDIC JARGON, THE BOOK'S ENTIRE PRINCIPLE CAN BE CONDENSED INTO A FEW, CONCISE, INSTRUCTIONS:

*FIRST, DEMONSTRATE THAT THE ACUTE, RECURRENT, OR CHRONIC SPINAL PAIN'S ETIOLOGY IS REFERENCED TO A SPECIFIC INTERVERTEBRAL DISC HERNIATION VIA A **PARTIALLY WEIGHT-BEARING DIAGNOSTIC CIRCUMDUCTION** MANEUVER. THEN, MANUALLY REDUCE THE HERNIATION BY EXECUTING, IN SEQUENCE, A **FLEXION-IN-TRACTION** CONTRALATERAL TO THE AREA OF PAIN REFERENCE, **THERAPEUTICALLY CIRCUMDUCTING IN TRACTION** TO EFFECT AN **EXTENSION-IN-TRACTION IPSILATERAL** TO THE PAIN REFERENCE AREA WITHOUT CONTRACTING THE PARASPINAL MUSCULATURE, AND **RE-WEIGHT-BEARING** WHILE **MAINTAINING HYPEREXTENSION**. THEREAFTER, PRESERVE THIS REDUCTION BY ASSIDUOUSLY AVOIDING **ACTIVE AND PASSIVE WEIGHT-BEARING FLEXION, MAINTAINING EXTENSION,** AND SELECTIVELY EXERCISING TO **HYPERTROPHY MUSCULATURE** SO AS TO DYNAMICALLY ALTER THE WEIGHT-BEARING LOAD ON THE AFFECTED DISC.*

THERE YOU HAVE IT! IF YOU ARE AS KNOWLEDGEABLE AS AN ORTHOPEDIST, THE "MAGIC" IS REVEALED. IF YOU CAN ACCOMPLISH THE ABOVE WITHOUT FURTHER ELABORATION OR EXPLANATION, THEN TRY IT AND SEE WHAT HAPPENS. IN MY CLINICAL EXPERIENCE, THE OVERWHELMING MAJORITY OF BACK PAIN SUFFERERS SUCCESSFULLY ACCOMPLISHING THIS WILL ACHIEVE RECOGNIZABLY DRAMATIC RELIEF IMMEDIATELY OR, AT LEAST, MUCH FASTER THAN ANY OTHER EXISTING BACK PAIN MANAGEMENT PROGRAM AVAILABLE TO DATE.

IF YOU FIND IT DIFFICULT TO UNDERSTAND THE ABOVE INSTRUCTIONS, THEN I SUGGEST YOU READ THIS BOOK AND LEARN HOW YOU CAN REGAIN THE LOST ENJOYMENT OF YOUR LIFE BY **MAKING YOUR BAD BACK BETTER** IN SIMPLE, EASY TO UNDERSTAND LANGUAGE AND ILLUSTRATIONS.

TEST YOURSELF

The prospective reader can rapidly determine if one's particular back pain is most likely caused by a disc problem amenable to *The O'Connor Technique (tm)* as well as quantify for themselves the probability of benefit. In the universe of back pain, one size does not fit all. The more your back problem correlates with affirmative responses to the following test, the more chance you have of successfully looking forward to a less painful and more active future using the methods described in this book.

PERSONS MOST LIKELY TO BENEFIT FROM THIS BOOK ARE THOSE WHO, FOR THE MOST PART, ARE OTHERWISE HEALTHY, NOT ELDERLY, HAVE NO KNOWN MAJOR SPINAL X-RAY ABNORMALITIES UNRELATED TO DISC DISEASE, AND HAVE BACK OR NECK PAIN THAT:

[ ] IS AGGRAVATED MOST OR INCREASED WITH CERTAIN MOVEMENTS, ESPECIALLY BENDING THE SPINE FORWARD OR TO THE SIDE.

[ ] INITIALLY BEGAN WITH AN INJURY WHEREIN FORCE WAS APPLIED TO THE SPINE WHILE IT WAS BENT FORWARD OR TO THE SIDE (SUCH AS LIFTING, AN AUTOMOBILE ACCIDENT, DELIVERY OF A BABY, OR A FALL) AND NOT WHILE BENT BACKWARDS.

[ ] IF OF LONG-STANDING DURATION, IS CHARACTERIZED BY LOW-PAIN OR PAIN-FREE PERIODS PUNCTUATED BY INTERMITTENTLY SEVERE EPISODES SOMETIMES LASTING DAYS, WEEKS, OR MONTHS.

[ ] OFTEN RECURS SUDDENLY WITHOUT TRAUMA OR EXERTION FOR SEEMINGLY NO REASON (SUCH AS COUGHING, SQUATTING, OR EVEN WAKING UP WITH PAIN AND LOSS OF MOBILITY AFTER GOING TO SLEEP WITHOUT ANY PROBLEM.)

[ ] USUALLY IS LOCATED IN THE SAME AREA(S) OF THE BACK.

[ ] FEELS LIKE SOMETHING IS SWOLLEN OR ENLARGED AT THE SITE OF THE PAIN.

[ ] OFTEN RADIATES TO THE SHOULDERS, HIPS, OR LEGS WITH A DULL, ACHING, SENSATION THAT IS HELPED DURING MASSAGE, HEAT, OR COLD, BUT IMMEDIATELY RETURNS AFTERWARDS.

[ ] CAN BE OCCASIONALLY ACCOMPANIED BY NUMBNESS OR TINGLING SENSATIONS IN THE ARMS OR LEGS, ESPECIALLY WITH CERTAIN MOVEMENTS OR REMAINING IN UNCOMFORTABLE POSITIONS.

[ ] DURING EPISODES, HAS POSITIONS OF COMFORT SUCH AS CERTAIN SLEEPING POSITIONS OR A NEED FOR SPECIAL SLEEPING SURFACES OR POSITIONS.

[ ] INCREASES WITH POSITIONS INVOLVING FORWARD BENDING OF THE SPINE WHILE PULLING, PUSHING, LIFTING, COUGHING, OR SNEEZING.

[ ] BECAUSE IT HURTS BENDING TO FAR TO THE SIDE, FORWARD, OR BACKWARDS, THE MOST COMFORTABLE STRATEGY IS TO CAREFULLY BALANCE THE BODY'S WEIGHT ABOVE THE PAIN SLIGHTLY FORWARD.

[ ] IS AGGRAVATED BY PROLONGED SITTING OR ESPECIALLY DRIVING.

[ ] IS SOMEWHAT RELIEVED BY LYING DOWN OR HOLDING YOURSELF IN A POSITION WHERE YOUR ARMS TAKE THE WEIGHT OFF OF YOUR SPINE.

[ ]   AFTER PROLONGED FORWARD BENDING, MAKES THAT AREA OF THE SPINE DIFFICULT OR SLOW TO STRAIGHTEN UP AGAIN.

[ ]   IS ACCOMPANIED BY A STIFFNESS OR DECREASED MOBILITY LEAVING YOU UNABLE TO LOOK OVER YOUR SHOULDER OR BEND TO THE SAME SIDE AS THE PAIN WITHOUT YOUR MOTION BEING STOPPED BY THE PAIN.

[ ]   CAN SOMETIMES BE PAIN-FREE IMMEDIATELY UPON WAKING FROM SLEEP BUT PAIN BEGINS WITH THE PROCESS OF GETTING OUT OF BED OR WITHIN MINUTES AFTER RISING.

[ ]   FEELS AS IF JUST MOVING THE "RIGHT WAY" WOULD RELIEVE THE "CATCH," BUT ATTEMPTS TO DO SO USUALLY RESULT IN INCREASED PAIN.

[ ]   IS AGGRAVATED BY REPETITIVE ACTIVITIES INVOLVING FREQUENT LIFTING, SQUATTING, LEANING FORWARD, OR STOOPING (e.g. VACUUMING, GARDENING, PICKING UP OBJECTS)

[ ]   IS AGGRAVATED BY SITTING WITH THE LEGS STRETCHED STRAIGHT IN FRONT OR PROPPED ABOVE THE LEVEL OF THE HIPS.

[ ]   IS WORSENED BY EXERCISES IN WHICH THE PAINFUL AREA IS BENT FORWARD SUCH AS ROWING, SIT-UPS, OR BICYCLING-TYPE EXERCISES.

[ ]   STANDING OR WALKING CAN SOMETIMES MAKE IT FEEL BETTER.

[ ]   HAS PROMPTED YOU TO GO TO A CHIROPRACTOR OR YOU HAVE BEEN TOLD TO TRY ONE.

[ ]   CAUSES A PINCHING SENSATION IN YOUR LOW BACK OR NECK WHEN LYING ON YOUR STOMACH OR LEANING FAR BACKWARDS AND/OR TO ONE SIDE OR THE OTHER.

[ ]   LIMITS YOUR ACTIVITIES OUT OF FEAR OF INCREASING PAIN OR CAUSING IT TO RETURN.

[ ]   HAS BEEN ASSOCIATED WITH FORCEFUL ACCIDENTS OR TRAUMA RELATED TO THE SPINE; BUT WITHIN MINUTES OF INJURY DIDN'T SEEM TO CAUSE MUCH PAIN, YET WITHIN HOURS THE PAIN PROGRESSIVELY WORSENED AND PERSISTED FOR AN EXTENDED PERIOD.

[ ]   IS OR WAS ASSOCIATED WITH A "POP" OR CRUNCH AT THE TIME OF INJURY AND/OR YOU HEAR CRUNCHING SOUNDS ASSOCIATED WITH PAIN OR ITS RELIEF.

[ ]   CAUSES YOU TO FREQUENTLY "CRACK" YOUR BACK OR NECK TO GET SOME SHORT-TERM RELIEF.

[ ]   IS HELPED, BUT NOT LARGELY RELIEVED, BY MEDICINES.

[ ]   HAS BEEN ATTRIBUTED TO A "DISC," "SLIPPED DISC," "DEGENERATIVE DISC DISEASE OF THE SPINE," "HERNIATED DISC," "ARTHRITIS OF THE SPINE," "MUSCLE SPASM," "STRAIN," "SPRAIN," "PULLED MUSCLE," OR "SCIATICA,"

[ ]   IS NOT ASSOCIATED WITH OTHER SYSTEMIC DISEASES (RHEUMATOID ARTHRITIS, LUPUS, ETC.), GENETIC DISEASES, OR PRIOR SURGERY.

[ ]   IS NOT ASSOCIATED WITH A LOSS OF FUNCTION IN ANY OTHER PART OF YOUR BODY, SUCH AS AN INABILITY TO WALK ON YOUR TOES OR HEELS.

[ ]   DESPITE CONSULTING HEALTH CARE PROVIDER(S), YOU HAVE NOT OBTAINED A CONSISTENT OR SATISFACTORY EXPLANATION FOR THE PAIN NOR BEEN GIVEN SIGNIFICANT OR SUSTAINED RELIEF.

HOW THIS BOOK CAME INTO BEING

It could be that **Nature's most efficient means of remedying a painful condition is to afflict a doctor with it.** Speaking from experience, if I weren't a doctor, I might have been permanently disabled from my own "bad back," addicted to narcotic pain medicines, or have undergone a painful, dangerous surgery without any reasonable certainty that it would have solved my problem; and, ten years later, I statistically would have been no better off than not having had the surgery. Instead, I can lift heavy objects as well as most of my peers, play most sports, do physical labor, sleep comfortably, and I am not in constant, incessant, unrelenting, pain. Most people with "bad backs" would give almost anything to be able live that reality. In a sense, the development of *The O'Connor Technique (tm)* is more a personal triumph than an academic achievement because I can function for the most part without pain; and when pain occurs I can rapidly stop it. Retrospectively, this triumph is tinged with a paradoxical tragedy, in that, had I the knowledge I have now, years ago, when my back first started hurting, I sincerely believe I could have prevented the damage I have sustained through ignorance and significantly reduced the severity of the dreaded *degenerative disc disease*. However, this belief is predicated upon my assumption that I would have followed the appropriate advice if it had been presented to me.

It is difficult to prove whether I would have put forth the effort to sufficiently protect my back without first experiencing the grinding pain of a disc herniation. I believe I would have because I distinctly recall, in my teenage years, attempting to seek advice upon the best posture to prevent the discomfort I was already, by then, experiencing and can distinctly remember being told by nearly everyone: "Keep your back straight," "Be sure to lift with your knees," "Don't rock back on your chair, sit up straight," etc. I did not, then, have the knowledge to understand that **straightening the naturally extended curvature of the Lumbar spine is physiologically and anatomically disadvantageous, lifting with the knees is insufficient advice to prevent lifting damage, and rocking back in a chair actually helps unload the spine.** Adhering to such traditional advice (as I did) served to aggravate the problem rather than alleviate it.

The triumph is that coming upon alternative knowledge, although late, has made my life much more pain-free and largely has prevented further damage and disability. This experience has at least convinced the skeptic in me that even the worst evil has a component of good. Since, had I not been stricken with this pain, I would not have been motivated to help eliminate this particular form of suffering.

I did not set out to write a treatise on back pain. The principle impetus for developing this technique came because I was in pain; and I discovered, to my dismay, that the pre-existing and currently widespread "state-of-the-art" back pain management methods were (and for the most part still are) woefully inadequate. I was forced by circumstance to self-apply the dictum: "Physician--Heal Thy Self." Having largely done so, in the writing of this book, I can share my hard-found ability to prevent pain and disability by educating people in the art of arresting back pain whenever and wherever it occurs, protecting, as well as strengthening their spines against future episodes.

The O'Connor Technique (tm) **did not come suddenly in a burst of creative bathtub genius; rather, it is the product of a physician (myself) living with a radiographically defined disc herniation (See Figure 1, showing my actual CAT scan) for greater than ten years.** I

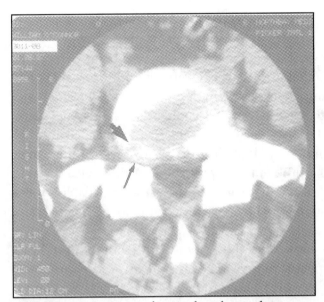

Figure 5 CAT Scan photo of author's disc conveniently oriented with Left/Right inverted so as to be nearly identical to the lesion shown in Figures 17 & 18 in Chapter 2 . Large arrow = piece of herniated disc material, small arrow=bulging capsule.

suffered debilitating pain after a flexion injury, was unable to gain any satisfactory answer as to the cause of the pain or a solution from my colleagues, and resorted to figuring out the problem myself by an intensive study of the spine and the existing available methods for reducing the pain.

In developing *The O'Connor Technique (tm)* and the mechanical solutions to back pain, I started from the basic anatomy and **analyzed it as a mechanical problem rather than a medical one**; then, through a combination of common sense, a study of what existing therapies were beneficial in myself, applied intellect, and good old-fashioned trial-and-error using my own back as an experimental model, I arrived at an elegantly simple, perfectly reasonable explanation of the source for what I discovered was a majority of spinal pain.

Working on myself, experimenting by seeing which techniques worked and which ones didn't, I was able to design and refine the most successful methods of putting my own disc back in place. Later, when I was certain that the effect was not a delusion, coincidence, or some serendipitous result from random activity, I began testing the method on nearly every patient that fit the criteria for a disc problem in my practice. I soon began to achieve very gratifying results in others. People were being helped immediately. They would come into the office bent over, in terrible pain, and nearly unable to move; then, they would leave walking upright without the pain. Carefully selecting patients with disc symptoms upon whom I could test the technique and very carefully using my technique to re-position their discs, I became convinced that this constituted a novel approach to the management of back pain that was predominately successful. As the technique evolved, more and more people were getting beneficial results. If one technique didn't seem to work, I re-examined the problem and altered the technique so as to be able to fine tune it to focus upon the specific areas of pain in the back or neck. I studied what motions and movements were successful in my own back and neck then utilized them whenever patients complained of the same symptoms.

I was understandably anxious in the beginning, after all, the fear of harming people was so much a concern that, at first, I was reluctant to try it on anyone except those who were exhibiting the least symptoms with the lowest probability of having a complete disc protrusion. The subset of patients in whom any manipulation might create an increased chance of nerve damage were carefully screened out from these early trials.

Later, I developed the means to avoid any active manipulations on my part. I was able to limit the clinical activity to those motions that the patients could reasonably have accomplished themselves with normal exercise-type movements. This insured that I did not induce any harm that would not have otherwise reasonably been assumed to have been inevitably occasioned by a return to normal activity. After I convinced myself that so many people were being helped and none were being harmed, I began to use it as a therapeutic trial. Persons with back pain were quickly assessed to rule out a neurosurgical lesion, then they were directed through what are later described in the book as "MANEUVERS." If they got relief, they could be assumed to only have had a disc as the problem because that was the only anatomical area being changed through motion. It came to be so successful and non-traumatic that, if it didn't give nearly immediate relief, I then had evidence to conclude that the problem was probably not disc-related; and I looked for an alternative source of pathology. Since the pain was so easily remediable by this method, which only works on the discs, I also soon found that an extraordinarily high percentage of back pain was attributable to disc pathology.

In both a literal and figurative sense, **I may have figured out the "combination" to a "lock" that has kept countless millions of people imprisoned in pain over the course of centuries**. I make no apologies for the manner in which I arrived at this revelation. For a time, I was both the researcher and the principal human subject.

The use of a single patient by an enquiring mind to scientifically study the anatomical and physiological responses of humans is certainly not without precedent in the history of medical inquiry. William Beaumont, an obscure army surgeon, took advantage of a rare opportunity to pave the way for the present understanding of the gastric process. He treated a gunshot wounded patient in 1822; but the patient was left with a permanent exterior opening in his stomach. He conducted a long series of experiments which he assembled in his classic work *Experiments and Observations on the Gastric Juice and the Physiology of Digestion*.[1] His findings pertaining to digestion made a great contribution to medical science and are just as valid and relevant now as when they were first understood.

I also came to the conclusion that the relief couldn't be sustained without intentionally teaching the method to patients so that they could practice the principles on a continuous basis. If I didn't teach them--I had no way of confirming whether education could sustain the relief. After several years of personally instructing patients and observing the results, I was able to prove to myself that the method could be taught successfully to the average patient and keep them pain-free--it worked!

HOW THIS BOOK CAN BE USED

Do not be intimidated by the implied complexity of this book nor act under the assumption that its concepts will require too much new learning in the absence of a guarantee for absolute benefit. *The O'Connor Technique (tm)* is really not that difficult to understand; and, after taking the preceding test, if it sounds like yours is the type of pain being described, you shouldn't mind the inconvenience of learning something new because your probability of benefiting is so high.

Even for the "normal" back, this book can be of immense value in keeping it that way. Barring some unforseen accident, anyone fore-armed with the knowledge of the spinal mechanical principles put forth in this book can expect to never suffer from back pain. However, if your back was normal you wouldn't have picked up this book in the first place; yet that does not limit the back pain sufferer who wishes to prevent the same fate from befalling their children or loved ones from passing this information on in a preventative manner. So, in the broadest sense, this book is potentially beneficial for everyone. Nevertheless, if you have proceeded this far, you can safely operate under the assumption that the probabilities are decidedly in favor of your pain and stiffness being relieved.

Despite this book's length, *The O'Connor Technique (tm)* does not purport to be a cure-all for all forms of back pain, nor does this book describe all the information I have acquired or that is available on spinal pain. Such would be beyond its scope and my intent, not to mention making a dry subject even more exhaustive and tiresome. Let's face it, back pain literature doesn't lend itself to enjoyable reading. Too, it is not intended to be the final word or an all-encompassing academic and research-oriented treatise on the spine. There are other medical textbooks that cover the general subject of back pain more fully and several back pain books available for non-medical people that lead the reader to believe that they provide such a service. None of them contain the presentation you will read herein.

This book was designed to provide a simple, yet competent description of what has previously been regarded as a mysteriously complex problem. When understood, any reader of average intelligence should be able to perform this physically manipulative method, on themselves, to improve their own back pain. These physical manipulations are called "MANEUVERS" because that is the classic term used in Western medicine to describe any intentionally planned movement which represents an alteration of human anatomical position.

The length of the book relative to how much you actually must read is misleading. **A person can realistically satisfy their own necessity by reading only a relatively small portion.** You may be relieved to know that much of the actual instructions in this book (the MANEUVER sections) are dedicated to specific regions of the spine that are painful for one set of patients yet are probably normal in others. **If a reader's particular pain is located in the low back, that should be the area of pertinence that the individual need focus on, to the exclusion of the exhaustive descriptions of how to perform MANEUVERS on other regions of the spine.** After all, if you don't have neck or thoracic pain, pouring over those areas' details is not an efficient use of time.

The extent of MANEUVER directions mostly satisfies my need to provide as maximally accurate a description as feasible of what movements and positions the reader needs to accomplish with precision; so, it is often repetitive. This is intentional. **It was not meant to be read like a novel; and no one is expected to read every part, unless they have pain in every region of their spine. Nonetheless, it can be read from cover to cover by those who intend to put the principles to work as educators or practitioners.**

Additionally, if you find one MANEUVER is successful, you needn't learn all the other MANEUVERS dedicated to the same spinal region unless you wish to increase your armamentarium. Many patients of mine are satisfied with simply learning one MANEUVER because their back pain events are so few and far between. Others, whose pain episodes are frequent or whose discs are particularly damaged need to learn a repertoire of MANEUVERS for "all occasions." If, after performing the first MANEUVER in the particular series proves unsuccessful or you wish to expand your ability to manage more frequent events in different settings and different manners, then it is recommended that you should learn more.

Feel free to skip through sections of the book. Simply because the most important Sections, the "MANEUVERS" Sections, fall in a particular order, **do not feel that you have to read the book like a mathematics course from start to finish. If you have only low back pain, you can overlook the Thoracic and Cervical Sections. If your pain is located only in the low back, you can feel free to go directly to the section of Chapter Five on LUMBAR (LOW BACK) PAIN MANEUVERS**; and, if you choose, simply elect to **try a MANEUVER pertinent to your particular condition immediately**. If it works for you and relieves your back pain, then that technique may be the limited extent to which you wish to engage spinal pain mechanics and all you really need.

The first MANEUVER of each section was placed at the beginning due to its intrinsic ease balanced against successfulness. For neck pain, one can go directly to the section dedicated to CERVICAL (NECK) PAIN MANEUVERS in Chapter Five; and do the first neck MANEUVER. For chest pain related to the back, go to the section on THORACIC (CHEST) PAIN MANEUVERS. If relief is instantaneous and you are satisfied with that, you needn't pour through the whole treatise. If you can do the MANEUVER effectively, you needn't bother with all the theory, mechanics, or anatomy unless you wish to gain a deeper insight into your back pain and the reason **why** the MANEUVER worked. As expected, if you are unfamiliar with some of the terms you encounter, you can always back up to the Sections in the book that cover those topics. I wrote it in a manner that accommodates that style of reading, assuming that if I relied upon the reader's mastery of the antecedent nomenclature too heavily the practical value of the work would be lost to the average, non-physician, reader.

By reading the section of the book dedicated to the PRINCIPLES common to various MANEUVER actions, you will understand what is happening during the MANEUVERS and better understand the actions relative to what is happening to your back when you make certain specific movements. However, it is not absolutely necessary that you understand them, you can still perform the MANEUVERS without this underlying justification. Largely, the supportive information is provided for those readers who are assisted by theoretical concepts and logical understandings during the learning process.

Too, assuming that the reader's time is valuable, an efficient, time-and-effort conserving means was provided to give the reader an opportunity to determine whether they want to expend the effort to read the whole work. You may think that it is too much of an inconvenience to read a book attempting to teach you something that appears so complicated that you may never understand it; but you shouldn't feel intimidated. **It really is not all that complicated**; and it was designed to be as understandable and readable as possible for lay persons. If some of the MANEUVERS seem overly complex at first, go slow and pay attention to the pictures. For the descriptive text, it may help to have someone read it to you while you go through the motions. Of course, this should be someone who legitimately cares about your welfare or has a vested interest in "**making your bad back better**."

Rest assured, it probably **will not be necessary for you to attempt to master all or a majority of the MANEUVERS,** although it is recommended that one read the entire MANEUVER description before attempting it. **One MANEUVER usually does the trick if it is the right one for your particular problem**. Chances are that the first MANEUVER in the section that concerns you will work; however, if one doesn't work, you can try the next. Similarly, if you can't perform one MANEUVER for some reason, there are multiple other options given. No expensive devices are needed.

I understand the necessity for this strategy because I got a dose of reality when one patient I had wasn't getting relief despite my repetitive description of MANEUVERS designed for a bed or couch. Despite being well-dressed, urbane, and articulate, it turned out that he had lost all his furniture when he had to quit work due to his back injury; but was too embarrassed to reveal his new level of poverty. As I instructed him in one MANEUVER he could do on the floor, an audible movement of the disc material was heard, he obtained instant relief during the demonstration, and left the office tearfully joyous and grateful.

In designing this book, I felt compelled to give as much a reason for **why** the method works as I was to teach the reader **how** to make it work; but that doesn't mean you have to know or memorize it. If the reasoning *why* this method works and the anatomical nomenclature is not of interest to you and all you care about is "the bottom line," you can elect to pass over the majority of the beginning chapters of this book. If you later run into something you don't understand, you can go back to the section in the book that deals with that subject and acquire whatever information you need to understand the process. There is usually a chapter heading for every concept with which the average person can be assumed to be unfamiliar.

In practical application, when I have a patient in pain, I usually give a brief description of the injury, pain, and resolution mechanism, then I teach them how to do the most appropriate MANEUVER. Usually that is sufficient, and it only takes me about thirty minutes to educate them in how they can get themselves out of pain. They do not need to be articulately educated as to the anatomy and physiology of disc units to understand how to solve their problem.

Just as my patients with low back pain needn't learn about the neck, it is inefficient to spend the time teaching them those MANEUVERS or waxing poetic on the supportive theory and mechanics. However, if you have the time and penchant, learning a little extra never hurt anyone. By gently trying a MANEUVER intended for another not particularly painful region of the spine, you may find a stiffness relieved that has been present so long that it no longer is recognized by the mind as a problem, yet when the MANEUVER is accomplished, you may recognize a new, more comfortable, feeling and an increased range of motion that you never realized you had previously lost. Among other things, this book does serve as an excellent **USER'S MANUAL FOR THE SPINE.**

If you are experiencing back pain for the first time or are in a particularly painful period, it would behoove you to go directly to the section on **ACUTE PAIN MANAGEMENT STRATEGY** for the immediate management of a back injury or acute exacerbation of pain.

Performing these MANEUVERS is in no way dangerous nor inappropriate for a normal, non-painful, disc or spine. There also exists a rational understanding encompassing the damaged spine that, **if your spine is so damaged that it cannot do simple, non-forceful MANEUVER-type movements that would reasonably be expected to be accomplished in a normal lifestyle, then you would probably be harmed anyway or caused to have surgery when you unconsciously made equivalent movements during your activities of daily living**.

There is an advantage to understanding and applying all the concepts in this book. **You can expect to become a "back pain mini-expert" in your own right.** You may be able to "play doctor" by instructing others in the techniques, or do parlor tricks and be the "life of the party." Above all, don't part with this book once you are out of pain. There is a good chance you will need it again in the future. Even if only your low back is a problem, there is a very high probability that you will eventually have disc pain return later (long after you have forgotten the MANEUVER directions) or develop it at other regions of the spine. In that event, you can turn to those particular MANEUVERS for relief and understand why I included them all in the same book.

IF YOUR PARTICULAR PAIN IS NOT HELPED BY *THE O'CONNOR TECHNIQUE (TM)* OR IF INDEED IT IS AGGRAVATED OR THE PAIN IS INCREASED, BY ALL MEANS, STOP PERFORMING THE MANEUVERS OR ACTING UPON THE ASSUMPTION THAT YOUR INDIVIDUAL BACK PAIN ORIGINATES FROM A SOURCE THAT IS REMEDIABLE FROM THE INFORMATION IN THIS BOOK. This book is designed to help the majority of back pain sufferers; it cannot hope to help everyone. In the event that your pain is worsened, be certain to seek medical consultation. If you have any doubt, even before engaging in any exercise program, consult with your own physician. He/she may understand something about your particular problem that would require a modification or discontinuance of the method.

OF PARAMOUNT IMPORTANCE, DON'T CONTINUE DOING ANYTHING THAT INCREASES PAIN. The old adage "no pain--no gain" or the demand that one "work through the pain" not only makes no sense but can result in serious injury if taken to the extreme. **TO REDUCE THE POSSIBILITY OF DOING FURTHER DAMAGE TO YOUR ALREADY DAMAGED SPINE, ESPECIALLY IF YOU HAVE SUSTAINED A SIGNIFICANT INJURY OR HAVE SYMPTOMS THAT RESULT IN WEAKNESS IN THE UPPER OR LOWER EXTREMITIES OR BURNING OR ELECTRICAL LIKE PAIN THAT SHOOTS DOWN THE LEGS OR ARMS, GO TO A DOCTOR, GET AN EXAMINATION, AND HAVE HIM/HER GIVE AN OPINION AS TO WHETHER MOBILIZATION OR EXERCISE IS SAFE OR NOT.**

The most accurate means to assure that exercise is safe is by obtaining an NMRI (Nuclear Mass Resonance Image) to determine if the disc material has escaped the disc's capsule and is impinging upon a nerve. If such is the case, performing any movement, including the MANEUVERS elaborated in this book, has a potential probability of not working; and the activity may theoretically be equated with the induction of further harm. Unfortunately, an NMRI costs over $1000. In lieu of sustaining that economic burden, you can acquire the clinical experience engendered in this book which will give you the prerequisite knowledge necessary to diagnose and treat yourself.

If the MANEUVERS are done correctly as described, there is little or no opportunity to cause additional harm because the forces generated are not greater than those which are generated in predictable normal activity anyway. Common sense also comes into play here. **IF SOMETHING HURTS MORE WHEN YOU DO IT--YOU STOP. The MANEUVERS taught in this book should only change the character of the pain, not substantially increase it. Any marked increase in severity of pain requires further diagnostic exploration before proceeding.**

Don't get anxious or immobilized by fear. When I speak of the fear, I suspect that in most instances it emanates from fear of increasing the pain and/or fearing that through incompetence you will make it worse. Addressing the first concern, you need not fear increasing the pain because this is not some entity that you have to rise up and confront with an all-or-none throw of the dice. With *The O'Connor Technique (tm)*, you are able to try a certain movement, test it to see if it causes a problem, if no harm is done, you can go on and test it further with little increments at a time to reassure yourself that no greater pain will be experienced.

Many people legitimately fear that they will be caused pain for no certain benefit. It is this attitude that keeps people from participating in everything from chiropractic to the best state of the art University level medical care--**FEAR OF PAIN**. There is no reason to look upon this method in that light. You can gradually approach this method with non-forced trials and ease into it without any fear that you will "go too far" and hurt yourself.

This brings us to the second concern: fear that, through not knowing what you are doing, you might end up hurting yourself more. Dispel that fear with your intellect. Too many people today are programmed to believe that they are incompetent to make decisions or take actions related to their own bodies and health. Just as many people make decisions that are not based upon knowledge but upon faith. This book neither asks nor expects you to do either. It only encourages you to understand your fear and overcome it by your own individual scientific method. You test a particular movement, **if it hurts--you stop**. You substitute your anxiety with the testing of hypotheses. You will ultimately decide if it is safe and effective by your outcome.

All things considered, the spine is a pretty tough structure. It takes substantial forces to truly damage an intact spine. It is unreasonable to believe that you would come to any greater harm by gently trying a few movements you probably would have made anyway during the course of your future. So, it makes better sense to try the movements in a controlled atmosphere wherein you can easily modify any circumstance that would otherwise be capable of causing you harm.

The opportunity for being helped dramatically with *The O'Connor Technique (tm)* is so great that it is worth taking an exceptionally small risk, if one exists at all, especially when you consider that, if the damage to the back is already so severe as to be increased through these non-traumatic MANEUVERS, you most likely would have to resort to surgery regardless of what you did or didn't do. It is highly unlikely that you are going to break anything unless it is already too broken to make much of a difference in the overall outcome . The vast numbers and percentage of people who, over the years, have reassured me that the method works in the absence of any damage attributable to this method, encourages me to relegate the possibility of further damage to the realm of the theoretical. I mention the remote possibility of further harm not only for

11

completeness sake, but to legally protect myself in these litigious times. I considered not publishing this information out of fear that someone will be harmed and attribute the damages to me in a lawsuit. However, the amount of benefit far overshadows any perceived risk of harm; and to not publish would lead to much more suffering.

Like all aspects of life, employing *The O'Connor Technique (tm)* is not without risk. So is getting out of bed, swinging with your head upside down on a swing, or riding an amusement park ride. We do not live in a perfect world. Of course, doing the MANEUVERS haphazardly, too rapidly, or attempting to violently manipulate a damaged disc could result in further damage.

There are obscure anatomical conditions that may make this method unsuccessful and even problematic for some individuals. Sometimes a person, especially if elderly, can be caused to pass out when their neck is stretched. This is probably related to the tension placed on the vertebral arteries that pass through the first cervical vertebrae.[2] So, there are an exceedingly small number of persons who may get light-headed when they attempt the method on their necks. Of course, the solution is to stop doing it if light-headedness occurs. **It's common sense--if a particular MANEUVER or position described in this book causes a problem (such as a change in sensation or strength distant from the site of pain), don't persist, consult a physician.**

Also, there are a certain very low percentage of people in the population born with separations in the bridge-like bones that connect the front portion of the vertebral bones with the back portion called spondylolisthesis or spondylolysis. This method may not help their back pain and could aggravate it.

I have no illusions that this particular method of back pain management will help everyone because there are an assortment of back pain causes that will probably not be helped by this method. There are various musculoskeletal conditions to which anyone can fall prey such as Spinal Stenosis (a condition where scars or bony growths close in the canal where the spinal cord or nerves travel), Sacro-ileitis (an inflammatory condition of the joint between the pelvic bone and the sacrum), Ankylosing Spondylitis (an arthritic condition that fuses the vertebral bones), Good old fashioned arthritis (Osteoarthritis) of any source, Bursitis, Myositis (muscle inflammation), Tendinitis (Inflammation of Tendons that join muscles to bones), Fibrositis or Fibromyalgia (an inflammatory condition that affects soft tissues surrounding and between muscles accompanied by fatigue, muscle aches, and morning stiffness), and last but not least--Fractures.

All of the above could mistakenly be confused with disc herniation disease; however, most of these pains are routinely handled by the medicines you will be taking for inflammation anyway so they, too, will serendipitously be helped by the complete method I describe. But don't let the sheer number of these conditions scare you into believing that a major undertaking will be necessary to figure out which one you have. **By far and away, the most common source of back pain and the highest percentage of it is caused by herniated disc disease.** Just because a whole panoply of conditions can cause back pain, that doesn't change the reality that **most probably you are dealing with a herniated disc condition by virtue of the preponderant statistical probabilities.**

There are other conditions that are the uncommon causes of pain that appear to be spinal in nature but are not true spinal pain. They don't relate to musculo-skeletal causes but fall into a separate category both due to their rareness and not really being associated with spinal tissue, per se. A partial list includes: Abdominal Aortic Aneurysm (a breaking down and expansion of the largest artery in the abdomen), Kidney Stones, Kidney infections, Inflammation of the Pancreas, Stomach Ulcers, Infections of the Uterus or fallopian tubes, Ectopic Pregnancy, Prostate Inflammations, Pleural Effusions (Fluid in the Lung Spaces), Colon Obstructions, Tumors or Cancers of the bone or tissues contiguous with the back. So uncommon are they, that I can't recall being fooled making these diagnoses in the past 10 years despite thousands of patients. In most cases, these diagnoses are so readily obvious to me, that I think most people with common sense, when they consider the absence of and presence of other associated symptoms, will figure out for themselves that the pain doesn't really originate in the spine.

In fact, the pain they cause is so different and readily distinguishable from disk pain (by both non-affirmative answers to the test given at the start of this book and by the method I describe under the heading of "SELF-DIAGNOSING YOUR DISC") that the distinction is usually obvious. I can even go one step further to say that **if you don't get relief from** *The O'Connor Technique (tm)* **then you may reasonably suspect that the pain is from some other source and go searching for an exact diagnosis through the usual and customary medical channels.** However, again, the majority of spinal pain originates from disc related causes so **don't assume that your best bet is to just let a doctor manage it.** Read this book and practice the techniques, if they don't work, you can, therefore, reasonably rule out mechanically treatable disc disease; and, then, the application of other diagnostic modalities and expensive imaging studies are more likely to be cost-effective and productive.

On the other side of the coin, **oftentimes doctors make diagnoses that attribute the pain to muscle strain, arthritis, ligament tears, etc. when in reality a herniated disc is really the ultimate source.** Too, a herniated disc can cause muscle spasm and the doctor is not technically wrong when making the diagnosis of muscle spasm. However, frequently, the underlying origin of the problem is the disc and until that mechanical pain is solved, little or no relief can be expected. The practical message here is that **even if you have been given an alternative, inadequate, diagnosis, in my experience, you still could probably be suffering from a herniated disc.** In light of that reality, trying *The O'Connor Technique (tm)* can provide the relief you seek in spite of a previously made, incorrect, diagnosis .

Far too many of the patients who come to me already have other diagnoses yet, in reality, have disc disease as the source of pain. I prove that contention by "fixing" them right then and there in the office, but rarely do they go back to the previous doctor to educate him/her.

This book and these MANEUVERS are directed to the majority of intervertebral disc pain sufferers who's damage is not so extensive as to require immediate surgery or so degenerated as to not have any functional disc remaining. In fact, once a person has been examined by a doctor and surgery is ruled out, there is little other hope for reduction of mechanical pain except by mechanical solutions. This book provides those mechanical solutions.

Once you have mastered the mechanical solutions, you may, at first, as I found necessary, have to use them on a constantly repetitive basis to get out of pain; but that small inconvenience is vastly preferable to constant pain. With time, however, you most likely will discover that you require exercising the pain-stopping MANEUVERS less and less. In my case, unless I "over do it" by too much lifting or sports, I only occasionally have to perform the MANEUVERS to stop the pain. Over the last several years, my Lumbar disc pain has drastically been reduced in frequency and severity. **It is my assumption and belief that my spine has responded to the intentional alterations in movement and mechanical forces by re-molding into a more stable and pain-free configuration.** I suspect my autopsy will be the only means of proving that contention--a prospect that my inevitable critics will relish.

Lastly, I feel the need to explain that the illustrations in this book are not always intended to be anatomically exact representations of human tissues or bio-mechanical actions. As the reader will learn, a few millimeters of distance at the level of the disc can mean the difference between pain and non-pain. The whole spinal disc unit is so small that it can be easily grasped in the palm of the hand. It is very difficult to represent comparisons between diagrams that differ only by a few millimeters of change. Therefore, some exaggeration of anatomy (especially distance and angles) is often necessary to convey an adequate understanding of the physical properties being discussed. I accept that knowledgeable medical professionals may be critical of these anatomical representations; but the book was not predominately designed for their use.

The bulk of the illustrations were drawn by myself, in part because these are new concepts that have never before been represented and the time and cost of employing a medical illustrator to give physical form to my concepts would have been prohibitive. The truth will out, I am not a world class artist; however, it is my opinion that it is more important to get the idea across rather than to stand on anatomical exactitude. However, this revelation by no means implies that the drawings do not accurately reflect physical reality because they, to the best of my understanding and ability, are intended to do as great a service to reality as to the readers' back pain.

1.   Lyons AS, Petrucelli RJ, *Medicine An Illustrated History*, 1987; Abradale Press, Harry N. Abrams, Inc. Publishers, New York:504.

2.   Pelekanos JT, et al, Neurology, 1990;40:705-07.

CHAPTER ONE: BACK PAIN IN CONTEXT

YOU ARE NOT ALONE

Excruciating back pain is so seemingly unique and awesome an experience that the suffering individual often assumes that they are the subject of a rare event or perhaps one of the few persons to ever sustain such a degree of agony. After all, if it were a common phenomenon, surely someone they know would have told them about it. The reality is that few people actually discuss it because, in so doing, it exposes a frailty or imperfection in themselves. The ego rarely allows this revealing a disclosure.

Surprisingly enough, **recurrent back pain is the most common complaint among adults approaching their physicians. It is second only to the common cold as a reason for office visits to primary care physicians.**[1] Low back problems **affect virtually everyone** at some time during their life. Surveys indicate that in any given year, **50% of working-age adults have back pain symptoms,** but only 15-20% seek medical care.[2] In one recent study, 41% of enrollees in a group health plan reported having back pain within the last six months. By the age of 70, **85% of the population will have had an episode of back pain.**[3] At any given moment, **15% to 20% of the adult population have low back pain.**[4] **Back pain is the leading cause of disability in persons younger than 45 years, and the third leading cause among those older than 45.**[5] A number of studies have indicated that **40% of all adults will experience sciatica (back pain with radiation down the leg) some time during their life.**[6] In the U.S., 13.7% of all persons have back pain lasting more than two weeks.[7] Lastly, **back problems are the second most common reason for non-surgical hospital admissions among adults under age 65.**[8]

If money spent on a problem gives some measure of its extent in our society, the staggering costs and lost productivity are sufficient to convince the back pain sufferer that they are, indeed, a part of something big. The annual costs of disability and treatment of back pain increased from $14 Billion in 1976 to $30 Billion in 1986. **By 1989, just the medical costs of back pain alone generated $14 Billion per year in the United States.**[9] The latest and most recent quote for the yearly costs related to back pain comes from the authors of the Agency for Health Care Policy and Research's publication. They estimate it costs the health system upwards of **$20 BILLION PER YEAR.**[10] In the U.S., back pain is responsible for an average of 12% of all sick leave,[11] **rivaling the common cold as a leading cause of absenteeism from work.**[12]

Back pain results in the loss of more than 93 million work days each year. It has been estimated that the **yearly medical costs for treatment of just Lumbar disc disease is nearly $5 Billion.**[13],[14] In the automobile industry, as much as 5% of a car's price pays for back injury claims, and among postal employees, 1 in every 25 cents of postage pays for back problems.[15] Tragically, back pain disables as many as 4 million persons in the United States per year.[16]

Misery may love company, but delineating the magnitude of the problem offers small consolation for the individual back pain sufferer in the throes of agony. However, as Karma would have it, if spinal pain were not such a ubiquitous, inadequately addressed, problem in our society, this book probably would never have reached your hands. You are holding this book precisely because *The O'Connor Technique (tm)* and the principles elaborated herein promise to favorably and dramatically alter the above statistics.

There is every reason to believe that, if put into wide-spread practice, *The O'Connor Technique (tm)* has the potential to revolutionize the manner in which back pain is treated. By arriving at both a novel understanding of spinal mechanics and the development of a mechanism to physically alter them, **most back pain can be successfully managed earlier and better than ever before.** Prior to the onset of irrevocable damage, the **deleterious consequences of neglecting spinal mechanical principles can be prevented, human movements can be directed to rectify anatomical discrepancies, and the environment can be altered to accommodate spinal anatomy** rather than the inverse. Even though the evidence is not available to fully support this claim, I personally believe that **practicing *The O'Connor Technique (tm)* regularly throughout the ageing process can prevent the crippling effects of kyphosis (the bent-forward posture of old age).** Finally, by applying the knowledge presented in this book, its readers can expect to extract themselves from otherwise contributing to the horrific aforementioned back suffering statistics.

THE PAIN

Few people who do not have "bad backs" can appreciate the excruciating torture that constitutes back pain, the inconvenient agony of lying on the floor in a fetal position knowing that any movement produces a sensation equivalent to a sharp wedge being driven into the spine, the exponential number of lifestyle restrictions it produces, and the depression accompanying the realization that your mind has youthful desires yet your body's actions are confined by limitations ordinarily reserved for the elderly.

Understanding that an exactingly intricate description of disc disease pain, reproduced here, can be seen as redundant, any reader who has experienced the pain is free to return to the TEST YOURSELF section for commiseration or confirmation that their back pain is truly disc related.

Many cannot sympathize or empathize with back pain sufferers because they have never experienced the awesome reality of a pain so intense that they cannot lift themselves off the ground, let alone walk. A pain so oppressive that the simple act of freely breathing is denied, forcing one to take shallow breaths to avoid any extraneous movements. They cannot conceive of what it feels like to constantly search for a comfortable position where seemingly none exists. People, especially health care providers, who have not experienced this pain have no conception of this "task-master's" incredible might. Back pain is so brutal and unforgiving that it exists only in the abstract to the uninitiated. Attempts to describe its magnitude by patients, if accurately done, are easily interpreted by others (physicians included) as an exaggeration for sympathy or histrionics for secondary gain. After all, nothing could hurt that bad!

Guess again unbelievers! I routinely hear stories from patients in which they describe being absolutely unable to move and only weakly able to call for help. One patient known to me sustained a fall in which she suffered a disc protrusion with spinal nerve root damage but the disc material recoiled back within the confines of the ligamentous capsule. Recently, she stood at the sink for an half an hour unable to change her position without agonizing pangs that shot through her back down to her legs. She had to be physically assisted to her bed by her mother. Adding literal insult to injury, she was adjudicated by the medical and judicial system to have psychological overlay that negatively influenced her ability to be helped, minor arthritis with a few osteophytes, and otherwise no evidence of significant back injury. Her tragedy was magnified by the "specialist" who couldn't admit in his written procedure note that he failed in his attempt to properly perform a discogram on her (he stuck her unsuccessfully with a needle at least half dozen times). He, then, cleverly worded his findings (something to the effect that "no disc pathology could be identified") which made it appear that she had no genuine pathology for the record. Therefore, no real physically demonstrable injury could be documented when she tried to sue the parties whose negligence was responsible for her fall. Compounding the physical pain she suffers, she also bears the psychic pain of experiencing that "the system" is so rife with injustice that it is hard for her to discern which is worse, the divine injustice of back pain or the societal injustice of a medical and courts system supposedly designed to prevent injustice.

As a consequence, any surgical option has been denied her because one doctor determined that her pain was largely psychological; and, yet another failed to diagnose it properly. The weight of these two opinions makes any surgeon reluctant to proceed without fear of a law suit should the results not meet expectations. Through my "hands on" manipulative technique, I could put her back "in", but she, as of my last contact with her was unable to keep it in for any length of time. It is obvious by the relief that she gets with MANEUVERS that she has a mobile piece of disc material that is difficult to stay centralized; however, she cannot get this removed surgically because she has been determined not to be a surgical candidate. She is caught in a painfully surreal Catch-22. The pain she has experienced exists on levels far exceeding the physical realm, and she is probably forever limited to that relief which she obtains through practicing *The O'Connor Technique (tm)*.

CONTEMPORARY PERSPECTIVE

At this juncture, I suspect I am "preaching to the choir" because if you have picked up this book, it is most likely due to a personal experience with back pain or knowing someone close to you who can't be faking that much discomfort so convincingly and consistently. Therefore, you probably know enough to understand that very little help can be expected from the current medical practices widely available to the back pain sufferer. After all, if you were largely satisfied with how you were treated, you wouldn't have felt the need to acquire this book in the first place.

Not only myself, but **other physicians categorize the current state of affairs as nothing less than "monstrous ignorance."** Dr. Paul Altrocchi, a neurologist in private practice told the Washington Academy of Family Physicians in 1987:

"In any group of people, we may find that 80% have had back pain at one time or another...yet **few fields in medicine abound with such a monstrous amount of ignorance and lack of understanding.**" The belief that the condition is a surgical disease is at the core of the myths surrounding back pain. This idea has come about because primary care physicians have for years, abdicated responsibility for these patients to others, he charged. "Back pain does not titillate our diagnostic minds, and it gives us complaining patients whose exams don't lead to a wonderful sense of exhilaration.[17]

It's odd how back pain has gotten the "short shrift" in terms of the devotion of effort on behalf of the medical profession to analyze it to the degree necessary to properly manage it. I am constantly frustrated by how much pseudo-science is applied to the making of inaccurate diagnoses and prescriptions for illogical therapy. This is not solely my criticism but emanates from numerous other sources capable of publishing their objectivity. For instance, the medical journal, *Emergency Medicine*, anonymously reveals an attempt to rationalize a decision to abandon the time-honored requirement demanding that the physician make an accurate diagnosis before initiating treatment.

BACK PAIN
Is a Definitive Diagnosis Necessary?

Precise identification of the cause of lower back pain can be a frustrating, expensive, and ultimately unrewarding pursuit, so focus your efforts on ruling out the most serious causes

Figure 1 Excerpted headline from the 1993 medical journal, *Emergency Medicine*

The article, "*BACK PAIN, Is a Definitive Diagnosis Necessary?*" begins:

Vague associations between symptoms, pathologic changes and the results of history-taking leave primary care physicians no choice but to send patients with lower back pain home with no specific diagnosis. Many attempt to plug the clinical gaps with a progression of imaging studies. That route, however, is costly and sometimes misleading. But is an exact diagnosis really necessary in all cases of lower back pain? A Seattle physician thinks not. He believes that the goals of the history and physical examination should be somewhat less ambitious, aimed

18

more toward the identification of more serious problems and the **practical disposition** (emphasis mine) of the patient

"The essential issues can be approached with the history and physical examination alone," says Dr. Richard A Deyo, professor in the departments of medicine and health services at the University of Washington School of Medicine. "Only a minority of patients require further diagnostic testing.[18]"

Sounds more like pragmatic **disposal** of patients to me. My wager is that the author has never suffered from a bad back, or he would be less likely to advocate diagnostic ignorance in order to search for a potential means to "dispose" of those who do.

Antithetically, the sagacious William Osler, M.D., in 1902, presciently answered this attitude by stating:

> "In the fight which we have to wage incessantly against ignorance and quackery among the masses and follies of all sorts among the classes, diagnosis, not drugging, is our chief weapon of offense. Lack of systematic personal training in the methods of recognition of disease leads to the misapplication of remedies, to long courses of treatment when treatment is useless, and so directly to that lack of confidence in our methods which is apt to place us in the eyes of the public on a level with empirics and quacks."

Whether originating from frustration, incompetence, or a desire to reduce medical expenditures, a willingness to abandon the necessity for a diagnosis reveals better than any other the current decision by medical intelligentsia to deviate from previous, held to be inviolate, standards. By way of comparison, if a patient with swollen ankles and shortness of breath asked a doctor precisely what was happening on a pathophysiological level, the doctor would, most likely, insist upon a battery of tests to make the diagnosis and justify its necessity with elaborate explanations involving sodium retention, serum renin levels, pulmonary wedge pressures, etc.; but just ask the doctor why, when you simply wake up in the morning, with no apparent trauma you have immobilizing neck stiffness or stabbing back pain, he will more than likely not give you a direct, competent, or anatomically sensible answer because it is as much a mystery to him as it is to you. The reality is that medical science has not really directed the equivalent amount of scrutiny to the back pain problem as has been devoted to other human diseases. When physicians attempt to educate patients as to the nature and means to a resolution of back pain in the absence of a diagnosis, they seemingly must be indulging in self-serving obfuscation apparently more illusional than realistically helpful.

An interesting study was recently done in which researchers educated physicians as to the state-of-the-art of back pain management; then, by telephone interviews of the patients these physicians subsequently treated, the researchers attempted to determine the success these physicians had in satisfying their patients desire to have their back pain "fixed." The results were devastatingly dismal. **The education program did not measurably affect outcome among any of the patients, including that subset of patients whose physicians had perceived themselves**

19

to have had the greatest benefit from the educational intervention![19,20]

I think this 1991 study, more than any other, exposes the failure of current medical management for low back pain. It would be comical if it were not underwritten in so much agony. Here, we are relying upon the most up-to-date minds in back pain management, educating society's supposedly best and brightest, only to learn that, despite 62% of the providers believing that they had "acquired increased confidence" that they could help patients and 50% believing that they had "learned more" about the scientific and psychosocial aspects of back pain management, as well as 50% "feeling more comfortable" treating patients with low back pain, **none of the patients got any better than they would have otherwise**. One has to just shake one's head and ask: "What is wrong with this picture?" It's almost reminiscent of the finest and best-educated doctors in the 18th Century priding themselves upon having attended educational seminars on purging and bleeding and believing themselves to have arrived at the definitive state-of-the-art.

To be fair, there are other factors contributing to this complicated equation. There is also a great deal of physician trepidation in tampering with the spinal column in these days of litigation. If a doctor were to stray too far from the standard therapies and a paralysis were to occur, the next person he might be talking to would be that patient's lawyer. Leaving well-enough alone and adopting a policy of "Less is More" (which is how the back pain gurus have interpreted and applied the overall message of the government's guidelines discussed below) doesn't appear so likely to result in nerve damage or paralysis for which an intervening physician can theoretically or legally be found culpable. No intervention, in that regard, is superior to one that might end the doctor in court when the outcome appears to be the same regardless of what any physician chooses to do. This philosophy updates the age-old physician's precept, "first do no harm," to the more contemporary, "don't do anything outside of the guidelines and you won't get sued." This attitude appears to be well-received by doctors and insurance companies; unfortunately, it leaves patients suffering--a condition which seems to result every time bureaucrats try to practice medicine.

I intentionally delayed putting this book together until the definitive "state-of-the-art" was formalized in writing by way of the government's new encroachment into medical arts referred to as Clinical Practice Guidelines: *Acute Low Back Problems in Adults: Assessment and Treatment*. Every physician in the country, one way or another, was going to be influenced by this promise to codify and justify back pain management (or better, "mis-management"); and I wanted to be sure that the state-of-the-art had been ultimately defined before I presented my method. I was not surprised to learn that nothing new is being really offered to the back pain sufferer by the government's incursion (or academia's dangerous collusion with same) into the realm of disease treatment.

Certainly, there was some advantage gained by assembling the country's leading experts in an attempt to define the way a patient should be routed through the medical system; and I would encourage the reader to **obtain the Agency for Health Care Policy and Research's free publications related to: *Acute Low Back Problems in Adults: Assessment and Treatment*, by calling the information clearing house at 1-800-358-9295.**

There are physician versions and consumer versions. They do at least a good job at defining dangerous back symptoms and signs as "Red Flags" indicative of a potential need for surgical intervention and differentiating these conditions from those amenable to **"conservative** treatment" (which, **in truth, amounts to something more akin to neglect** if one follows their advice). Nevertheless, the guidelines do serve an excellent function for my purposes. Their availability makes it unnecessary for me to reproduce all the work necessary to compile the existing literature or describe in detail the state-of-the-art in back pain management so that the readers may assess for themselves the available alternative methodologies. The reader can easily turn to those guidelines to determine what constitutes a potentially serious spinal condition. Any person satisfying those "Red Flag" criteria should probably not rely too rapidly or readily upon this book for their salvation until they have been reassured that they do not have a serious surgical condition. If so, they should insure that they present themselves to the most appropriate physician for evaluation before proceeding with <u>any</u> therapy. After exhausting all of the remedies outlined in the government pamphlets and provided through the current medical system, then, the reader may feel free to return to this book for advice and relief.

In delineating the current thinking on back pain, the guidelines prove, if only to my satisfaction, that no current literature seems to have arrived at as well-founded an explanation for the origins and solutions of spinal pain than is engendered in *The O'Connor Technique (tm)*. The careful reader of the government guidelines will note that in all their recommendations in favor of or recommendations against specific alternative methodologies, not a single one follows from "strong research-based evidence." Therefore, it would seem unlikely that anyone could criticize myself for advocating my method; since the justification inherent in the government's currently recommended modalities has arguably equivalent research-based scientific support as my own.

Actually, I should be content with that state of affairs. If all the answers were already available, there would have been little need for this book. No new revelations would be possible if the mysteries had been previously elaborated and the puzzle solved by someone else. One nice outcome of the government's compilation of information is that manipulation therapy during the first month of symptoms was given some semblance of credibility by categorizing it as being justified with support by "moderate research-based evidence." Since no mention was made of self-manipulation (which, if one were to characterize *The O'Connor Technique (tm)* in its application by lay persons to their own back pain, it undoubtedly should be classified), it must, therefore, constitute a novel and unique classification.

Unfortunately, the manner in which these sort of governmentally-sanctioned pronouncements are received by the medical community tends to lend them an aura of "the final word" or becoming "written in stone," leaving little or no room for innovation and an excellent means for a third party payor to refuse to pay for alternative medical strategies. One must understand that when the government decides to accomplish something, the impetus is politically motivated and controlled. With back pain, it appears to have gone something like this: **The politically powerful and influential insurance companies would like to see less money spent on back pain. They monetarily support and acquire politicians who can control bureaucrats who then selectively employ and seat on committees only those professionals who espouse the desired medical philosophy that coincides with their monetary strategy. That way, the resultant conclusion appears to have been arrived at in an unbiased manner by objective experts. It's an excellent societal management technique used by the ruling class for centuries to give the illusion that the very best is being done for the masses.**

I fear that this current, government-sanctioned, justification for doing little or nothing for the majority of back pain sufferers a majority of the time will prevail; since, already, **"*The new thinking*" on low-back pain concluding that "*less is more*" is severely limiting the use of needed imaging techniques by giving third party payers an elegantly documented means of denying approval for those modalities.** I happen to especially advocate the use of imaging studies to document the reality of disc disease for diagnostic purposes, to ascertain the position of a displaced disc fragment, and to insure safety prior to ordering exercise-based physical therapy or active forceful manipulation. **None of these governmental inquiries bothered to count all the people who got worse when they were sent out for manipulation or "work-hardening" exercise training in advance of a competent diagnosis.**

Contrary to the prevailing recommendations, I have found imaging studies prove very self-helpful for insurance purposes. Immediately after an accident or other forcefully damaging event, I believe it behooves the sufferer to gain as accurate a piece of injury evidence as possible, since often, the only means of proof that can be obtained to justify a claim must be gathered while the damage is fresh before the disc migrates back into its central location either as a consequence of manipulation or random activity. On this issue, I heartily disagree with their findings and recommendations based upon the knowledge I have acquired through my own, albeit independent, experience.

The fact of the matter is, *The O'Connor Technique (tm)* can be equally as effectively applied by an office-based physician to carefully but non-forcefully immediately alleviate acute as well as chronic back pain by a hands-on manipulative re-positioning of displaced, protruding or herniated disc material. Even after I teach them and they have shown successful ability, some patients nevertheless require intermittent assisted manipulation when they cannot get their own disc material back in place with *The O'Connor Technique (tm),* requiring the repeated services of a trained practitioner. However, the government's Clinical Practice Guidelines "recommend against" a "prolonged course of manipulation." Does this give third party payers the justification they need to deny these services after an arbitrary period of time has elapsed? Does this imply that even prolonged courses of self-manipulation are not recommended? The originality of *The O'Connor Technique (tm)* calls some of the most "modern" thinking into question. Principally, does what the government certifies as "ok" exclude all else and legitimize a denial of services or reimbursement?

I have been performing the type of manipulations arising from my unique understanding of back pain mechanics for several years now and have also arrived at a very simple assistant-mediated method which applies the principles of *The O'Connor Technique (tm)* and may be practiced by any trained person to whom a back pain suffer turns for relief. This should probably be relegated to physicians or chiropractors so long as they are sufficiently educated to determine which patients are candidates for the technique and which ones should be referred to surgeons for last resort management.

HISTORICAL PERSPECTIVE

In some respects, using non-surgical, physically manipulative, means to mechanically alter the spine may be retrospectively looked upon, in part, as a long-lost art probably practiced by

Medieval Arab physicians. The *Canon of Medicine* (Figure 2) by Abu Ali al Hussein ibn Abdallah ibn Sina (shortened to Avicenna, A.D. 960-1037), appears to have been instructing the 11th Century reader in a not unrelated method of back pain relief. It seems to me a method remotely related to *The O'Connor Technique's (tm)* application of traction accompanied by manipulation was most likely practiced a thousand years ago. In the absence of an anatomical foundation, these ancient practitioners may have been utilizing some of the basic components of what today I have independently developed as *The O'Connor Technique (tm)*. In the upper illustration of Figure 2, a board appears to be being used to forcefully hyperextend the Thoracic spine. In the middle illustration, an extension technique is being combined with weighted pressure to forcefully hyperextend the Lumbar spine. In the bottom illustration, the practitioner appears to be utilizing a mechanical traction device combined with an extension technique. It is not unreasonable to assume that the purpose was to mechanically remedy the same age-old problem that has plagued mankind since he began walking on two legs--the pain of a herniated disc.

In Indian Yoga, the practitioners

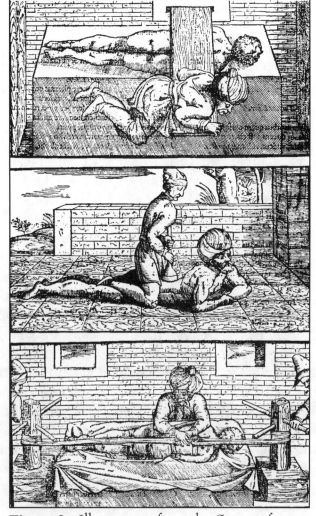

Figure 2 Illustrations from the Canon of Medicine by Avicenna

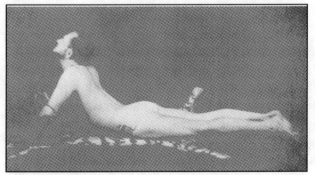

Figure 3 Swami Kriyananda adopting the Cobra (Bhujangasana) posture [With permission from: Yoga Postures for Self-Awareness]

appear to have realized centuries ago some benefit to be gained from adopting certain extension postures (Figure 3). Their efficacy was attributed to allowing energy to pour through opened nerve channels[21] and the effect, presciently claiming to exercise back muscles, **"adjust any slight displacement of the spinal column, and relieve any backache caused by overwork,"** constipation, flatulence, and utero-ovarial (sic) complaints.[22]

Comparing Figure 3 with the McKenzie-type posture in Figure 4, seems to bear out this speculation; however, McKenzie (a New Zealand physiotherapist who devised a back pain program in wide-spread contemporary use)claims that he arrived at his method of centralizing disc material by accidently leaving a patient in a similar posture for a prolonged period on his examination table only to discover that the patient's back pain was resolved when he returned to the room. McKenzie further advanced this fortuitous finding into an exercise program with which many patients get relief from back pain.

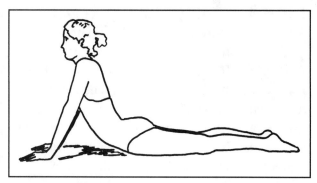

Figure 4 McKenzie extension exercise posture (Adapted from R. McKenzie)

However, *The O'Connor Technique (tm)* exponentially advances upon this age-old wisdom from the perspective of a medical doctor who has first-hand knowledge of the anatomical, physiological, practical, as well as theoretical aspects of back pain. This book seeks to impart this newly found wisdom to the back pain sufferer. ***The O'Connor Technique (tm)* rationally discards the harmful and logically incorporates the beneficial aspects of both the William's and McKenzie techniques into a unified method that succeeds far beyond the limited benefits of either method taken individually**.

I make reference to the McKenzie exercises because my initial reasoning that evolved into *The O'Connor Technique (tm)* started with a different theoretical explanation of the origination of spinal pain than that proposed by McKenzie and because the manner in which McKenzie extension exercises claimed to centralize pain was inconsistent in alleviating my and others' low back pain.

As an interesting and factual aside, before I came to the understanding engendered in *The O'Connor Technique (tm),* I was helping some of my patients with a modified version of the McKenzie method (and meeting with limited success in stopping my own pain) and in my typical evangelical nature I presented it to my cousin who had all the symptoms of a chronically reducible disc herniation (that is, a piece of disc material that periodically went "in" and "out".) When he attempted McKenzie extensions, he said they only hurt him more; and he related that the only way he could get relief was by lying on his side, assuming a fetal position, and forcefully pulling his head as close to his knees as possible. This was a technique similar to that described by William's as effective; but I found that confusing because he was doing the exact opposite of the extension techniques and getting more relief. There had to be a rational explanation for why he got relief while accomplishing a bio-mechanically opposite activity. That caused me to return to the proverbial "drawing board" for the explanation of this conundrum.

When I independently looked, *de novo*, at the mechanical principles underlying the causes of back pain and examined them in terms of both the forces and actions resulting from those forces, I concluded that "over-stretching damage" to soft tissues of the spine (alleged to be the source of pain according to McKenzie[23]) were not the principle originating source for spinal pain. Rather, the pain comes from actual displaced disc material putting pressure on the ligaments surrounding the disc and disturbing the mechanical functioning of the disc unit. I assumed that this disc material had to have been displaced due to forces applied to the disc unit, and I reasoned that **by reproducing the mechanical forces that caused pain in a reversed sequence, one could alleviate the pain using the individual's anatomy as the tool to apply those forces**. Lo and behold, it worked to alleviate my own back pain much more successfully and efficiently!

I ran into inconsistencies and more conundrums but held steadfastly to the belief that the mechanical processes of spinal pain were capable of being understood and reversed. When I found contradictions to my original hypotheses and events in the real world that didn't fit my early beliefs, I reasoned out explanations. Where modification of my opinions were necessary by virtue of their being inconsistent with my observations or what patients told me of their experiences that weren't consistent with the mechanics as I saw them, I was caused to revise my method to accommodate reality. I don't feel this book perfectly answers the entire enigma of back pain, because I would be the first to admit that I do not have all the answers. However, I have solved enough of the mysteries to go public with what knowledge I have so as to be of enormous benefit to countless suffering people.

SCIENCE AND ART

This book is based upon the premise that **there is nothing meta-physically mysterious about back pain**. It is not only the result of fate but of function as well. By and large, **once the mystery is revealed, the "secret" becomes common place and like all mysterious entities, it then becomes less frightening and manageable.**

I have attempted to make this book readable for both the average person and referenced for the academic or professional. Despite my credentials as a physician and a University professor, I have elected an alternative method of presenting this to the academic world and documenting its success without controlled, peer-reviewed, "scientific" studies. Many academic professionals would prefer that new medical information originate from an orthopedist or neurosurgeon at the University level. In practice, educated as well as uneducated people fall into the intellectual trap of believing that the state of human knowledge has risen to such complexity that nothing can be of true value unless it originates from teaching institutions where knowledge is codified, structured, and monopolized. Such is not necessarily a fact.

Don't misunderstand, I have deep respect and admiration for the theory and practice of science; however, there arise situations wherein the scientific process, as we have come to institutionalize it today, makes it sometimes inadequate for the study of human phenomena by its demand for absolute exactitude. If anything, the Heisenberg Uncertainty Principle (a theory holding that the more one attempts to study a phenomenon, the more one changes it simply by the observational act's interfering with the true nature of the phenomenon) applies to some of the demands made upon the absolute adherence to scientific theory with respect to back pain because the process of observation is neither exact nor foolproof. I believe the manner in which back pain has been approached in this century fell victim to this reality.

The mechanically manipulative approaches taken by massage therapists, chiropractors, and ancient healers were often dispelled in their entirety by the medical establishment without looking to see if they had any basis in reality or attempting to discover the reason why they worked when successful.

In truth, **I carefully observed a human phenomenon, acquired an in-depth understanding of the previously existent information base, found it inadequate, proposed countless hypotheses, tested those hypotheses, abandoned the non-reproducible components, formulated a theorem, then compared my observations and experiences against that theorem by testing, re-testing, and re-working the details.** Admittedly, the knowledge came to me as much as by trial-and-error as what would be considered pure scientific inquiry. In spite of that, I am to the point where I feel I have arrived at a "truth" that constitutes a competent solution to an age-old-problem.

It also so happens that I have been in the unique position of having a population of back pain patients upon whom I was able to practice my technique and modify it accordingly **without exposing patients to any mechanical forces or risks greater than that which would be expected from normal day-to-day activities**. My own back also conveniently provided me with a willing and ever-present study group of one; but medical history is replete with major advances coming from competent observation of a single patient. Unfortunately, often, it seems, for anyone to be able to make even the simplest medical statement, it has to have been the product of a major, costly, project involving blinded study groups, control groups, and rigorous examination for statistical significance. I (as well as a large contingent of medical experts) have arrived at the conclusion that back pain has so many variables involved in its study that it is not always amenable to the usual methods of scientific inquiry.

For instance, if one were to attempt to compare so much as a single facet of *The O'Connor Technique (tm)* with some other method in a controlled scientific fashion, it would be nearly impossible to eliminate what is called "bias." One could never be certain that the person educating the patient populations did so properly and identically nor that the recipient of the information absorbed it uniformly or completely, was motivated to succeed, or remembered the details sufficiently to be successful. In advance, the researcher would have to have sufficient confidence in the method to be convincing to the patient (or else the advice might not be followed) and at the instant that was achieved, he would be guilty of injecting bias into the study. His inherent confidence in the method can be expected to alter his results by a projection of sincerity; otherwise, one would have to argue that patients could not be able to perceive nor would be affected by insincerity when the researcher had no idea whether his instructions would lead to benefit. Such constitutes the "art" of medicine as it applies to research.

I understand that, in medical science, sometimes as much as a third of the people get better as a result of the placebo effect. If another researcher were to be firmly convinced in the superior efficacy of an alternative method, a larger percentage of people might get better simply upon the strength of that researcher's conviction that what he is doing will work. Also, in those people who were destined statistically to improve regardless of the treatment, they would be more likely to attribute the improvement to the alternative method regardless of its merit; otherwise the researcher would have had to have pretended to be neutral.

Also understand that many patients throughout medical history have gotten "better" despite therapies that ultimately were shown to have done more harm than good. Medical historians have ample examples of therapies that were so "effective" that they lasted for centuries only to be later shown to be worthless or actually more damaging. One would have to be biologically arrogant in the face of infinity to assume anything other than medical "science" still being in it's infancy today. Future historians will probably have a comedic field day with what is currently acceptable medical practice.

Regardless, I can assure the reader of one fact, my life and the lives of countless numbers of my patients have been substantially bettered as a direct result of applying the principles of *The O'Connor Technique (tm)*. I have not failed to keep documentation on those patients that have walked into my clinic literally **crippled with pain who achieved instantaneous relief when guided through the method and have been able to sustain that relief for prolonged periods**. Certainly, not everyone achieves this dramatic level of relief; however, the overwhelming percentage of those people who I can define as having herniated disc material as the source of their pain do achieve remarkably favorable and reproducible results.

So as to test whether or not some would have achieved that relief anyway with a more well-established therapy, I withheld my method from a number of people and sent them through the usual orthopedic and neurosurgical routes. When they returned without relief, I then used *The O'Connor Technique (tm)*, and they were able to become pain-free. Now, I can't, in clear conscience, persist in this practice because I would be denying them a valuable treatment for no apparent gain. This situation is reminiscent of the experiments that had to be stopped because the placebo control group was suffering so much that it would have been unethical not to give them the real treatment.

I have no doubt that *The O'Connor Technique (tm)* can be **superlatively effective in getting injured workers back to work faster, alleviate pain and disability more efficiently, and keep physically active people away from surgery more often and for longer periods than any existing back pain management program**.

I have been developing this method for at least eight years and have been enormously successful with the patient population at my clinic. I know that the **pain relief is not coincidental because it is too often dramatically immediate and most often in such close proximity to the start of therapy that no other explanation is suitable**. I have followed these patients long enough to know that the relief is sustainable and recognized by the patients as valuable because they are so firm in their conviction that the method worked.

If a demand arises for documentation of this method's success, I can simply return to the medical records for the appropriate analysis to prove my assertion. My records would be open to any researcher who legitimately wishes to verify or refute my claims. I am so convinced that *The O'Connor Technique (tm)* works that I am reluctant to engage in the standard, costly, and time-consuming effort it takes to formalize the proof that is often demanded of others similarly situated. In reality, however, the success of this method will be demonstrated or refuted when large numbers of people begin to be helped by the techniques and the demand for the book makes it obvious that the principles are genuinely therapeutic.

It is understandable for the potential reader to question the veracity of claims made by myself in this book. I've met with this attitude from celebrities who have back problems that are easily attributable to discs. They understandably believe that there couldn't possibly be a better method than that prescribed by their own highly paid, University-affiliated specialist. Who can blame them? Their condition has been described to them in articulately specious terms, and they are convincingly reassured that they will be better in a reasonable period of time because the

27

doctor is privy to the statistic that the majority of back pain is resolved within two months regardless of the method used. This statistic holds for *The O'Connor Technique (tm)* as well; however, **anyone using my method will find that usually the relief is instantaneous. There is no reason to wait weeks, months, or forever for random activity to possibly accomplish what my method does immediately and intentionally.** Unfortunately, unless they have had the misfortune of being previously treated with some other method; they have nothing with which to compare my method.

For the individual or the study group, the obvious criticism of my intellectual process here would be: "How do you know that they wouldn't have gotten better anyway just as rapidly with another method?" The answer I must resort to is my personal and professional experience both prior to my understanding the principles and after. Before I could genuinely help them, I was occasioned (like the over-whelming majority of doctors today) to watch them heal at their own pace, go from neurologist, to neurosurgeon, to physical therapist without definitive relief and continually get the same non-answers, veiled but never spoken assumptions of malingering, and with a frustrating inability to enjoy life as they knew it.

I distinctly recall one of the first patients upon whom I tried my method. He was a young man in his twenties unable to stand without a cane who bitterly complained about how his life was ruined and how he wanted to work but was sentenced to poverty because he couldn't function with his back pain. He had been denied surgical relief because of no documentable nerve damage and his young age, but that didn't change the fact that he was, for all intents and purposes, crippled. We both figured that he had nothing to lose. So, I gave my MANEUVERS a try on someone other than myself for the first time, and he actually walked out of the office without need of his cane. Within a month of following my instructions, he was able to seek work again. A few days later, I asked him if he thought my technique was responsible for his recovery or if he thought he would have recovered without it. He didn't attribute his relief to chance nor consider his relief anecdotal (as I am certain my skeptical colleagues might readily point out). He was as convinced as I was that my method had achieved success where all else failed him.

Since then, I have been utilizing *The O'Connor Technique (tm)* on everyone in whom I can define a discogenic (originating in the disc) source for back pain. I have made numerous modifications, toyed with some mechanically assisting devices, made certain that nothing posed a risk to the spinal cord or nerves with numerous imaging techniques, and followed numbers of people over long periods. The results have been so favorable that I had to publish the method.

I predict that in a short time, the method will become established therapeutic practice and evolve as things like that do. A therapist-assisted modification of this technique (like I do in my clinic) can be taught to the orthopedist, the primary care physician, or, yes, even the chiropractor so that within the space of an average office visit, the MANEUVERS can be administered to patients and immediate pain relief achieved where applicable.

I have evolved *The O'Connor Technique (tm)* in the clinical/therapeutic environment to a point wherein mostly what I do with patients is verbally give them directions on the exam table and assist them in making their own movements in a controlled and protective setting. Their retention of the sequence allows them to practice the same techniques in the privacy of their own home, on household surfaces, at no cost, and whenever immediately necessary. I know this can be accomplished and taught to patients rapidly and effectively because I have repeatedly succeeded in this goal in my practice too often to attribute their immediate or rapid recoveries to happenstance.

I solidly understand that incorporating the principles and practicing the techniques described herein offers no guarantee that either I or the reader will not eventually have to resort to surgery. I accept the potential for my back to possibly get progressively worse as age-related changes occur, and the reader should consider likewise. Notwithstanding that concern, since I began using *The O'Connor Technique (tm),* I have most certainly not gotten worse and have decidedly improved at a number of spinal levels that have to be considered "diseased." Even though I have definitely improved, I accept that I have a good chance of re-injuring my back. With the prospect of relentless aging viewed as inevitable, I have every expectation for the on-going process to worsen, but I can say that I am certain that without understanding this method, my condition would have already progressively worsened to the point of surgery or incapacity. For nearly a decade, I have been able to avoid surgery and significant disability. Even if that were all this book could offer most back pain sufferers, I would consider it a resounding success.

Needless to say, I believe this method can do more than simply help people with existing back pain. **If this method is practiced early enough in the course of disc problems, the relentless degenerative process can be forestalled and suffering prevented to the point of elimination, provided that the readers take personal responsibility for their problem and make the necessary modifications in their activities of daily living to positively affect their destiny.**

ALTERNATIVE THERAPEUTIC MODALITIES

There are certainly other back pain therapies available; and I would invite the reader to try them. They are usually divided into conservative and surgical modalities. For an overview of the available modalities, I again refer the reader to the above referenced AHCPR literature or any practitioner.

In short, the conservative model usually involves any number of physical therapies which can be summarized best in a single sentence:

> "There's no evidence that typical physical therapy in the form of ultrasound, hot packs or heat make any difference at all. Asking a patient to spend a lot of money on various approaches is unwarranted."[24].

I couldn't have said it better. In fact, if I'd have said it first, the reader might think I was self-servingly trying to coax people into believing that my method was the only path to relief.

The purpose of this book is not to evaluate the merits of all the available therapies; however, it would be incomplete unless I gave some direction to those who's back pain is not alleviated by this method and are forced to seek other relief from pain. I do not believe that my method will solve everyone's pain; so, for those instances, I have a duty to offer some of my perspectives so that at least some pitfalls can be avoided. After all, I have been forced by my own back pain to consider all the options. Who better can lend that personal touch to the experience?

SURGERY

If the reader is considering the alternative surgical option and turns himself over to a surgeon for a solution, I must first reveal a sobering statistic. In a study by Weber[25], 280 patients were evaluated over a ten year period. At the end of one year, 90% of surgical patients reported a satisfactory outcome compared with only 60% of the conservatively treated group. However, 25% of the conservatively treated group over the ten year period resorted to surgery. At ten years, this difference disappeared, indicating that **surgery is initially helpful but the outcome at the ten year point is largely the same with or without surgery**. Revealing another interesting statistic, 40% of conservatively treated patients are not satisfied as much as ten years later. This would seem to indicate that, **over the long term, state-of-the-art management (surgical or conservative) fails to satisfy at least 40% of back pain sufferers**.

When comparing the efficacy of non-surgical versus surgical management of disc disease, **no significant difference in recovery of function has been reported between patients whose herniated discs resolved spontaneously and those whose herniated discs were surgically removed.**[26] However, when using my method, the relief achieved cannot be considered spontaneous. It will come, if it does, as a consequence of directed therapy, the proof being in the rapidity of relief, in most cases. The future will determine how successful *The O'Connor Technique (tm)* is when it is compared against surgical intervention; my conviction is that it will be found superior in the long run.

It is with this thought that I temporarily abandon discussion on surgical remedies until the reader has had a chance to acquaint himself with the terminology of the disc, its anatomy, and pathology. At this point, my intention is to give an alternative to surgery and only after having exhausted the opportunities offered through *The O'Connor Technique (tm)* should surgery be realistically considered. Therefore, in Chapter Seven, a more thorough presentation of the surgical options is made and we will here direct our attention to the non-surgical, physical therapy alternatives.

COMPARATIVE PROGRAMS

Although there are several back pain books on the market and numerous physical therapy programs, *The O'Connor Technique (tm)* **is not just another back pain book filled with various exercises that no one can realistically be expected to do when in the throes of a back pain episode or for that matter maintained daily for the rest of one's life.** It differs substantially from any other previously described program in that it advances an entirely novel method of back pain management. The major difference between *The O'Connor Technique (tm)* and conventional, traditional, exercise therapy is that **this technique doesn't simply hand out a number of instructions that are assumed to be helpful without giving a rational, specific, physiological and anatomical justification**. In my opinion, the back and neck exercises advocated by pre-existing literature and prescribed by most physicians as "physical therapy" have no true direction or sense to them because among other failings, they are not diagnosis-specific nor do they consider the physical realities of the individual. Doctors prescribing them, today, attempt to "sell" the impossible "one remedy that cures all". While ignoring the necessity for specificity, upon which they so often pride themselves when dismissing any therapy which originates outside of academia, they, in essence, commit the same fault for which they so often criticize alternative therapists. If you don't believe this, ask the doctor who has prescribed physical therapy for your back pain exactly what mechanical principle he/she is relying upon and what specific instructions he/she is giving to the physical therapist relevant to your particular back pain. Then, compare that answer to the explanation you would get if you sought the same answers from this book. My bet is that you will find a much more cogent and sensible rationale in this book's prescription.

That is not to say that some physical therapy programs don't have successful outcomes. In fact, this method is a "physical therapy;" and it would be absurd to argue that physical therapy has no benefits. However, just as throwing virgins into volcanoes had been shown to effectively stop the Polynesian lava flows, so too, the exercise programs of the past tell you to do certain things that from time to time appear to be effective. If they are practicing the current state-of-the-art, their "effectiveness" is more likely the consequence of random chance and probability than directed, intelligent, common sense effort. After reading this book, I can pretty much guarantee that the reader will agree with me.

It makes very little sense when a disc is "out" to commit the same, identical, movement (under the auspices of an exercise) that put it "out" in the first place, even in small increments. Unless of course, they wish to verify the principles of homeopathy in which a small amount of poison that produces given symptoms is a means of curing a disease with the same symptoms. I don't think so. I think that even a little damage repeated many times cannot be expected to lead to consistent improvement.

One patient, I recall, described a series of neck exercises that she ritualistically performed every morning which seemed to make her functional yet did not even approach what could be looked upon as relief. They consisted of sequential side-to-side and rotatory movements of the neck. She was suffering from an off-center disc to the left in the C2-C3 level. So, every time she tilted her head to the right, she actually aggravated the problem. The relief she did seem to get was only because her ritual ended with a twisting movement after a left-sided flexion. Had she not coincidentally or by unconscious trial and error finished with that physical set of forces she would have received only pain for her effort. In her case, it only gave a modicum of relief which was to say she was in pain most of the time. When she began applying *The O'Connor Technique (tm)* she immediately, that is, the next day, began appreciating what it was like to live without pain again.

The O'Connor Technique (tm) relies upon a few basic, easily understood, principles, within the parameters of which any spinal activity can be evaluated as favorable or unfavorable. For instance, **this method does not allow intentional WEIGHT-BEARING FLEXION of the spine at the painful site**. For the Lower Thoracic and Lumbar spine pain sufferer, that eliminates any type of sit-up type exercise often advocated in other back pain management programs and literature wherein a supposition is made that increasing abdominal tone is essential to the restoration of a normal spine.

Take, for instance, the Williams exercises designed by the same-named orthopedist, repeatedly recommended through the years by countless doctors, and still in wide-spread use since at least 1974 for low back pain.[27] **They would have the back pain sufferer repeatedly engage in WEIGHT-BEARING FLEXION of the spine which causes a disc condition to actually get worse.** I've yet to figure out how they ever gained popularity in the medical profession. I suspect they were and are still offered as a "something" in place of the alternative "nothing." They apparently are statistically tantamount to ignoring the problem because the patients tend to eventually get better whether they are practiced or not. Nevertheless, they were and seemingly are still one of the standards of practice, since they continually and repeatedly are recommended in the current literature as well as by many primary care physicians, orthopedists, back pain educators, and physical therapists. Chiropractors rarely offer them because if anything worked at home, it might serve to keep patients out of their offices--they are seldom given to cutting their own economic throats. Besides, Williams exercises have never been proven to be effective.[28],[29]

In a limited regard, as it pertains to extension exercises, I would contend that *The O'Connor Technique (tm)* can be seen to be consistent with some components of most other back pain exercise programs. **Exercise, in and of itself, is not bad; but it becomes maladaptive when it is not rationally based.**

If the exercise program doesn't insure that no further damage is done by the process, then it is counter-productive. The absurdity of any exercise prescription given to an acutely injured back patient is made manifest any time that the doctor cannot accurately diagnose the lesion and insure that the exercises will not increase the damage. In the case of extension versus flexion exercises, a certain percentage of patients will get relief with either method owing to the varied disease states encountered by chance and probability; however, simply because a quantifiable number of people get relief doesn't justify increasing the pain of a probably larger percentage of those in whom a given exercise is decidedly inappropriate.

The test of any medical therapy is that it proves to be safe and effective. **The currently available exercise regimens prescribed in other programs for low back pain, in part, can be seen as effective if they contain extensor strengthening components, but cannot be considered safe if they include WEIGHT-BEARING FLEXION.**

The closest analogy I can draw to what is being given to back patients today with most physical therapy prescriptions is the same as if a patient were to walk into a doctor's office stating that he had a "blood pressure problem" and having the doctor offer two different pills. One pill makes the blood pressure go up and the other brings it down. The doctor then plays an "eenie-meenie-miney-moe" game and randomly gives the patient one of the pills. A higher understanding and logic tells us that most people are going to need the pill that brings down the blood pressure, and about fifty percent of the time the doctor will be "right." Unfortunately, an equal percentage of patients will not only be not helped but even harmed, by the wrong pill.

Certainly, after the pill takes effect, determining whether the patient's blood pressure goes up or down will offer some measure of information as to whether the truly correct decision was made; but that policy necessitates that the answer comes only after the prescription is administered and its expense and consequence is felt. In the context of a back pain exercise prescription, the incorrect choice is felt in both the patient's increase in pain and the nonproductive dent in his wallet. This book is predicated upon the assumption that these are two consequences that most people would rather do without if there is a better way of proceeding.

I would hope that most intelligent patients would argue the inadequacy of the analogy from the perspective that the doctor should have most certainly first measured the patient's blood pressure to determine the true nature of the problem before initiating a prescription. In the context of back pain, the doctor would, similarly, have been expected to first determine the precise nature of the back pain's origin before writing his prescription. However, one must understand that the principle means a doctor has of correctly diagnosing a disc problem (in the absence of applying *The O'Connor Technique's (tm)* methods to determine if the back pain's origin is discogenic) is with an objective measurable imaging study. Those have been deemed too expensive by the current "back pain intelligentsia" in the absence of clinically obvious nerve damage; and, even when they show a disc bulge, the artificially erudite clinicians will most likely quote a study that claims such a finding is present in too many supposedly asymptomatic people to be the source of the pain. So, the "eenie-meenie" game is played with exercise prescriptions because there is usually a failure to diagnose the disc as the source. Then, currently acceptable exercise regimens are prescribed without the knowledge necessary to logically presume how, or if, they will be successful.

I refuse to play that game. **This book gives the readers explicit means by which to determine for themselves what logic-motivated type of movements or exercise program should be employed and the physiological time an exercise program can begin based upon mechanical reality.**

I would argue that **the currently advocated exercise regimens are one of the major reasons why our present back care management strategy is in such obvious disarray.** Williams' and McKenzie's exercises have had years to competently address the problem and reduce back pain; yet they still leave the back pain sufferer today with the same statistically dismal chance for relief as they had for years in the past. One reason is simple: **They often actually reproduce the forces that caused the injury and ask the sufferer to repeatedly perform them.**

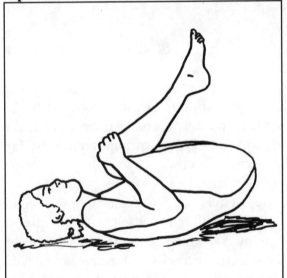

Figure 5 Exercise involving painful discs in flexion and bearing the weight of the legs while abdominal muscles are contracted.

Too, they usually are prescribed in a progressively increasing and complex series so as to give the illusion of scientific accuracy; when in actual practice, if you are not the ideal candidate, the more you do, the worse you will get. Like so many of my patients, I tried them before I developed my alternative. I, too, abandoned them because they hurt too much and seemed to make me worse.

In the chapters discussing WEIGHT-BEARING FLEXION, the demonstrations why these type of exercises can be harmful are discussed and the specific exercises that should be avoided are described. Here, it is sufficient to say that those components of the McKenzie or Williams exercises that involve WEIGHT-BEARING FLEXION should not be done under any circumstances.

Also, unfortunately for the large population of back pain sufferers the McKenzie method is felt by some clinicians to be inadequate:

"To carry out the mechanical spinal assessment described by McKenzie requires considerable education and clinical experience; clinicians must learn the many variations and combinations of spinal movements that enable accurate assessment of a wide range of patients...Regardless of the type of onset, the well-trained clinician can identify the correct direction of end-range spinal bending that centralizes and abolishes the pain in the majority of patients."[30]

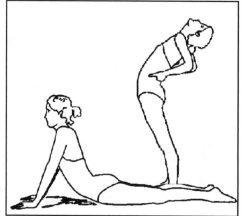

Figure 6 McKenzie exercise instructions that injudiciously promote weight-bearing on the affected disc

The O'Connor Technique *(tm)* differs substantially from the McKenzie technique because, among other reasons, it **does not require considerable education or clinical experience and can be performed by the average person rather than requiring a "well-trained clinician"** because it is designed to address, in a comprehensible manner, the overwhelmingly most common cause of back pain--disc disease due to disc herniations. It **can be easily understood by non-medically trained people** because it is based upon a few principles that once understood can be applied to nearly every activity of daily living to prevent back pain; and, above all, **costs nothing**. Alternatively, one can always count on spending a lot of money if one must rely upon a clinician with "considerable education and clinical experience" as described above.

I feel the need to delineate that there are multiple distinctions of substantive significance between *The O'Connor Technique (tm)* and McKenzie's method. The first seems to come from McKenzie himself. Clinician's who have recently heard him speak[31] state that he argues against the distinction of having created any "McKenzie Technique" since the method relies upon the individualized creation of specific exercises for each different patient depending upon the patient's pain pattern. By that, **it does not lend itself, by his own admission, to popular use by lay persons**. It requires a complex series of tests administered by a clinician who designs specific exercises which require a great deal of sustained exacting activity.

I am compelled to also point out that McKenzie, in his book, advocates the practice of actual exercises, which to my mind are not absolutely necessary to relieve back pain. **Of utmost negative significance, the McKenzie exercises ignore the resistance generated by the weight of the body part(s) above the lesion in designing the selective exercise.** One may note that in each of the terminal components of the McKenzie exercises, (See Figures 5 & 6), the Lumbar disc units are bearing the weight of the body parts above them. This practice is antithetical to my understanding and recommendations because it can aggravate symptoms, increase pain, and lead to disc damage (extrusions) that otherwise wouldn't have occurred if practiced without proper insurance that the disc material is properly positioned before attempting them.

Figure 7A shows a particularly contraindicated exercise promoted by both Williams and McKenzie. The posture recommended by McKenzie in Figure 7B should, likewise, never be allowed, let alone advocated, in a patient with low back pain due to disc herniation. The reasoning for not performing these exercises and those shown in Figure 8 will become manifest later, but suffice it to say that anyone with disc disease practicing these exercises can expect to increase and prolong their discomfort.

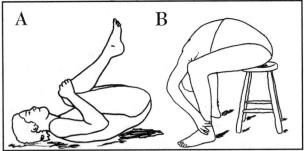

Figure 7 Flexion while weight-bearing serves to aggravate pain

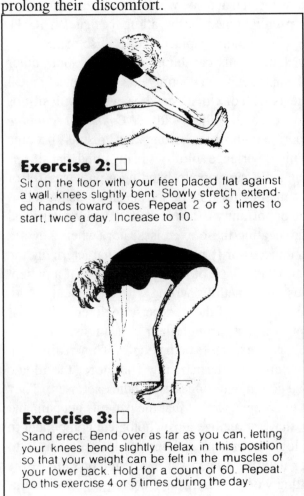

Exercise 2: □

Sit on the floor with your feet placed flat against a wall, knees slightly bent. Slowly stretch extended hands toward toes. Repeat 2 or 3 times to start, twice a day. Increase to 10.

Exercise 3: □

Stand erect. Bend over as far as you can, letting your knees bend slightly. Relax in this position so that your weight can be felt in the muscles of your lower back. Hold for a count of 60. Repeat. Do this exercise 4 or 5 times during the day.

Figure 8 Examples of physician-recommended exercises excerpted from a handout that are usually painful and never advocated in this book

No true exercise involving **WEIGHT-BEARING FLEXION** of the involved painful segment of the spine is recommended or allowed with *The O'Connor Technique (tm)*. You see, prior "wisdom" a la Williams has drawn a connection between lax abdominal tone and back pain. Probably, this association arises from the recognition that a substantial percentage of back pain sufferers have "pot-bellies." Increasing abdominal tone (by performing sit-ups or sucking in the gut) has the effect of flexing and straightening the Lumbar spine. According to William's and much of the current philosophy, a straightening of the spine is the ideal to be sought in an attempt to "stabilize" it. Therefore, they conclude, strengthening and increasing the abdominal musculature's tone *must* improve the condition of the spine. I view their reasoning as faulty and this opinion is supported by studies which make it increasingly clear that Lumbar extensor strength is more important than abdominal muscle strength in patients with low back pain.[32],[33]

Instead, I am forced to argue the opposite! Keeping the spine "straight" may even predispose to greater harm. Biological systems do not always satisfy teleological

35

argumentation because what appears to be the obviously logical conclusion to a set of understandings may turn out to be wrong. In biological systems, it is better to attempt to explain reality by starting with a known fact and using logic to explain the fact rather than the opposite mentation--trying to use logic to arrive at a biological fact. More often than not, this turns out to be an exercise in wishful thinking rather than science.

Human biological systems are complex, and simple logic doesn't always apply because there are many unrecognized variables that can modify the conclusions that would otherwise appear obvious. In this instance, I can prove for myself that certain exercises can be actually harmful for persons with disc disease. I know by viewing my CT scan that I have a herniated disc at the L5-S1 level to the right. When I do a sit-up or toe-touch as advocated in Figure 8, I get pain; and I can feel the disc material go "out" and pain radiates to the right hip/buttock region. I can get out of the pain with one of my MANEUVERS, and I can feel the disc material go back "in" followed immediately by pain relief. The pain is located at a site wholly consistent with what the CT scan indicates. My conclusion, based on enlightened observation, is that WEIGHT BEARING FLEXION exercises are pain-inducing due to their displacement of disc material.

There is an exceedingly small probability that all this can be explained by some other mechanism; however, I find that difficult to substantiate when I apply the same mechanical reasoning to the overwhelming majority of my patients with disc disease who get pain with sit-ups and toe-touches then, they find immediate and repeated relief with *O'Connor Technique* MANEUVERS. Thereby, these personal experimental observations and results become reproducible, constituting "scientific evidence." This experience solidifies in my mind that sit-ups are contraindicated. I happen to find this reasoning far superior to handing a patient a set of painful exercises and concluding that the patient is a malingerer if he or she doesn't practice them.

However, my experience has not yet had the opportunity to affect the many physicians and physical therapists, acting on faulty logic, from advocating these exercises; nor, when they are refused to be performed by patients who find them unnecessarily painful, from characterizing the patient's reluctance to engage in them as emanating from a lack of motivation. Too, if a patient refuses to exercise, then they assume that there must be something wrong with the patient. With their ego-logic, it is inconceivable that the sit-up component of their exercise regimen is in error because that is not what they have come to accept as a fact through their educations. You see, clinicians are didactically taught that the classic back pain exercises help people. They reason that they must have produced a beneficial or they wouldn't still be taught. Therefore, the illogic follows: *because* patients improved, they must have gotten better *because* of the exercises. They seem unable to modify their belief structures so as to accept as a fact that the patients get pain and could actually be hurt from that exercise. Rather, they rationalize a psychological component to explain the patients' behavior. I find that type of logic erroneous and unfair. It doesn't seem to dawn on them that the patients who did get better may have been getting better ***in spite*** of the exercise prescription; and, for those that were getting worse, it may have been ***because*** of them.

Also, as alluded to above, when lifting or squatting, **the other programs make nearly universal recommendations to keep the back "straight."** Realistically, when a person with a disc problem attempts to follow this advice, lifting is still painful because when squatting, in order to keep the body's center of gravity over the feet, the back naturally goes into flexion when the buttocks gets close to the heels and the hands get close to the ground. When a person attempts to keep simply a "straight" back while initiating the full squatting posture to lift, the thighs press against the abdomen forcing the Lumbar spine into a flexed position (especially if they have something more than a model's abdominal girth.)

The O'Connor Technique (tm) **advocates employing a judicious EXTENSION prior to lifting and the locking of the involved area into an intentional EXTENSION posture during lifting** so long as pain is not reproduced. If the pain is reproduced, then a series of specific MANEUVERS are taught to stop this pain so that the EXTENSIONS can be accomplished safely and intelligently. The justification for these deviations from the usual and historical advice will become apparent later, but suffice it to say: **This is not just another "same old, same old, back pain book."**

NOT AN EXERCISE PROGRAM

In fact, *The O'Connor Technique (tm)* is **not predominately an exercise program** at all. Although the value of proper exercise to keep the back musculature in good tone cannot be underestimated as a preventative measure, it is not necessary to exercise pain away. Pain is alleviated by a few simple movements called "MANEUVERS." **The only actual exercise advocated in this book is designed to preferentially strengthen specific muscle groups to alter the mechanical forces placed upon the involved discs after the pain problem has been solved.** For those who can't see themselves being sentenced to perpetual exercise, the exercise component can be ignored and the majority of benefit can still be realized by just doing the MANEUVERSs (some of which are so simple as to be incorporated into the act of exiting a bed or putting on your shoes in a different way.) The reader will not be expected to exhaust himself especially while in pain. In that sense, this book can be looked upon as **THE LAZY (WO)MAN'S GUIDE TO BACK PAIN.**

This method teaches the back pain sufferer a means to capitalize upon simple body mechanics to re-position the discs to relieve acute (immediate, short term) pain and to alter the forces of the spine acting on the discs so that the disc can be re-positioned and eventually made less likely to become painful in the future.

Other programs (especially those in vogue now) would have the participant repeatedly exercise and "work harden" the spinal and associated musculature in order to "stabilize" the Lumbar spine. Their latest advice recommends mobilization as early as possible. The problem is that **they fail to elaborate or define specific, safe, effective, and painless mobilization techniques.** This book provides those techniques and avoids any muscular stresses to the spine until the mechanical problem is solved. I find it cruel to mobilize an acutely painful back with the traditional methods especially if they make no effort to avoid weight-bearing flexion. The average physical therapist employing the state-of-the-art work hardening techniques seeks to find (largely through trial and error) a few exercises the back pain sufferer can perform and force them to repeat and increase the intensity of those exercises until exhaustion or pain arrests the process. All the while, they teach the sufferer to keep the back positioned in the "straight" or "neutral" position. The so-called "neutral" position being described as having the upper body directly above the hips with the Lumbar spine in neither flexion nor extension when performing any body movements. This is all well and good in theory; but, in practice, it is nearly impossible for the average person to maintain the degree of muscular energy that is required to keep the back constantly "straight." Later, the muscle tone that they demand cannot be achieved or maintained without exhausting constant daily work-outs. Realistically, the vast majority of people do not have the inclination or time to exercise daily. Those people who do have that inclination and keep their bodies in excellent tone and shape with regular exercise usually don't suffer from back pain anyway. This book, in that sense, makes no demand for a change in exercise lifestyle.

Adding to that, most other programs and physical therapy regimens ask people who are in or just recently coming out of acute pain to risk further agony by **exercising** within two days of the injury! Most people are smart enough to avoid exercising because they know that, often, exercise was what brought on the pain in the first place. As you will probably be convinced later, **exercising while the disc is herniated or prolapsed really shouldn't be accomplished**. As soon as it is "in," is a different story. Any actual exercise intended to strengthen muscles acting upon the spine is too painful to accomplish until the herniated disc has been anatomically re-positioned where it belongs. Even if one were to make a constant conscious attempt to maintain the postures advocated by most programs while sitting and standing, it is largely impossible to accomplish these even most of the time due to the pain accompanying the displaced disc material. The result is that the person's back pain persists; and, when they continue to complain, they are accused of not maintaining the postures and exercise levels consistent with sufficient motivation to get better. What their persecutors don't realize is that the positions that they advocate are realistically impossible to maintain without first insuring that the disc is not still herniated or prolapsed.

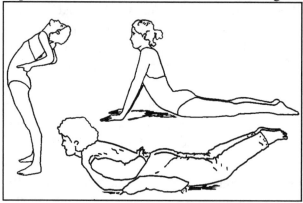

Figure 9 McKenzie exercises adapted from his text

This rationale, as you will hopefully come to understand, substantiates a legitimate criticism of The McKenzie exercises. Figure 9 shows the terminal components of several exercise postures advocated by McKenzie that comprise principle elements of his program. In and of themselves, they are not necessarily bad (in fact, you will find similar positions demonstrated in this book); however, the inappropriate sequence of their application, as directed by his method, can make them actually painful and damaging to a large percentage of patients with disc disease a significant proportion of the time. In order for them to be helpful, a person must be able to tell whether the disc is "in" or "out," where the displaced disc material is located (or they might be at best ineffective), and they must be applied at a specific time for rational reasons. To my admittedly limited understanding, McKenzie gives his students and readers none of this; therefore, anyone advocating these exercises lacks the necessary specificity for them to hope to be successful except under limited circumstances.

Please understand, my intention is not to denigrate McKenzie. These exercises do help a certain specific subset of back pain sufferers, giving clinicians limited legitimacy to advocate them; but, it cannot be assumed that patients who don't get relief must not be doing the exercises. If you don't exercise, the psycho-logic of some physicians flows--you must not be motivated to get better. It then follows that the lack of motivation is the source of the problem rather than the pain being too great or the method of treatment being inappropriate and ineffectual.

The logic becomes most damaging to patients with legitimate pain and disability when they interface with "experts" who are so certain that their methods of treatment are without fault that they have come to conclude when a patient fails to get better that it is the patient's fault instead of the disease process or the consequence of inadequate, poorly directed, exercise prescriptions. I have suffered these "experts" parading around conferences expounding the assumption that what they are presenting and practicing constitutes the definitive method. They responded to my inquiries into the logic of their method with defensive indignation and justify their methods with only the implicit superiority of their personalities and credentials. Don't misunderstand me, I have a great respect for medical professionals--except when they fail to accept that their methods may be fraught with inadequacy or refuse to advance their own knowledge by resting upon what they are usually unwilling to acknowledge exists as a grotesquely incomplete understanding. Unfortunately, this attitude inhibits the acquisition of new knowledge; and, in that atmosphere, I am offended by their arrogance.

Another fallacy (which is currently being touted in the back pain treatment circles usually accompanying the mischaracterization of a person in legitimate pain as being poorly motivated) is that when people don't get better in keeping with the averages, they have a good probability of having a psychological component to their back pain which is interfering with the therapeutic process. This causes me to advise: **When your doctor drags out a psychologist or psychiatrist to participate in the management of your back pain yet you know you are in real pain and that it is the pain itself causing the depression, anxiety, or hopelessness, it is time to re-evaluate the successfulness of your current therapeutic regimen and the wisdom of your physician or his HMO**. You can usually spot this coming when the doctor begins addressing the "lack of progress" in your treatment and starts talking about the potential for "the mind to play a role in the perception of pain." At that point, you should carefully read this book if only to reassure yourself that you are not crazy; and you may legitimately conclude that your medical provider has nothing more to offer you.

These supplemental diagnoses range from depression to malingering or "secondary gain." Now, I sincerely believe that many humans are prone to these problems; but not nearly with the frequency for which they are evoked as an explanation for failing to markedly improve. In this day-and-age of workman's compensation and employer-paid benefits, a designation of having failed to improve seems to be equated with nothing less than returning to full physical labor employment.

I actually get angry when attending back pain conferences wherein a major portion of the program focuses upon the psychological and psychiatric components of chronic back pain. Certainly, after suffering intractable back pain a person will most likely become anxious, depressed, and often temperamentally disappointed when met with unconvincing or contradictory opinions or when the same unhelpful pablum that they have heard before is regurgitated by yet another "expert specialist." The minute the doctor senses this attitude, he can defensively evoke the psychological component and allege that it is a mental problem that is preventing the patient from getting better. In this way, they place the "cart" way before the "horse" and attempt to convince the disability evaluator, your employer, or even yourself that your mind is what is the matter--not your back. At least one premise that this book operates upon is that in the overwhelming majority of instances **the psychological component is a consequence of the pain, not the source**. For that reassurance, I hope the reader will be at least grateful.

I have come to the above conclusions having experienced first-hand the excruciating, frightening and confusing pain of a Lumbar disc herniation. Within several days of that experience's onset, I guarantee, I was not willing to go out and exercise because, by then, the pain had subsided only just enough to walk around without assistance. I would reject now, as I would have then, the proposal that I begin exercising the back muscles so soon after the injury as one contemporary philosophy advocates.

I am convinced that this rejection would have been judiciously noted in my medical record (as I have seen so noted in my patients' records) and used later to argue the existence of a lack of motivation if, or better, **when** the treatment failed. In my case, despite being a resident physician in a teaching hospital with orthopedic, physical medicine, and rehabilitation teaching programs, the treatment was nevertheless benign neglect based upon the misleadingly grand assumption that 70% of back injuries recover in 2-3 weeks and 90% of back injuries resolve within six weeks no matter what is done. By doing nothing, at least they couldn't be accused of making the problem worse. However, if I knew, then, what I know now, I have no doubt that I would have been able to get out of pain immediately, and could have prevented a majority of the problems that came later due to ignorance.

Hopefully, with the intention of eliciting a sigh of relief in the reader, for the most part, **the movements advocated in *The O'Connor Technique (tm)* are not true exercises**. So, **I refer to them as MANEUVERS**. Exercises are designed to build, strengthen, or increase the endurance of muscles. The movements described in this book are intended to centralize displaced disc material. Once the disc material is centered, it is not absolutely necessary to persist in such movements. In fact, if these MANEUVERS are over-done, the risk of irritating tissues and inducing inflammation could be increased.

For instance, **when the back is put into hyperextension and moved excessively or repeatedly as in a push-up type McKenzie _exercise_, the joint surfaces of the vertebral bones are exposed to excess wear to which they are not accustomed**. This can cause arthritis. Additionally, the edges of the vertebral bodies (that portion that constitutes the outer circumference of the vertebral body) nearly rub bone on bone together especially in the ageing back with osteophytes (bone spurs) and disc height loss due to degeneration. Ordinarily these are not necessarily painful unless arthritis is present. However, when they are caused to rub together continuously, such as in the case of repeated exercise, an inflammatory situation can be produced similar to any activity in which joints are repeatedly over-stressed or pressured in the extreme ranges of their motion.

The beauty of *The O'Connor Technique (tm)* MANEUVERS is that they need only be accomplished when disc material is de-centralized and in the presence of pain. When a disc is de-centralized, "out," or herniated, it can be felt to be so upon self-examination (you will learn how to do this in the Chapter on DIAGNOSING DISC DISEASE); and only then need the movements be practiced.

GETTING BETTER AS A PROCESS

MAKING YOUR BAD BACK BETTER is, among other things, an ongoing continual process of altering your activities of daily living in a non-inconveniencing manner. Take heart, though, any inconvenience can be seen to be vastly overshadowed by the benefit. The process begins by accepting that your painful back is "bad," imperfect, damaged, broken, and/or impaired. The permanent nature of a disc problem is revealed in the studies showing that **40% to 85% of back pain patients will have recurrences within a year after their initial episode.**[34],[35] The underlying problem doesn't go away. I contend this statistic need not be the fate of a person who accepts that their back has a problem and actively uses *The O'Connor Technique (tm)* to prevent a future occurrence.

Like any person who has encountered a disability on the long road of life, in order to overcome it, it is necessary to accept it as a disability (just ask any alcoholic who has been through Alcoholics Anonymous) because it is impossible to accommodate to something that you do not accept as real. Therefore, **I would ask the reader, herewith, if you have back pain significant enough to have altered your lifestyle (even for a short period of time), that you accept the fact that your back is "broken" and that you technically have a permanent underlying disability.** If you recognize this early on and you re-arrange your lifestyle to accommodate to the disability, then you will have less probability of injuring your back in the future to the extent that you are in perpetual pain or require an operation to come anywhere close to being normal again. I am certain that, had I known the onset of my back pain meant that I had actually torn the back's non-healing structural elements, and that, if I were to sustain another flexion injury, it could mean a lifetime of pain, I would have been less likely to have participated, later, in those activities that put my back at additional, unnecessary risk.

Part of the reason I am writing this book is not only to relate how a person can get out of pain by a never-before-elaborated method but **to communicate the type of information people require to prevent a similar tragedy as my own from occurring in their lives.**

Had I known that my discs were weakened as a eighth grader from hauling two five gallon pails of water through Ohio farm snow drifts twice a day to bring water to our cow I would have been less likely to have launched an ultimately insignificant career in high school wrestling. During wrestling, had I known that the reason why it was necessary during warm-ups to have my back "cracked" to increase my flexibility and decrease my discomfort was because I unknowingly was getting relief by undergoing a traction/extension maneuver to centralize my own discs, I most probably would not have gone out on a mat to again lift another squirming human being over my head from a seated position. I had no idea, then, why my back hurt; and I made no effort to alter my activities even though I had found it necessary to avail myself of the services of a chiropractor at the young age of 17 years.

I had no knowledge as I aged that the small injuries I sustained as a youth were permanent and my back was a flexion accident just waiting to happen. I had no clue then as to the significance of my first flexion-type back injuries while in the military. I had not the knowledge I have now. Had I had it when I was preparing to jump off the diving board, as high into the air as I could, to do a cannon ball and land with my back in maximum flexion, I know I wouldn't have done it. Off hand, I would categorize the avoidance of cannon-balling as a non-inconveniencing life-style change. Incidentally, that was the first incident in my life where the back pain was so intense that I was unable to get out of a swimming pool.

If someone had explained the mechanisms of disc damage to me before I bounced down a mountain in a ski racer's tuck, I wouldn't have spent the next several weeks in agony. This was the second incident of excruciating back pain I could recall. **Had I the knowledge contained in this book, I would have deferred the wrestling, the cannonballs, and the downhill ski racer image of myself.** That is not to say that I still don't wrestle around for fun, dive, or downhill ski. I, and **almost anyone with a bad back armed with the knowledge in this book, can do just about whatever they want to, within reason**; but, **if they do it with the fore-knowledge that their backs must be guarded from flexion, kept in extension, and with particular purposed avoidance of weight-bearing flexion, they can accomplish these activities with relative confidence and safety**.

The presence of extreme pain cannot be the only motivating factor because, by then, it may be too late to prevent extensive damage. If you wait till you have pain to allow it to protect your back, the opportunity to prevent the damage is passed. After reading this book, you can let your newly acquired intellect decide what constitutes a wise move. If you are capable of assimilating the knowledge and experience of others and not the type of person who requires actually experiencing a negative event from which to learn, you will do well with your back.

If this book does significantly help you and you are convinced that the source of your pain is indeed a displaced disc, please don't adopt a maladaptive attitude towards yourself. If I may be given the latitude to wax philosophical, one must not look upon any constraints on your behavior as punishment, as a shackle or enforced prison. Not as a disgruntled malcontent should you look at your body. Regardless of its failings and imperfections, it is still the temple of your soul. It's the only housing your being has for the present. It is what it is for whatever reason.

You would do well to accept this "disability" as though you are a child issued your first set of prescription lenses, or as an elder your first prescription medicine which will be taken for the rest of your life. You must understand that Fate is an inscrutable mistress. She may dictate through your back that your chances of sustaining a flexion injury are enough to encourage you to walk away from a boisterous argument that years prior you would have confronted and otherwise put your life at risk. Believe it or not, as a teenager, I distinctly recall recognizing that my back pain would preclude my relying upon a career involving physical labor. That realization led me to invest more in my mind and, rather, cultivate my intellectual capacity.

I'm not advocating adopting a "Pollyanna" perspective, I'm just exposing you to the reality that you will never know (until perhaps the last second of your life) if your back pain was ultimately a beneficial happening. From all immediate perspectives it appears singularly disastrous; however, you never know, it may save your life someday. Funny thing is about Fate, you may never even know how or if your back saved your life. I know that my other disability, my glasses, saved my life. In an impulsive teenage heroic mentality, I had applied for the Warrant Officer Flight program in 1969 so that I could be a helicopter pilot in Vietnam. The prescription lenses that I cursed every day of my life excluded me from "going out in a blaze of glory" at the ripe old age of twenty years.

Certainly it is depressing to realize that your body is disabled to the extent which accommodations must be made for the rest of your life. Just talk to someone with an amputation or a stroke survivor, you will find that the successful ones simply accepted their "disability" and went on with the rest of their lives by making the necessary modifications to their lifestyle. However, there is good reason to expect that your back will eventually get and stay better especially if *The O'Connor Technique (tm)* is adhered to. The reader can breeze forward to the chapter on "Hope" to reassure themselves that there is some light at the end of the back pain tunnel so long as you can **bring your spinal education level up to the point where you can understand the terminology and practice the methods designed to accomplish the few principles enumerated in this book.**

Applying *The O'Connor Technique (tm)* **supplies a means whereby a person who is predisposed to back pain by genetics, comes to it by occupation, prior accidental trauma, or pregnancy, or has had a previous event of back pain (and wishes to prevent future ones) can alter their behavior with a process designed to protect their spine before the onset, during the period of pain, and subsequent to it.** In this manner, *The O'Connor Technique (tm)* can be said to be able to **prevent back pain** and **change the Fate of one who practices it**.

The principles are especially relevant to those who are wise enough to foresee the probability of acquiring back pain, decide not to expose themselves to that risk, and are willing to change their mechanical behavior to accommodate this desire. It requires wisdom to prevent future pain because rarely is it possible to convince someone, even with the best of proof, that an untoward event would have happened if it didn't or never does happen. That is what makes preventive medicine so difficult for some to accept as valuable. After all, they contend, one could theoretically be expending a great deal of extra effort trying to prevent an event that may never take place; however, when the reader gets pain relief using a maneuver in this book, it is easily seen how the maneuver is based upon spinal mechanical principles that make the maneuver successful. It is from consistently applying this same mechanical logic that the process of preventing future pain is designed. The more effort generated towards obeying and applying the principles, the less probability one has of committing the mechanical errors that lead to back pain and disability.

The permutations and levels upon which this preventive strategy operate are farther reaching than just immediate pain. For instance, knowledgeable of spinal realities, **new mothers can use this process to insure that motherhood doesn't turn into an experience that taints the life long relationship with their new child.** To estimate the value of that benefit, imagine a scientific experiment wherein every time one study group of new mothers bent over to pick up their baby they get a jolt of pain stabbing them in the back. It takes little imagination to predict how such a scenario could potentially breed a subtle psychological form of resentment directed at the child and dis-flavor the relationship as the mother subconsciously associates the infant as the origin and source of the pain. Applying the principles of *The O'Connor Technique (tm)* serves to prevent this potentially devastating ramification of pain.

I am firmly convinced that, had someone communicated the wisdom contained in this book to me as a juvenile when tossing hay bales to the point of exhaustion, as an adolescent while slouching for hours in my school chair, or as an adult trying to squat like an Asian while in Vietnam (mistakenly thinking it to be a natural and therefore biomechanically advantageous position), I would have understood how and why these activities were making and made my back worse; and I would not have persisted in them. In that sense, had I the wisdom to apply this intellect, my Fate would have been irrevocably altered by simple preventive medicine.

Armed with and applying this wisdom now, as a physician, when patients walk into my office in pain, I determine through a brief history and specific physical examination whether a disc is acting as a source of the pain, apply my technique in a manipulative manner, and they walk away with immediate relief after the application of gentle movements which could only result in a disc's re-centralization. In all those persons who obtain relief, the specificity of the therapy's efficacy proves the diagnosis. The objective evidence is that, after the application of *The O'Connor Technique (tm)* the patient can again move without the stabbing wedge-like pain in their spine with which they entered my office. With that experience, they are much more motivated to accept and apply the preventive philosophy I then impart to them. **It has proven to be an intensely gratifying experience to know unequivocally you have taken a person out of pain, unequivocally given them a means of preventing its return, and changed their Fate, forever. The reader of this book can expect to do the same for him or herself.**

I have no illusions that this self-applied "physical therapy" process will help everyone. However, I am so convinced of its efficacy, that those that it doesn't help have reasonable cause to assume that they have some other condition like those listed above or the disc is in such a difficult position that it cannot be self-manipulated back into place .

Fortunately for most physicians but unfortunately for their patients, they don't have personal experience with a disc problem upon which to base their belief systems. That, in the presence of never before being exposed to this technique nor the mechanical theory of disc movement upon which *The O'Connor Technique (tm)* is based, leaves them with little to rely upon except the customary, random, back mobilization exercises which, by the laws of random activity, do eventually help a percentage of people. Because some studies indicate that 95% of acute back pain resolves in 2 months no matter what modality of therapy is utilized, many practitioners simply give analgesics (pain medicines), anti-inflammatory medicines, some bed rest instructions, an admonition not to lift, some largely worthless exercises, and rely upon time and the law of averages to do the real work. *The O'Connor Technique (tm)* is refreshing in that it removes randomness from the process by selecting out those who most probably have a disc herniation as the source of their pain and mechanically re-positions the disc material so as to immediately resolve the originating component of the pain and teaches the process of keeping it in.

BECOME YOUR OWN CHIROPRACTOR

Chiropractors for years have explained their technique as one in which the manipulator "adjusts" the spine. The theory (as explained to me on numerous occasions when the nearly identical "spiel" is repeated in offices, at street fairs, etc.) holds to a belief that the spinal vertebrae can go out of "alignment." The chiropractor usually demonstrates this condition with a spinal model whereupon he rotates one of the vertebrae so that one edge of a facet (the joint type structure that constitutes a posterior aspect of the vertebral bone and acts to keep one vertebral body directly above or below the next) rests on top of another which then stays in that position until he re-rotates the spine in the opposite direction and the vertebrae falls into place. This action is to what they give credit as the source of their ability to relieve spinal pain, not to mention any other malady to which the body falls prey. I'm not certain whether even they truly believe it or not, however some seem pretty convinced and convincing. Maybe they are just repeating the same rationalization over and over (despite a knowledge that it cannot really explain the spine's mechanics) because they have to give *some* reason to justify a rapid and violent jerk to the torso and the wallet. However, it could be that they do have a knowledge of the true mechanics of the back yet understand that, if they reveal it to others, the majority of patients will figure out how to accomplish the same effect on themselves and eliminate the chiropractor along with his compensation.

Most physicians with a knowledge of spinal anatomy and function cannot accept the reasoning many chiropractors give as an explanation because it is blatantly obvious to them that the forces necessary to allow a vertebrae to assume that "misaligned" configuration would have to tear all the ligaments designed to prevent that action from occurring. Too, the degree of the misalignment has to be of such magnitude as to have occurred due to forces far beyond those reported as precipitating the painful event. Certainly, trauma on par with an auto accident could create such stresses; however, it is highly unlikely that 1) the interarticular ligaments could sustain such injury and still allow the spine to function at all, 2) that such a mis-alignment would not be obvious on X-Ray, and 3) once the vertebral column was re-aligned it would scar down and prevent further misalignment unless equivalently violent forces were again to act. This discrepancy between theory and observed reality, compounded by the seemingly arbitrary assignment of repetitive future alignments that appear to be more monetarily motivated than physically beneficial, probably is responsible for the failure of most medical doctors to accept chiropractors as therapists.

On the contrary, **I possess the objectivity to recognize that chiropractors do help some people**. Statistically, about a third of the people they manipulate get relief; however that only meets the batting average of a good placebo. Since there are only three possibilities that can result from any given therapy; the patient 1) gets better, 2) gets no effect, or 3) gets worse. I assume that the percentages for each option are about equal. When chiropractors go through their routine, they simply spin a three sectioned wheel of probability. The times that I have been "manipulated," it didn't seem to matter what my problem was, the treatment was the same. My back did feel a little better afterwards, some of the stiffness was relieved as the successive crunching was accomplished. But the problem was not addressed in any long-lasting or permanent manner.

This should not be taken to mean that they do not actually accomplish something that physically helps other individuals. I am only saying that I think they are attributing the relief, when it results, to a mechanism that they admittedly (in the literature) do not understand. Therefore, they should not take credit for their successes as a science since it is not the product of consciously directed action based upon intelligent thought processes. The possibility also exists that they are leading people to believe it is a different mechanism for some alternative reason, acting under the assumption that, if the true mechanics were explained, the patient could do the equivalent movement at home to themselves and, thereby, not need to repeatedly visit a chiropractor.

Their ability to help people then, to my assessment, becomes a process of simple therapy-mediated (as opposed to diagnosis-mediated) patient selection, whereby, those with minor disc herniations that are amenable to the chiropractic forces generated when the back is literally "wrung" by force, are helped. Those that do not have such simple lesions are eliminated with respect to the probability of future benefit. This causes me to contend that a certain set of patients actually do get true short-term relief because, in the twisting action of chiropractic manipulation, the disc is effectively (albeit violently) shoved back nearer to a more central position when the ligamentous structures holding the vertebral bodies together are tightened in a partially unweighted position. Regardless, it is not because someone figured out what was mechanically disordered through a diagnostic process and formulated the ideal therapy. It is more the product of myopic (in contradistinction to "blind") luck whether a person is helped or not.

It is technically fraudulent to classify chiropractic as a "science;" however, this is not to say that twisting a person's spine in a standard manner will not carry some level of success. Manipulative therapy is described by chiropractors as "the art of restoring a full and pain-free range of motion to joints in order to counteract the harmful local and distant effects of hyper- or hypo-mobile joints that have wide-ranging consequences on other parts of the body." They deliver a "high velocity but low amplitude thrust" that, usually, if successful, causes a usually painless, audible noise. In so far as I am concerned, the audible clunk, or crepitation that is heard is the fibrocartilaginous material crunching past other fibrocartilaginous material within the disc space. I have good reason to believe that it is the same sound often heard during the performance of *The O'Connor Technique (tm)* MANEUVERS.

A 1989 study reported that "the public seemed to be more satisfied with chiropractors' level of understanding of the problem of the spinal patient's problems and more confident with the diagnosis and management when compared to family practitioners"[36]. These data suggest that the family practitioners were not able to provide as clear or rational an explanatory model of the problem as chiropractors. **Considering that chiropractors themselves readily admit that they cannot explain how manipulative therapy actually functions mechanically, anatomically, or physiologically, these studies imply only that chiropractors are more expert at perpetrating misrepresentations than family practitioners.** It demonstrates to me that chiropractors do not help alleviate back pain better **but simply are better able to "con" patients into believing that they know what they are doing, and family practitioners are equally as ineffective but more honest in their responses.**

A societal casualty of this study's misinterpretation is the published conclusion: "**The message here is pretty clear: since most patients are going to get better regardless of the treatment they receive, how we (physicians) treat the pain is less important than how we make patients feel about their care.**"[37] To hear that sort of conclusion evidences to me the **sorry state of 1990's back pain management** and a more obvious finding. It would appear that **physicians are willing to concede that chiropractors are better at deceiving the public than they are and that doctors should learn to engage in similar practices so as to deceive patients equally well if not better. Such logic makes me lose faith in the competence of those researchers entrusted with the duty to adequately interpret scientific data and draw competent conclusions.**

In my opinion, the message should be something more akin to: physicians are doing a horrible job of helping people with back pain and rather than learn how to dissemble better than chiropractors, they should redouble their efforts to find a method that actually

helps people rather than creating an illusion of expertise while letting the patient walk out the door with only the law of probabilities on their side.

The O'Connor Technique (tm) can elegantly satisfy that need without resorting to hand-holding hocus-pocus. If you achieve substantial benefit from this book, I would suggest you give a copy of this book to the health care provider who failed to adequately alleviate your pain, so that they can, as rapidly as possible, begin to engage in meaningful discourse and treatments before they degenerate into chiropractic coddling. In the long run, true trust might be developed.

In deference to the field of chiropractic and to present a balanced picture, there are several controlled trials that provided evidence that chiropractic manipulation has a beneficial effect for low back pain, especially for select subgroups of patients; however in a study of 35 randomized trials of manipulation, only 5% showed an improved short term outcome, again though, selection biases and lack of standardized diagnoses make even that success profile subject to interpretive bias that evidences one already largely known marketplace fact: Some people do get relief from chiropractors.

What is problematic about their "theory" and practice is that they promote the belief that they can treat any number of unrelated diseases and that a long term management plan is necessary that causes a person to return again, and again, and again, for complete treatment success. In fact, they cannot consistently or scientifically fulfill those representations. Getting people to believe that a long-term, repetitive, practitioner mediated process is necessary accomplishes at least one thing--it insures a steady income for the chiropractor. Leading the patients to believe unrelated allergies or ear infections can be remedied by crunching on a spine, in my opinion, constitutes fraud and any chiropractor that strays into this realm should be abandoned in favor of one who sticks to helping the percentages of patients that they do help with spinal pain.

It is my belief that, in the future, when the principles of this book are widely studied for confirmatory validation, the chiropractic beneficial effect will be anatomically demonstrated to be slightly similar. In those few patients who have ideally-placed pieces of displaced disc material in the Lumbar or Cervical regions the herniated disc material can be serendipitously repositioned centrally by the wringing action of tightening the ligamentous peripheral lamina of the annulus fibrosus rapidly and forcefully during the twisting-type chiropractic manipulation very similar to the means described in the CHIROTATIONAL TWIST Section of this book. If this doesn't produce instant relief or if the lesion is in the less rotatorily mobile thoracic spine, another manipulative technique is employed in which the spine is put in slight traction by positioning; then a sharp, forceful push with the palms is given to the spine which induces an immediate hyperextension. This, too, is similar to the non-weight-bearing extension principle described in the EXTENSIONS Section of this book which physically squeezes the disc material anteriorly, so long as the disc material isn't positioned too far peripherally. If so, the pinching can squeeze off a partially extruded disc segment; and turn it into a fully extruded or sequestered fragment. Therein lies the harm they can do.

Their limited success rates can be explained because there are only certain small percentages of displaced discs configured ideally to be helped by conventional chiropractic manipulations and, I would argue, that these are the only patients who are benefited and, then, only for the short term. This commits those select patients who "swear by" instead of "swear at" chiropractors to a lifetime of repeated remissions requiring costly subsequent treatments. **Until**

the advances made by this book are put into widespread practice, without chiropractic treatments, these patients would still suffer; so, chiropractors do provide a legitimate service.

It is humorous (if not absurd) in this supposedly scientific era to recognize that chiropractors themselves admit that they can't (despite years of education) competently describe or explain adequately the means by which their method works; however, I do not deny them their successes in the above described context. The charade begins to be exposed when, before accomplishing the manipulation, scarce real efforts are made to truly diagnose those who definitely will be benefitted by the treatment. Too often, there is scant effort directed to select out those who most probably will be further injured by the process because that would be turning away "business;" however, in all fairness, I have treated a number of chiropractic referrals because the chiropractor did legitimately recognize a nerve impingement before initiating treatment.

In order to make the proper assessment, I can see no other way for them to safely persist in these practices unless they apply the theory and practice of this book or resort to routinely using CAT Scans, NMRI's, or Myelography to determine, in advance, the precise location of the disc material relative to the spinal nerves prior to the application of exogenous force. However, it would be unrealistic for them to attempt to convince patients to spend hundreds of dollars to insure that their manipulations are safe; so, they must just keep "cranking" on backs to see what happens. In an almost Darwinian selection process, only the "fittest" survive their culling and the rest are left to Nature's sometimes cruel alternatives.

You see, in order to achieve their limited success rates and therapeutic results, it is necessary for chiropractors to generate a certain high level of torque force to be effective on that percentage of backs that they do help. It is the act of applying that equivalent level of force injudiciously that gets them into trouble. Most apparently don't disseminate statistics upon how many patients leave the office in greater pain than when they entered.

Instead, most patients are given basically the same gibberish about a nebulous "subluxation" causing an aggravation of nerves having effects on any number of distant, anatomically unrelated organs or tissues, lain on a table, and given the same hand-on-shoulder and hip-twisting of the spine procedure given to everyone else who walks in the door. This may be accompanied by some different hocus-pocus with measurements of the legs, levels of the shoulders, or expensive (largely useless) X-rays. This practice wouldn't be so bad if they didn't usually buy-up old X-Ray machines with higher radiation outputs than are allowed to be sold today and unnecessarily expose their patient's sexual organs which are particularly sensitive to radiation damage. One needn't accept my word on this score, according to a recognized authority on the spine, Dr. Richard A. Deyo: **"Spine films are of little use in making a diagnosis, and they are costly and expose patients to significant radiation directed right at the genitals."** One would do well to consider the risk/benefit ratio of spinal X-rays before consenting to them.

My knowledge of the spine gives me reason to believe that a wrenching maneuver of the spine could quite reasonably result in a worsening of the patient's condition. If the herniation has progressed to the point where the disc material is on the verge of or has actually escaped the joint capsule, then the action of twisting can squeeze the fragment further into the canal resulting in a sequestered fragment or, worse, can shove the fragment into a nerve root. This can change a condition from not necessarily a surgical condition to a surgical necessity.

No statistics of which I am aware have documented the number of people who have had borderline discs turned into surgical cases due to forceful manipulation. In fact, it would be very difficult to do so because it would require an NMRI or CT scan in advance of going to a chiropractor. Then, after the damaging event, the patient would have to have a repeat NMRI or CT to document the disc material's movement. Such a study would also have to demonstrate that the disc did not get worse on its own. Such a study would require the coordination of a chiropractor and a neurosurgeon such that the chiropractor anticipated that he could make a particular patient worse and, immediately after he does, sends him to a neurosurgeon. Alternatively, thousands of patients going to chiropractors would have to have a CT or NMRI immediately prior to and after such an event. The former would never occur because no reasonable chiropractor will expose himself to the potential lawsuit resulting from a condition he knew he made worse in the presence of an anticipation to do so and the latter would be so expensive as to be prohibitive. So, the requisite science to provide this information does not appear to be forthcoming in the immediate future.

The O'Connor Technique (tm) doesn't fall into this trap because, **largely, through self-manipulation, the patient is able to control the direction and level of force at all times**, which they can automatically stop before it becomes too painful to cause damage. No rapid torque is required to achieve the same results in nearly all the people who would otherwise be actually helped by chiropractors. In that sense, **the reader of this book can, more safely, become their own chiropractor and more.**

Personally, with those patients I manipulate in the office, I could not bring myself to do such a forceful manipulation without knowing the anatomy of the problem for fear that I could possibly make the patient worse. A simple X-Ray would not accomplish this necessity because it doesn't image soft tissues and the non-bony disc material does not show up on an X-Ray. The CT and the NMRI do so, but they cost around $1000. No other imaging study short of a myelogram (a painfully invasive X-Ray that places dye into the spinal canal) would show the proximity of the disc material to the nerve root and thereby ascertain manipulation's safety.

So, chiropractors largely approach the condition blindly or at best with such poor acuity that, to me, constitutes a potentially dangerous form of individualized human experimentation. If they perform the same manipulation on everyone, the ones that get better will come back, and those that are hurt worse presumably won't. When the people who do get worse don't come back, the chiropractor assumes they are better if he is an optimist, but rarely will concede that they may have gotten markedly worse unless he is taken to court.

Luckily, the low back is relatively forgiving when it comes to the damage a chiropractor can potentially do; but, when chiropractors attempt to manipulate the neck, especially in the elderly, the vertebral artery's actual passage through a hole in the transverse processes of the cervical vertebrae and/or the tension put on the carotid artery can lead to a stroke.

A recent report presented at a stroke conference sponsored by the American Heart Association, at which several specialists said they had treated patients' arteries torn during sessions with chiropractors, described "probably the best documented cause of rips--what doctors call dissections--is chiropractic manipulation of the neck." At the conference, Dr. William Powers of Washington University in St. Louis said "every neurologist in this room has seen two or three people who have suffered this after chiropractic manipulation." It was also stated that 85% of cases result in at least mild impairment according to a Stanford survey.[38]

The O'Connor Technique (tm) differs substantially from chiropractic in that no forceful movements or manipulations are necessary or advocated. **Success in alleviating pain does not rely simply upon the actual movement or forcefulness of the effort with** *The O'Connor Technique (tm)* **but with the proper sequential combinations of movements** that are revealed herein. **Forcefulness is not necessary to open a lock if one knows the combination.** The patient performing the MANEUVERS controls the amount of force and can stop the maneuver at anytime pain occurs. The time taken to relax necessary muscle groups and allow the components of the annulus fibrosus to accept traction is an individualized process that the individual determines. In those cases where this technique would be equivalently as successful as chiropractic, the same end is achieved; but the cost is almost non-existent with *The O'Connor Technique (tm)*.

With *The O'Connor Technique (tm)*, **most persons who do routinely get relief from chiropractors are taught to do their own "manipulation" and given the power and means to prevent future pain themselves.** Even if chiropractors knew what they were doing they would be unlikely to share their "secret" because that would reduce the number of people coming back for treatment, after treatment, after treatment. For this reason, **it will probably be a long time before chiropractors embrace the theory and practice of this technique and may be reluctant to teach it since to do so might put the majority of them out of business.** In fact, it would not surprise me to see a rather boisterous reaction to any large-scale promotion of *The O'Connor Technique (tm)* from some components of the chiropractic establishment.

HOPE

At times, it may seem to the back pain sufferer that there is little or no hope for ever being "normal" again. Some readers may say to themselves, "If I have to go through all this every day of my life, I might just as well have the whole thing fused surgically and live with a stiff low back."

I would strongly argue that this is the wrong attitude. **Surgery should only be viewed as the very last resort for unremittant, debilitating, pain or vertebral instability when neurological function is compromised or at risk of being lost.** Later in the book, you will learn that, **even for people who undergo a fusion surgery or discectomy, the predisposition for additional degenerative disc disease still exists at other (especially adjacent) levels of the spine. Without intentional intervention, the damaging forces acting upon the discs will still be present and capable of inducing further future disability and pain.** Quite often, the surgery is only a partial discectomy and the same disc continues to degenerate. Just because you have one disc repaired, doesn't mean that your problems with your spine are solved. Quite the contrary, if **you don't alter the mechanics, there is every reason to believe that other discs will fall prey to the same forces that damaged the original one.**

In fact, my observation has been that an inordinately **large percentage of persons with Lumbar disc disease eventually present with similar Cervical or Thoracic disc problems and visa versa**. This leads me to conclude that there must be certain genetic predispositions to faulty disc mechanics and that the ramifications of some inherent structural protein difference results in a weakness of ligamentous capacity that is reflected in one person's ability to sustain the same amount of force without damage to the disc whereas another person under identical circumstances ends up with a damaged disc. I suspect it has something to do with the tensile strength and elasticity of their collagen fibers (the proteins that compose ligaments and cartilage) and that there are certain genetic subsets of persons who are destined, by virtue of their hyper-elastic collagen, to have an increased probability of disc disease regardless of whether or not they sustain major, forceful injuries. This trait may make them evolutionarily more likely to survive by giving them the "wirey" capacity to wriggle free of their enemies; but the gains they achieve in elasticity leave them deficient in tensile strength. If this is true, these people (of which I think persons with hyper-flexible joints and/or scoliosis may be an extremely affected subset) may be prevented from what otherwise appears to be an inevitable fate. However, it is too early for me to make that speculation formally; and this book is not the appropriate forum. Suffice it to say, I have enough information to advance the suspicion and hypothesis because I have observed scoliosis induced by disc disease. Time and wide-spread use of *The O'Connor Technique (tm)* will determine whether this suspicion is correct. Until then, persons with early scoliosis are free to make and act upon the assumption that the origin of their disease process rests in hyper-migratory disc material and use *The O'Connor Technique (tm)* to try to prevent disfiguration. They certainly are unlikely to come to any additional harm by practicing these techniques; and I would enjoy learning if they appear to be successful, so that a comprehensive, scientific study could be rapidly assembled to test that hypothesis. The number of scoliosis patients I currently, or ever, will see in my practice is so small as to be negligible--someone else will have to study that question.

Contrary to political rhetoric, all men are <u>not</u> created equal. However, that is not to say a person with a predisposition for a bad back is inferior to someone with an intact spine because having extra-flexible collagen may impart some other selection advantage and survival value. Judging from the multitudes with bad backs alive today, it seemingly doesn't carry any Darwinian selection disadvantages. Perhaps the increased flexibility carries with it an, as yet unrecognized, selection advantage, the usefulness of which becomes less significant after offspring are successfully reared.

However, **it does not follow that simply because one has a bad back that it is the result of an inexorable genetic failing. One needn't adopt the fatalistic attitude that their Fate is immutable or that they are pre-destined to suffer or I would not have written this book.**

Hope does exist in the peculiar capacity the human organism has for accommodation on an intellectual and structural level. Understand that acting upon knowledge can favorably change fate, and the body is not a static entity. It is constantly being broken down and rebuilt on a microscopic level. Although, to the unenlightened, when viewing a skeleton it seems to exist as a hard, rigid, structural frame that is unchanging in life as much as it is in death. Quite the contrary, even this rigid bony structure is constantly being broken down and reformed at the cellular level. This rebuilding can be modified depending upon the stresses applied. Obviously, there are certain structures that, once broken, cannot be rebuilt to their original functional capacity. There are certain conditional restrictions upon the ability of the human organism to repair damage. Yet, **over time, the pre-programmed capacity of the body to modify its structure can be capitalized upon to expect eventual healing and return to a near-normal functional activity level.**

51

A major constituent of *The O'Connor Technique (tm)* is a fundamental methodology that optimizes the capacity of the human body to intellectually and physically adapt to spinal damage as well as maximize effective repair. These components are referred to as **FLEXION AVOIDANCE, MAINTENANCE OF EXTENSION, DYNAMIC POSITIONING, and PREFERENTIAL STRENGTHENING/SELECTIVE HYPERTROPHY.** With these and other innovations in back pain management, *The O'Connor Technique (tm)* **has taken a great step forward in reducing the healing time, decreasing the duration of back pain events, and preventing or reducing the frequency of future episodes.** Separate sections in the book specifically address these components and throughout the book wherever pertinent, they are reiterated in contexts where appropriate. **The reader who understands and practices them can expect to have true hope for a largely pain-free future.**

1.   Bigos SJ, Deyo RA, Romanowski TS, Whitten RR, The new thinking on low back pain, *Patient Care*; July 15, 1995:140-172

2.   Bigos S, Bowyer O, Braen G, et al. *Acute Low Back Problems in Adults.* Clinical Practice Guideline, Quick Reference Guide Number 14. Rockville, MD: U.S. Dept. of Health and Human Services, Public Health Service, Agency for Health Care Policy and Research, AHCPR Pub. No. 95-0643. December 1994.

3.   Korff, et al., *Pain* , 1988, 32:173-83.

4.   Reis S, et al., Low Back Pain: More than Anatomy, *The Journal of Family Practice*, 1992;35(5):509.

5.   Deyo RA, Mayer TG, et al., The painful back: Keep it moving, *Patient Care*, October 30, 1987:47-59.

6.   Frymoyer JW, Helping your patients avoid low back pain, The *Journal of Musculoskeletal Medicine*, May 1989:83-101.

7.   Frymoyer JW, Helping your patients avoid low back pain, The *Journal of Musculoskeletal Medicine*, May 1989:83.

8.   Graves EJ. *Diagnosis-Related Groups Using Data from the National Hospital Discharge Survey: United States--1985.* Hyattsville, Md: 1987. US Dept of Health and Human Services publication 87-1250.

9.   Miller S, Total Fitness Program Best for Low Back Problems, *Family Practice News,* June 1-14, 1989; 19(11):37.

10. Op.Cit. Endnote #1;p.140-172

11.   Cole HM (ed.), Diagnostic and Therapeutic Technology Assessment (DATTA), *The Journal of the American Medical Association*, Sept 19, 1990, 264, (11):1469--1472.

12.   Sack B, Acute and Chronic low back pain: How to pinpoint its cause and make the diagnosis, *Modern Medicine*, Sept. 1992;(60):58-92.

13.   Vlok GJ, Hendrix MR. The Lumbar disc: evaluating the cause of pain. *Orthopedics*, 1991; 14:419-25.

14.   Deyo RA, Loeser JD, Bigos SJ. Herniated Lumbar intervertebral disk. *Ann Intern Med*, 1990;112:598-603.

15.   Predicting Outcome in Back Pain Patients, *Family Practice News*, Oct 1-14, 1986:1-36.

16.   Frymoyer JW. Back pain and sciatica. *N Engl J Med*. 1988;31;82-91

17.   Anon, Family Practice News, August 1-14, 1987.

18.   Anon, Back Pain Is a Definitive Diagnosis Necessary?, *Emergency Medicine*; February 15, 1993:131-134.

19.   Cherkin D, Deyo RA, Berg AO, et al, University of Washington, Seattle, and other centers; Evaluation of a physician education intervention to improve primary care for low-back pain I: Impact on physicians. *Spine*, Oct 1991;16:1168-1172.

20.   Cherkin D, Deyo RA, Berg AO, et al, University of Washington, Seattle, and other centers; Evaluation of a physician education intervention to improve primary care for low-back pain I: Impact on patients. *Spine*, Oct 1991;16:1173-1178.

21.   Kriyananda, *Yoga Postures for Self-Awareness*,(1969) Ananda Publications, San Francisco, CA, USA.

22.   Yogiraj Sri Swami Satchidananda, *Integral Yoga Hatha*, (1970), Holt, Rinehart and Winston, New York, USA, p. 49.

23.   McKenzie, R, *Treat Your Own Back*, Spinal Publications LTD., P.O. Box 93, Maikanae, New Zealand, p.9.

24.   Mooney V, quoted in Backache: What Patterns of Pain Pinpoint the Source?, *Data Centrum*, April 1984;1(4):25-37.

25.   Weber H, Lumbar disc herniation: a controlled, prospective study with tens years of observation. *Spine*. 1983;8:131-140.

26.   Saal JA, Saal JS, Herzog RJ. The natural history of Lumbar intervertebral disc extrusions treated non-operatively. *Spine*, 1990;15:683-6.

27.   Williams PC. *Low back and neck pain causes and conservative treatment.2nd ed, Springfield, Ill:Charles C Thomas, Publisher;1974.*

28.   Leblan K, et al. Report of the Quebec task force on spinal disorders. *Spine.* 1987;12:S1-S8.28.

29.   *Op.cit.*, Bigos, Endnote #2.

30.   Donelson RG, Identifying appropriate exercises for your low back pain patient. *The Journal of Musculoskeletal Medicine*; December 1991:14-29.

31.   Weed D, *Chiropractic Care*, The Specialists Neck and Shoulder Injuries Lecture, August 31, 1995, Fairfield, CA.

32.   Ross EC, Parnianpour M, Martin D, The effect of resistance level on muscle coordination patterns and movement profile during trunk extension. *Spine.* 1993;18:1829-1838.

33.   Flicker PL, Fleckenstein JL, Ferry K, et al. Lumbar muscle usage in chronic low back pain. *Spine.* 1993;18:582.

34.   Valkenburg HA, Haanen HCM. The epidemiology of low back pain, in White AAIII, Gordon SL (eds) American Academy of Orthopedic Surgeons Symposium on Idiopathic Low Back Pain, St. Louis, CV Mosby Co, 1982:9-22.

35.   Troup JD, Martin JW, Lloyd DC, Back pain in industry: A Prospective Survey, *Spine* (1981) 6:61-69.

36.   Cherkin D, MacCornack FA. Patient evaluation of low back pain care from family physicians and chiropractors. *West J Med*, 1989, 150:351-5.

37.   Hockberger RS, Meeting the Challenge of Low Back Pain, *Emergency Medicine*; August 15, 1990:99-127.

38.   Associated Press, Report on the causes of stroke fingers chiropractors, *San Francisco Sunday Examiner and Chronicle*, 2/20/94:A5

CHAPTER TWO: PHYSICAL REALITY

SPINAL ANATOMY

In order to comprehend the concepts presented in this book it is essential to acquire a clear understanding of the vertebral column's basic anatomy. Since this book is not intended to be an all-encompassing re-creation of the great anatomical textbooks, I have chosen to limit discussion to only those anatomical terms and features that have a direct bearing upon the understanding of *The O'Connor Technique (tm)*. For a more extensive elaboration of spinal features, the reader is directed to any medical school anatomy textbook by which they choose to be bored.

Don't be intimidated by a few new terms. It takes only a few minutes to quickly learn them and be able to employ them in the context of the ensuing discussions. I have intentionally limited the technical aspects of the book to a minimum because it is more important that the layman understands what is going on than for me to be able to market this book as the definitive reference on the spine to my physician colleagues. If, at first, it is hard to keep the terms straight, just refer to the diagrams every time you need to refresh your mind as you read on. I have made a distinct effort to repeat and clarify whenever technical terms are used that aren't readily known by most people. So, don't get bogged down trying to memorize all the names of the body parts because you erroneously believe that you must commit them to memory before you can understand the remainder of the book. Keep reading, look at the diagrams, and refer back to the definitions whenever you are not certain about a particular term or technical name.

Unfortunately, unique things have unique names and to understand a novel topic, you must be prepared to learn a few new words. Referring to a particular anatomical structure as "the little thing in the back," would only denigrate the accuracy of what is presented here and make things more confusing. So, just don't look upon it as a burden, and settle in to learn a few new words if you already don't know them. Assuming that the reader is not immediately technically oriented, I have made an effort to repeat the definitions in the text so that as it is read, the positional anatomy is clarified until the reader is sufficiently familiar with the terms.

DIRECTIONAL TERMINOLOGY

The following terms are frequently used in medical terminology to describe anatomical directions. They can be used to describe the entire body or any of its parts. One should have a familiarity with them in order to fully understand the concepts, positions, and movements described throughout the book:

SUPERIOR--means in the direction of the top of the head or the top of the body. Saying "up" is often inaccurate because if a person is lying on their back, "up" is really anterior, so using the term "superior" is superior because it is always references towards the head's aspect of the anatomical part in question. The whole body or any part can be moved superiorly if it moves in the direction of the head.

INFERIOR--means in the direction of the soles of the feet and situated below or directed downward. It can also refer to that part of the body or body part closest to the feet (such as "the inferior aspect of the chin"). The whole body can be moved inferiorly if it moves in the direction of the feet.

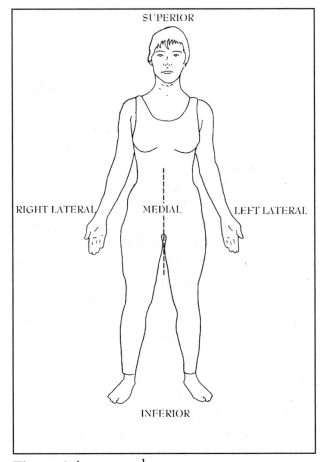

Figure 1 Anatomical terms

LATERAL--refers to the sides of the body. There is a left and right lateral (side) aspect to just about every anatomical part as well as the body in general. When the term lateral aspect is used it refers to that component of anatomy away from the midline of the trunk. When something moves laterally, it moves away from the midline.

MEDIAL--refers to the center or midline of the body or body part. When an anatomical structure is said to be medial, it is more towards the midline of the torso. Often, the term, medial aspect, is used and that refers to that component of anatomy closest to the midline of the trunk. Something moves medially if it moves towards the midline.

ANTERIOR--means toward the front of the body. One can move a body part anteriorly by moving it towards the front of the body. A body part can have an anterior aspect, that being that component closest to the front of the body. From the word "ante" which refers to something "up front," before, or at the beginning, such as in antebellum (before the Civil War) or like what you do before you play a hand of "penny-"ante" poker. You put up a penny up front as a bet.

POSTERIOR--means toward the back surface or rear of the body, such as getting kicked in your "posterior." It can reference a part of the body in relation to another such as the vertebral bone parts that are closest to the back surface of the body are referred to as the posterior elements. One can also move a body part to the posterior by moving it towards the back surface of the body.

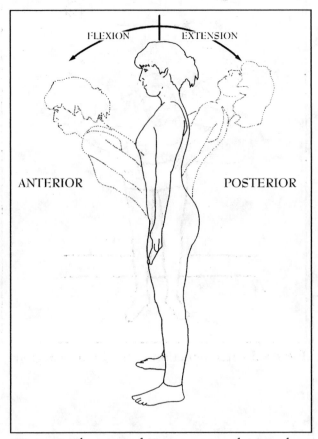

Figure 2 Flexion and Extension at the Lumbar region from the Neutral anatomical position.

FLEXION--from "to bend" in Latin. Any time you decrease the angle made by two bones you "flex" at the joint which joins those two bones. In the case of the spine, bending forward produces the action of anterior flexion when viewed from the side. When viewed from the front, a person can bend to the side and the spine can be said to laterally flex or bend. Spinal Flexion in this book refers to any movement that bends the spine anteriorly whether the spine is in the neutral position or while in an extended posture flexes to return towards the neutral position.

EXTENSION--the opposite of flexion, from the Latin for "stretching out" and therefore is an increase in the angle formed by the axis of two bones. This can refer to the body being brought back to the neutral, resting, anatomical position from a flexed position, or going from the neutral anatomical position towards the posterior.

If a person bends backwards or posteriorly, the spine is said to perform EXTENSION, regardless of any other position the body may be assuming at the same time.

The spine can be in flexion and extend to the neutral position or be in the neutral position and extend to the posterior. Also, the spine can be in EXTENSION and extend maximally beyond the usual range of motion into HYPEREXTENSION.

CIRCUMDUCTION--from the Latin "to draw around." This is actually a combination of the movements previously described. It consists of a smooth series of movements (Shown in Figure 3) starting with anterior flexion, leaning into lateral flexion, lateral extension, and posterior extension in that specific sequence. In this example, the circumduction takes the upper body in a clockwise direction. However, it could start at any point on the circle, go only part way around, or even go in the opposite direction; and it still would be considered circumduction. If this action is performed at any level of the spine, the portion of the body above the point of movement will be brought anteriorly and laterally, then posteriorly and then medially, resulting in the superior aspect of the anatomy to gyrate around in a circular pattern. Since the inferior aspect of the spine below the point of motion is fixed in this example, the upper section moves through its range of motion carving out the form of an inverted cone in space.

SUPINE--that position in which a person lies flat with the face, abdomen, and toes pointing up.

PRONE--that position in which a person lies flat with the face, abdomen, and toes all pointing down.

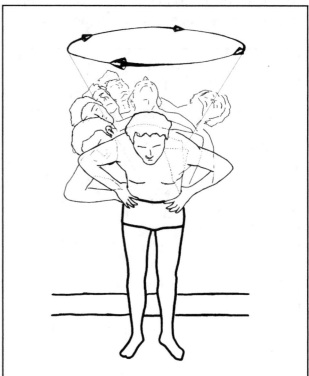

Figure 3 Circumduction at the Lumbar region.

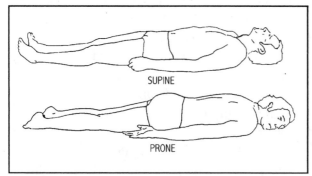

Figure 4 Prone and supine positions

58

STRUCTURAL ANATOMY

The spinal column has classically been divided into several structurally and functionally distinct sections, the cervical spine, the thoracic spine, the lumbar spine and the sacral spine. Largely, this book deals with the cervical, thoracic, and lumbar sections since the sacral section is functionally fused and offers little opportunity for mechanical manipulation except where it interfaces with the lumbar spine at L-5, which is probably the most problematic area in the spine because it is the first mobile segment above the rigid pelvis. (See Figure 5)

It is important here to note the curvature of the spine. It is not a straight linear structure when viewed from the side (or the "lateral" view). The major curves are seen at the cervical and lumbar regions where the majority of flexibility is also present.

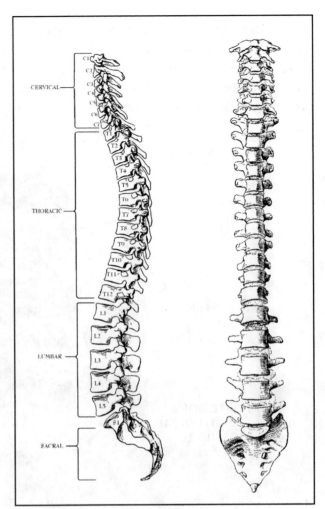

Figure 5 Vertebral Column

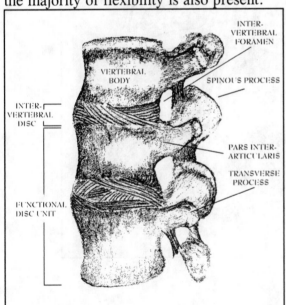

Figure 6 Vertebral Column Segment L3-L5.

One can look upon the spinal column as an incredibly strong central support structure upon which the trunk and upper body rest similar to a long series of bony spools separated by cushions. The spools being named the vertebral bodies and the cushions are the intervertebral discs (or simply referred to as the "disc"). A functional disc unit is comprised of the vertebral bone above and below an interposed disc (see Fig. 6).

59

The anterior portion of the vertebral column (spools with cushions between them) is a weight bearing, shock absorbing, flexible structure capable of amazing feats of strength. The posterior portion is composed of bony bridges and spikes that protect the spinal cord and nerves, acts both as a moment arm and as a fulcrum, and guides the movement of the functional unit while maintaining the vertebral bones' positions relative to the each other. As can be seen in Figure 7,

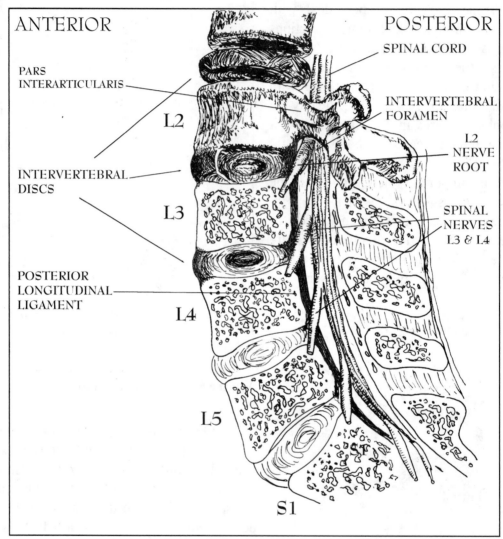

Figure 7 Cut-away lateral view of Lumbar Spine

the anterior and posterior components join at the *pars interarticularis* to create a canal through which the spinal cord travels and sends its major branches, the spinal nerves, out through spaces called intervertebral foramens. The superior aspect of the intervertebral foramen is composed of one *pars interarticularis* and the inferior border is composed of the vertebral bone adjacent and inferior to it.

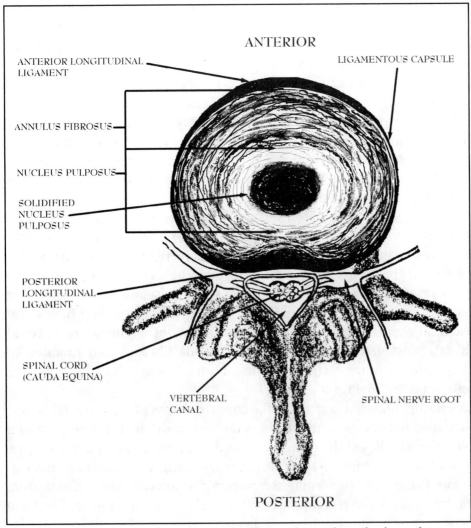

A view looking down on a cross-section of the vertebral bones can be seen in Figure 8 so the reader can understand the relationships between these structures. Especially important is the close proximity of the discs to the spinal nerves. If a disc ruptures posteriorly, it can be easily seen to be capable of impinging upon a spinal nerve root and damaging it, resulting in paralysis and anesthesia.

Figure 8 Cross-section of Intervertebral Disc from above looking down

For the purposes of this book, the posterior elements can be largely ignored. Not that they do not serve as sources of pain such as arthritis (because they contain joints) or sprains (because they have ligaments holding them together); but, **in the largest part, the mechanical pain experienced in the spine originates from a degeneration of the stress-dissipating and pressure containment structures known as the intervertebral discs**.

Of course, the intervertebral disc (usually referred to simply as the "disc") is not the only structure that dissipates stresses placed on the spine. With flexion, extension, rotation, or shear stress, the load distribution on the entire functional unit is shared by the intervertebral disc, anterior and posterior longitudinal ligaments, the facet joints and the capsule, and other ligamentous structures like the ligamentum flavum and the interspinous and supra spinous ligaments, which attach to the posterior elements of the functional unit. Those **anatomical structures other than those directly contiguous with the disc are largely unamenable to mechanical manipulation and don't usually get into trouble without major trauma** (by major trauma, I refer to falls off of roofs or major motor vehicle accidents as opposed to minor trauma like lifting garbage cans); therefore, they are outside of the scope of this book. They need not be focused upon in this book because to do so would just be confusing and distract the reader from the major goal of understanding that **the most common source of a "bad back" is damage to the disc itself.** However, that is not to say that the other problematic entities are insignificant or incapable of producing misery, it is just that the other causes of back pain are both individually and cumulatively in the distinct minority. **In fact, if one doesn't achieve relief from practicing the principles of** *The O'Connor Technique (tm)***, it is unlikely that a disc is the source of the pain; and I would encourage that category of patient to seek help elsewhere armed with the reassurance that they have probably eliminated disc disease as the origin of their pain.**

The spool-like vertebral bodies are held together with tough ligaments that connect bone to bone. On the front (anterior) surfaces lie the anterior longitudinal ligaments and at the back (posterior) surfaces lie the posterior longitudinal ligaments. These two major ligament systems which traverse the spine lengthwise blend at the disc spaces between vertebral bodies with other laterally situated, ligamentous structures of the spine (the lateral intervertebral ligaments) that also run longitudinally along the axis of the spinal column. All these ligaments merge together to circumferentially enclose the more cartilage-like central regions of the disc, forming what is often referred to as a **"capsule"** at the disc level. **This capsule consists of dense, strong fibers that are firmly bound to each adjacent vertebral body. These sheets of ligamentous material blend with the peripheral, most dense, portion of the annulus fibrosus and function to contain both the more gelatinous inner sections of the annulus fibrosus and, in turn, the more liquid nucleus pulposus** (See Figures 8 & 9).

This ligamentous capsule, in combination with the concave shapes of the vertebral bones' surfaces, **keeps the more internal components of disc material positioned in line with and centrally between the vertebral bodies of the spine.** When the body bends forward (flexes), the postero-lateral ligamentous lamina (layers) and the posterior longitudinal ligaments straighten, tighten, and assume a more linear axis, preventing the posterior aspects of the vertebrae from totally separating or coming apart while retaining flexibility. The anterior ligaments perform likewise for the anterior when one bends posteriorly (extends).

Other ligaments which are attached to the processes of the vertebral bodies also function to hold the entire apparatus together; however, they are not as pertinent to the principles of this book because the **posterior longitudinal and the intervertebral capsules' ligamentous structures are the fibers which house and keep the cartilaginous disc material from moving posteriorly.** Were it not for these ligaments, the discs would have no structural elements to maintain the central disc material positioned correctly between the vertebral bodies. Figure 9 shows these ligaments with their normal structure on the right and their damaged structure on the left.

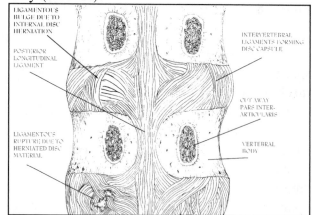

Figure 9 Posterior view of vertebral ligaments with *pars interarticularis* cut away.

When these structures are damaged, they no longer prevent the central disc material from moving posteriorly, the profound significance of which will become apparent later.

The ligamentous tissues that form the disc's capsule are well-supplied by nerves-- both stretch and pain receptors. This nerve supply enables the brain to know where in space (relative to the other bones) a given bone is positioned, enabling a human to stand erect and balance the portion of the body above the hips with his spine. In contrast to the outer, peripheral, ligamentous structures, the material deep to the capsule, the annulus fibrosus and the nucleus pulposus, do not have a nerve supply (See Figure 10). **So, disc pain, when it is present, comes from structures other than the more liquid "cushions" or any other structures deeper than a few millimeters from the surface of the disc.** This fact leads some to conclude the common misconception that a patient cannot have pain from their discs. On the contrary, **when the disc material that should remain secure within the center presses upon or distorts the ligaments that surround the disc, the pain can be exceptionally intense.**

More on pain later; but, for now, it is helpful to understand that the numbered spinal nerves exit the spinal column at the level of the disc inferior to the same numbered vertebral bone. So, the Second Lumbar (**L2**) nerve and its root (See Figure 7) passes out of the spinal column at the level of the disc below the Second Lumbar Vertebrae through the *intervertebral foramen* partly formed by the inferior component of its *pars interarticularis* (also known as a pedicle). The *intervertebral foramens* are round spaces (between one pars interarticularis and the next) created by the spinal bones through which pass the spinal nerve roots (See Figures 6&8). The spinal nerves supply motor and sensory functions to their corresponding segments of the body. The proximity of these structures to the intervertebral disc is important because **if the central disc material herniates and protrudes it can irritate or trap the spinal nerves resulting in pain, loss of sensation, and/or paralysis wherever the effected nerve roots supply innervation.** The pattern of this pain is classically described in terms of what structures are supplied by the nerves: dermatomes (areas of skin), myotomes (muscles), sclerotomes (bones, joints, & ligaments) to which the individual nerves for each major spinal nerve travel.

It is technically interesting to know what each spinal nerve innervates so that when pain is felt or function lost it can be localized to a particular spinal nerve and, hence, a doctor can determine which disc protrusion is compressing its corresponding nerve. Such detail is too complex for the intended readers of this book. The reader is free to research any of a number of medical textbooks for this additional information; however I have found this level of expertise confusing and unnecessary to understand the concepts of *The O'Connor Technique (tm)*.

What is important to understand is that each numbered spinal nerve sends a branch (the *recurrent sinuvertebral nerve*) to the ligaments that surround and contain the disc immediately inferior to the same numbered vertebral bone. The pain and sensory fibers of the discs travel in these nerve branches (See Figure 10). The *recurrent sinuvertebral nerve* is significant because if pain comes from a disc's ligamentous capsule it travels in that nerve. Pain impulses from this nerve can be interpreted by the brain as coming from the larger, numbered, spinal nerve in which it travels as one of many other different nerves. The implications of this anatomical design peculiarity will become more apparent later, but suffice it to say, here, that **this phenomenon can explain why pain in the disc can masquerade as pain in the extremities and why muscles**

distant from the actual site of disc pain can go into spasm even though the muscle itself has not been a c t u a l l y traumatized. More on this subject when pain is discussed.

It is very pertinent to the understanding of *The O'Connor Technique (tm)* to have a view of the disc in the mind's e y e . T h e intervertebral discs' spherical centers are composed of a gelatinous liquid cartilage material

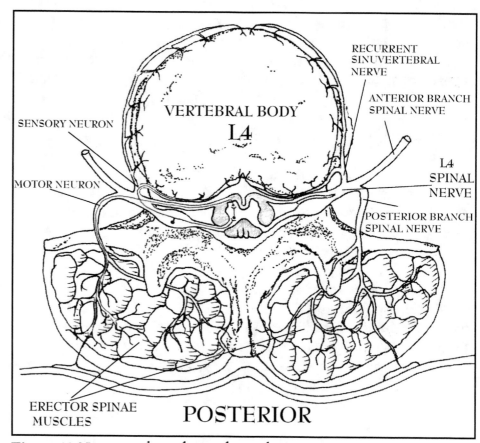

Figure 10 Nerve supply to disc and muscles

identified as the nucleus pulposus surrounded by an intermeshing laminated concentric fibrous structure known as the annulus fibrosus. The annulus fibrosus is designed with fibrocartilaginous

and fibrous protein tissue arranged in concentric layers, each of which attach one vertebrae to the other (See Figure 11). As one moves, anatomically speaking, from the nucleus pulposus to the periphery, the tissues become more dense, stronger, less elastic, less fluid, and more ligamentous until reaching the outermost layers. There, the tissues actually become a tough, capsular ligament.

The laminations of the annulus fibrosus are arranged in bands of tough elastic tissue whose fibers run at oblique angles to the adjacent layers to form a shock absorber (See Figure 12), built like a gelatinous/liquid surrounded by layers of Chinese finger traps.

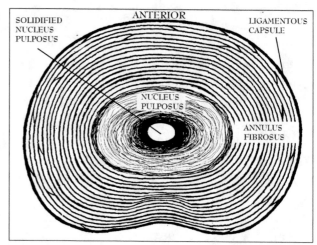

Figure 11 Cross-sectional view of Intervertebral disc viewed from superior

64

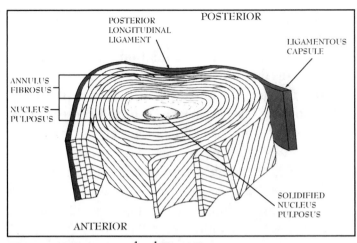

Figure 12 Intervertebral Disc Laminations

As vertically (axial) directed forces are placed upon a disc's liquid center (nucleus pulposus) it deforms by flattening along a horizontal plane. In this way, the pressure is absorbed and contained by the laminations of the annulus fibrosus. The fibers of the annulus fibrosus are firmly secured to the vertebral bones and mingle with the lateral ligamentous structures as well as the anterior and posterior longitudinal ligaments.

To experience an accurate representation of this structure's consistency, the reader can go to a meat market that stocks large ox tails. Feeling with a finger the center portion of the largest ones and, often in older animal's discs, you can appreciate the liquid character and the central hardened material by pressing the center of the circular white solidified segment. A nearly identical structural design is located in the human disc. By manipulating the hard center structure, one can appreciate how it can be moved with alterations in pressure supplied by the finger. When one bends the spine, forces are placed upon the disc that cause the part-liquid/part-solid, disc material to be equivalently moved.

FUNCTIONAL ANATOMY

The **nucleus pulposus in combination with the annulus fibrosus affords shock absorbency function to the disc** and allows the functional disc unit its dynamic flexibility. With compressive forces, the nucleus pulposus stretches the annular fibers somewhat like a jelly filled tennis ball would flatten when a weight was placed on it. Flexion or extension of the functional unit occurs in part because of the horizontal shift of fluid within the disc, resulting in the expansion of the annular fibers posteriorly or anteriorly, respectively. The elastic nature of the annular fibers tend to oppose and contain the movement of the nucleus pulposus, thereby, tending to restore the functional disc unit to its resting state when the compressive forces are relieved. **Sadly, as the disc ages, this elasticity is gradually lost and the capability of the disc to recoil from compressive forces decreases.**

Fibro-cartilaginous structures like those comprising the annulus fibrosus have some measure of elasticity; but their fibers are largely fixed in their maximum length and, if stretched beyond that, especially if done rapidly, they can fracture or fragment. **When these types of tissues tear or break, they (as a rule after childhood) do not repair themselves.** Even the peripheral ligamentous structures do not heal by re-making equivalent tissue (as is often incorrectly assumed) but are replaced by scar. Unfortunately, the scar tissue is never quite as strong as the previously intact ligament. The ramifications of this fact will become painfully

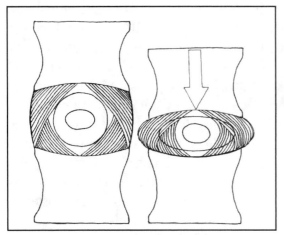

Figure 13 Disc as Shock Absorber

apparent as an understanding of disc "disease" unfolds later.

Thus, **the combination of the annulus fibrosus and the ligamentous capsular structures surrounding it functions to contain the shock absorbing, weight-bearing, liquid center, yet at the same time, allowing an incredible amount of flexibility**. If one wishes to appreciate just how flexible, dynamic, adaptable, and amazing a structure the *homo sapiens* vertebral column is, just watch an Olympic gymnastics competition and compare the flexibility seen there with the strength displayed in the weight-lifting sessions. For all its supposed faults, the vertebral column still garners an awesome depth of respect from this author.

The intact spine is no anatomical or physiological wimp by any stretch of the imagination. The lower lumbar discs can sustain loads of **1,000 Kilograms** (2,200 lbs) when stressed with pure compressive forces.[1] In a rather narrow-visioned perspective, many "experts" criticize the evolutionary design of the back by asserting that the vertebral column has not adequately developed evolutionarily to support man's upright posture. I would argue that it is doing a fantastic job, and a more adequate structure-for-function relationship doesn't exist within the parameters of biological design.

Thinking about it from an evolutionary survival standpoint, humans do not really need their back after they have reproduced and successfully raised their children to the age when they can fend for themselves. That's just about the time the discs start to age and break down. I think Evolution and/or God designed it pretty well considering what it is capable of accomplishing. It is only when humans are no longer useful (from a Darwinian perspective) does the spine fail.

Reportedly, aboriginally-living peoples experience a much lower prevalence of disc disease. The peaceful, archetypal, hunter-gatherers infrequently need put the forces on the spine sufficient to herniate discs. Only when man <u>socially</u> "evolves" to the level wherein he routinely builds structures out of heavy materials, fights one another, eats so much excess food that he becomes twice the weight he was designed to accommodate, or performs feats of athletic largess beyond the limits for which it was intended, does he destroy the integrity his spine. Our problem is not inferior spinal construction, the design is perfect for "Gardening in Eden." **Our problem is that the evolution of our tools and their use has not caught up with the design specifications imposed by an otherwise perfectly suited creation. Thus far, unable to find "the right tool for the right job," we have resorted to using our backs as tools--mostly in pursuit of purposes for which they were not constructed to accommodate. One can hardly charge Nature with the sin of imperfection when it is our own chosen misgivings at fault.**

This point is exemplified, and the reader can gain an appreciation of the magnitude of the forces applied to the disc, by an enterprising researcher who once convinced a number of average-sized study subjects (70 kg male volunteers) to allow him to stick needles in their intervertebral discs. He attached the needles to a pressure measuring device and put the people in varying positions. He found that the load on the lumbar disc varied from between 25 kilograms (55 lbs) when lying down to over 250 kilograms (550 lbs) in the seated, forward bending position.[2] (Figure 14)

Interestingly, simply sitting generated load magnitudes equal to standing stooped forward in moderate flexion (about 150 kg). Sitting with the back in flexion was worse, generating about 180 kg of load force. The greatest load was experienced when the subjects held a weight while seated and flexed. This position developed disc loads in excess of 275 kg.--that's **over 600 pounds of force!** This explains why even the simple task of lifting a garbage can may result in putting your back "out" as well as why driving occupations carry such a high risk for disc disease. When driving, one is essentially sitting in a forward flexed position while the bumps and vibration of the road intermittently magnify the stresses at high frequency.

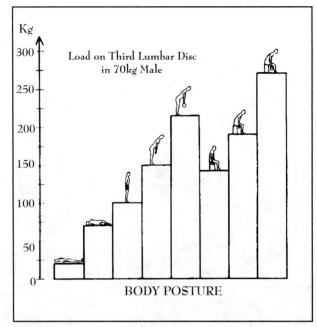

Figure 14 Disc Loads in various postures (From Nachemson, Acta Orthop Scand, 36:425, 1965)

When these numbers are expressed as percentages of the pressure experienced at the disc while standing (See Figure 15), one can see that the simple act of flexion increases the hydraulic pressure of the disc by fifty percent. Sitting and flexing increases it to one hundred and eighty percent. The significance of these pressures and their increases with flexion will become manifest later when this pressure is felt on the capsule in the form of pain.

Note also that the supine position does not completely remove pressure from the disc, and it remains at 25 percent of the standing pressure. This is an important consideration because if a man weighs 150 lbs., there is still 55 lbs. of pressure acting upon the disc unit in the absence of traction. The significance of this will become apparent later when one considers

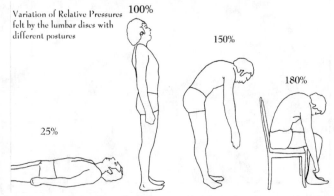

Figure 15 Disc pressures represented as a percentage of standing pressure

other back pain programs' exercises or the activity of chiropractors in which the supine position is utilized.

These discs, being unique structures, break in a unique, pressure-induced, manner by herniating. When a disc is said to *"herniate"*, that technically means that a portion of the nucleus pulposus or other disc material has pushed through an anatomical structure meant to otherwise contain it. Many physicians refer to a herniation only when disc material is pushed through the outer capsule. This misuses the term because, then, they cannot rationally reconcile the painful events

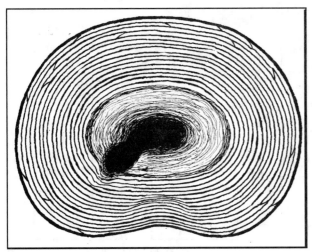

Figure 16 Cross-sectional schematic of disc looking down from above with herniated liquid Nucleus Pulposus

preceding a full protrusion or extrusion with their conception of a "herniation." In fact, a herniation in the absence of a protrusion is very capable of causing pain.

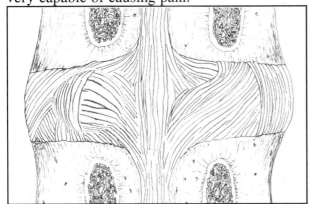

Figure 18 Posterior view of disc bulge to left

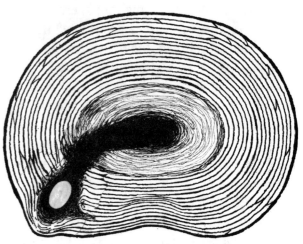

Figure 17 Cross-sectional view of disc bulge to left

In this book, a herniation is used in the universal, medical, definition as being **anytime a portion of the anatomy protrudes through an abnormal body opening**, even if that body opening is only a few innermost layers of the annulus fibrosus (See Figure 16).

When a disc is said to "bulge," or "protrude" that should be taken to mean that the central material herniates or pushes through the annulus fibrosus to such an extent that it presses upon the ligamentous capsule causing it to deform and bulge outward (See Figures 17 & 18).

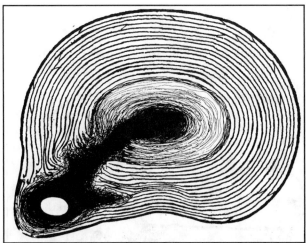

Figure 19   Disc prolapse to left with solidified nucleus pulposus herniating through capsule

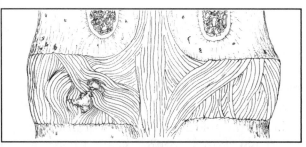

Figure 20 Disc Prolapse to Left viewed from posterior

When a disc is said to "prolapse," that is usually taken to mean that the disc material has herniated through the capsule (See Figures 19 & 20).

When a disc completely herniates through the capsule it "extrudes," the ordinarily central material tears through the ligamentous, peripheral, capsular structures and often enters the spaces adjacent to the spinal column (See Figure 21).

Additionally, as a disc suffers multiple damaging events such as these, at many and varied sites within the discs, it can be said to "degenerate." When this is the case, the bulk of the inner structural integrity is lost and the annulus fibrosus and nucleus pulposus can become a poorly functional conglomeration of broken fibers and pieces of cartilaginous debris. This "degenerative disc disease" usually comes later in life and is sometimes so severe as to have only the capsule functioning to connect one vertebral bone to the adjacent one.

The concepts in this book apply to all these levels of damage but more so to that period of time when a total degeneration of the disc has not yet taken place. Even though this places limitations on the ability of *The O'Connor Technique (tm)* to benefit all disc related problems, nevertheless, the time in which relief can be expected is substantial and the principles still can be applied to relieve pain.

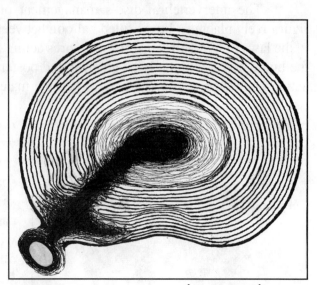

Figure 21 Disc extrusion with rupture of capsule

DISC HYDRAULICS/MECHANICS

Since the majority of back pain emanates from problems related to the intervertebral disc, a discussion that is centered around the inter-relationships of anatomy, physiology, and mechanics is most pertinent. The effect of forces acting upon the spine which generate pain can be understood best by considering what physically occurs when forces are applied.

When a person is standing erect, the entire weight of the upper body above the pelvis is supported by the lumbar spine. Look at a skeleton, when the ribs end, the lumbar spine is the only structure left to support the weight. That means better than half the weight of the human body is resting upon the vertebral column in the upright position. This force is directed from above on every vertebral disc, compressing it. The bones are rigid, but the consistency of the discs more approach that of a liquid. The bones don't physiologically compress, but the discs do.

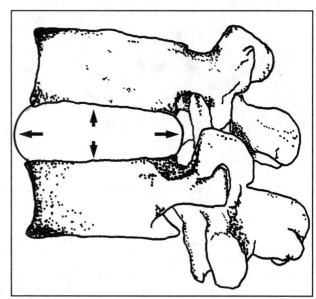

Figure 22 Balloon depiction of disc unit pressures in neutral position

The intervertebral disc's management of compressive forces can be demonstrated by figuratively placing a liquid filled balloon between two vertebral bones (Figure 22). It is known in the laws of hydraulics that the pressures acting on a liquid are equal on any surface upon which the liquid acts. With both the anterior and posterior surface areas nearly the same, the pressure acting upon them is roughly equal when the material within the disc is largely a liquid.

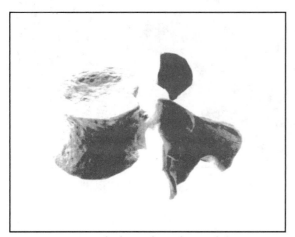

Figure 23 Bowl-shaped surface of disc area of vertebral body

Now, consider what is happening when the body bends directly forward in flexion with weight on the vertebral column. The posterior aspects of the vertebral bodies separate and the space between them widens, increasing the surface area upon which the pressure acts, and causing the liquid center to bulge posteriorly. **So, when the enormous pressures, as delineated above, are applied to the disc in anterior flexion they are felt by the posterior aspects of the annulus fibrosus and the capsule** as in Figure 24.

When in flexion, the anterior component of the dish- or bowl-shaped (See Figure 23) disc containing surfaces of the vertebral bodies close

70

while the posterior aspects of the bowl-shaped surfaces of the vertebral bodies open. In the anterior, the pressure is contained by two bony walls that have come together. **In the posterior, the pressure is received by relatively weaker, stretched, ligamentous structures, causing the contents of the nucleus pulposus to protrude towards the back (posteriorly and peripherally as in Figure 24).**

Like clapping jell-o with half-open cupped hands, the anterior aspects of the vertebral bodies are closed so the nucleus pulposus is forced posteriorly by the pressures exerted when these similarly bowl-shaped surfaces close. The "jello" has no alternative than to be squeezed out through the widest opening--the posterior.

Under the tremendous forces generated during a flexion event (as in lifting a heavy weight), the nucleus pulposus, its hardened center, and the more gelatinous components of the annulus fibrosus are all caused to forcefully move and expand posteriorly. The central disc material is caused to move away from the anterior compression force generated by the weight of the superior vertebral body pressing down on the bony surface of the inferior vertebral body. The vertebral bodies above and below the disc have concave surfaces which direct the central disc material posteriorly.

This central disc material (especially when it is not liquid as in an older person)

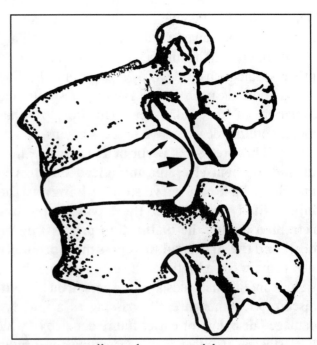

Figure 24 Balloon depiction of disc pressures in FLEXION

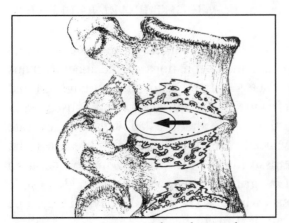

Figure 25 Movement of nucleus pulposus in WEIGHT-BEARING FLEXION

often must move under the influence of these dish-shaped pressures and has no where else to go except posteriorly during WEIGHT-BEARING FLEXION especially during traumatic or forceful events. It cannot move superiorly or anteriorly because it meets the bony surfaces of the vertebral bodies. The anterior component is closed by virtue of the flexion, and there is only one place for the hard central disc material and the liquid component to travel--**peripherally and posteriorly**, that is, away from the anterior compression induced by the

WEIGHT-BEARING FLEXION. **The damage to the disc occurs when these forces are so**

71

great as to exceed the strength of the materials meant to contain them.

DISC HERNIATION PATHOLOGY

As these forces act upon the posterior elements of the fibro-cartilaginous laminations, the individual fibers are caused to deform and bow posteriorly outward. This, combined with the stretching occasioned by flexion's separation of the posterior surfaces, rapidly takes these ligamentous structures to their full length. During rapid and excessive forces (such as in falls or heavy lifting) these fibers stretch beyond their tensile limit and tear. The first tears occur in the more central regions of the annulus fibrosus that have no nerve supply (so the damage is often not perceived) and that have no capillary blood supply (so that the cells of the inflammatory process cannot go inside to lay down scar or healing granulation tissue). These events constitute the initiation of the radial tear (Figure 26) and, thereupon, the degenerative process begins.

These tears can occur at an early age and, in and of themselves, go unnoticed due to the annulus's lack of a nerve supply; however, the injury (if it occurs after the blood supply has retreated during the maturation process) never heals and the structural weakness most probably will remain for a lifetime. It seems strange, but a

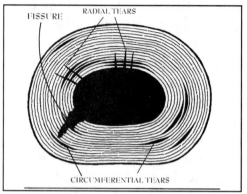

Figure 26 Radial and Circumferential tears in a youthful Annulus Fibrosus

significant fall that lands a young person on his buttocks in flexion and causes no more than a mild discomfort, although easily passing as a few days with a sore back, can, in fact, set up the damaged disc unit for easier future damage of which the individual has no conscious awareness. Nevertheless, the tear is there, waiting for a future traumatic WEIGHT-BEARING FLEXION event to result in advancing it to a frank herniation.

If the forces are sufficient, in injuries after an individual matures, the desiccated and hardened nucleus pulposus can itself fragment or cause the laminations of the inner annulus fibrosus to shatter and fragment. These materials once separated from their contiguous and attached cartilaginous structures become cut off from their nutrient supply and subsequently harden (when cut off from their water supply). Later, they can further break down and degenerate into what has been described as "crab meat" in advanced cases. They can also break off and become loose bodies within the spaces created by the fissuring and the tearing. This degeneration can become so severe that the disc loses its structural integrity causing one vertebral body to slide relative to the adjacent one. This results in a "listhesis" which can be painfully beyond the scope of this book's ability to manage and necessitating a surgical fusion.

More commonly, these loose bodies, especially the hardened nucleus pulposus, upon the successive, forceful flexion events, can be forced further peripherally and extend the tearing. If the forces are directed linearly along the path of a prior injury and towards the periphery, this creates elongations in the existing radial tears (See Fig 27A,B,C) and extensions of circumferential

72

tears (See Fig. 27 D), if the forces are created during a forcefully traumatic circumduction-like event such as twisting while lifting.

If the anterior compressive forces are generated more to the right side of the body, the opposite side of the posterior portion of the disc bears the brunt of most of the expanding force,

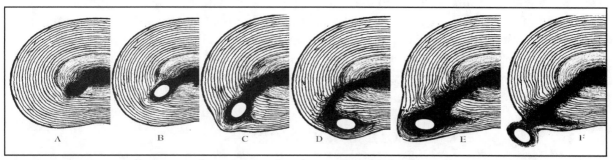

Figure 27 Sequential process of successive disc herniation leading to a sequestered fragment

that being the left side of the posterior aspect of the disc. This explains why a lifting injury caused by a heavy weight on the right side of the body causes the disc to be prolapsed or extruded more to the left. The above series of injuries (Figure 27) would have had to have been due to a flexion injury towards the right. It is not so much the twisting component of a lifting injury that results in damage, it is the fact that the more compressive force generated on one side of the body communicates more lateral force to the opposite posterior side where the ligaments are stretched to their maximum length already and cannot tolerate this force.

There is another reason why discs tend to herniate to one side or the other rather than directly posterior. As that force is felt more and more postero-laterally, the resistance of the ligamentous structures become weaker due to the gradual diminution of the posterior longitudinal ligament's fibers as they anatomically become thinner at the lateral aspects of the discs. This is why a person should never attempt to lift a heavy weight off to the side of the body or twist while lifting (this action is well-documented to be the cause of frequent disabling back injuries). Also, twisting while lifting is damaging because the rotation of one vertebral body relative to another stretches the fibers more and predisposes them to breakage easier because a ligament that is already stretched to its limit is much more likely to rupture when force is applied than one which still has some play in it.

This phenomenon explains why it is a good recommendation that, when lifting, the weight should be placed as close to the midline of the body as possible and lifted directly upwards. In that way, the disc units are not in flexion, and the annulus fibers are not stretched by twisting or posteriorly directed pressure. Instead, the weight is sustained ideally by the shock absorber function of the disc while it is in line with the vertical axis of the spine. Therefore, if a weight has to be moved to a place to one side or the other, it is better to move the entire body by repositioning the legs rather than leaning to one side and twisting to accomplish the same task.

As described above, these forces have been measured by pressure transducers and they are quite phenomenal. They are tolerable in the young, flexible, well-hydrated discs of youth as evidenced by the nearly incomprehensible ability of a child to sustain falls in which they land on the buttocks with the spine flexed forward yet seemingly suffer no untoward consequences. The equivalent fall would most likely cripple an adult because, as a body ages, the liquid center of the nucleus pulposus becomes solidified as the cartilage component loses water with age and actually forms a solid disc-shaped structure. Also, up until the age of eight years, there are small blood vessels supplying the more centralized disc material which help heal it when it is injured. These are gradually obliterated as a person ages. By the time growth has stopped, the nucleus pulposus and the inner regions of the annulus fibrosus no longer have an active blood supply. Thereafter, only the outer most ligamentous structures have a blood supply and the rest of the disc must obtain sustenance from the diffusion of tissue fluid across the cartilaginous end plates.[3] The central disc material becomes solidified and hardened with age probably due, in large part, to its loss of nutrient blood supply.

COMPRESSION FORCES

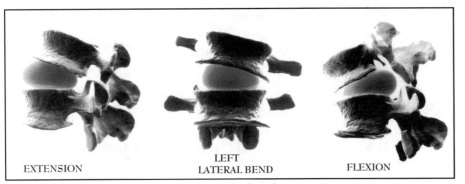

EXTENSION   LEFT LATERAL BEND   FLEXION

Figure 28 Balloon depiction of disc hydraulics

It is important to fully understand the compressive forces acting upon the disc. Here, visualize, again, the two vertebral bodies separated by a balloon filled with water to reproduce the disc unit, illustrating the hydraulic and mechanical forces. As the top vertebral body is angled in any direction, such as in a flexed, extended, or lateral bending posture, it compresses one side of the balloon and the opposite side opens, causing the balloon to bulge to the open side. The balloon model accurately depicts the forces that act upon the discs because its liquid center, too, has no where else to expand except away from the compressive forces. As one flexes, extends, or laterally bends the spine, the forces are directed nearly identically to that displayed by the bulging of the balloons in Figure 28. An equivalent mechanical and hydraulic activity is occurring at each intervertebral disc whenever the spine bends away from an exactly vertical alignment. **This is an important concept to understand because the direction towards which the nucleus pulposus bulges during traumatic events determines the direction and axis of the annulus fibrosus tears as well as the direction and axis that the nucleus pulposus contents would travel to herniate.** For instance, if a fall or lifting accident were to occur when the spine was flexed more to the left, the herniating forces would be aimed towards the right posterior, and that would be the direction that the consequent radial tear would take as the contents of the nucleus pulposus herniate through the lamina of the annulus fibrosus.

Likewise, the magnitude of the force placed on the disc would determine the extent and depth of the nucleus pulposus's movement; and, therefore, the degree of tear and/or consequent herniation. Lifting a small weight might not cause the nucleus pulposus to move much at all; however, a heavy weight can be seen to squeeze it with a lot of force and cause a lot of damage.

Archimedes said: "Give me a place to stand, and I will move the earth." In the design of the spine, Nature's reply has been: "Move the earth incorrectly, and I will make it so painful you cannot stand." In order to understand the enormity of the forces that can be generated within the disc, one must look at the disc system's relation to the spine in terms of the fulcrum and lever. The same principle that operates a nut-cracker or a claw hammer works against the disc when the forces are applied improperly during the act of lifting or falling in flexion.

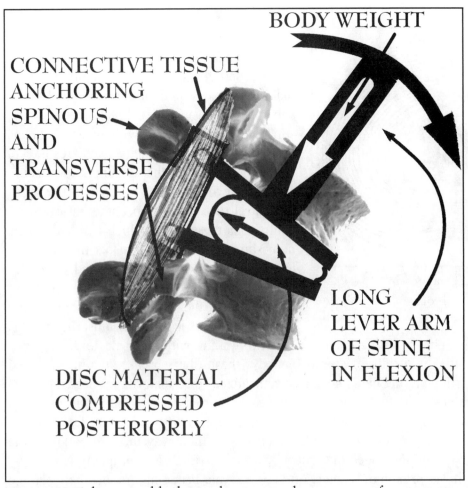

BODY WEIGHT

CONNECTIVE TISSUE ANCHORING SPINOUS AND TRANSVERSE PROCESSES

DISC MATERIAL COMPRESSED POSTERIORLY

LONG LEVER ARM OF SPINE IN FLEXION

As seen in Figure 29, the disc system can be analyzed in terms of fulcrum and lever systems. When lifting in flexion, the muscles and ligaments of the posterior elements of the spine that perform extension and limit the range of anterior flexion serve as an anchor point because after they reach their maximum length, they can stretch no further. To insure that the ligaments of the posterior elements of the spine are not torn and that the body doesn't fall forward during the lifting process, the muscles contract,

Figure 29 Fulcrum and body-weight generated compressive forces acting upon disc in WEIGHT-BEARING FLEXION

serving to further anchor and act as a compressive force added to the weight of the body bearing down on the particular disc.

This connective tissue (muscle, tendon, and ligament combination) is depicted as a schematic muscle superimposed upon a rigid bar. The spine above the disc acts as the long lever arm of the fulcrum system. It can be imagined how with one end point of the "T-bar" (which is the entire vertebral bone above the disc) relatively fixed, the rest of the "T" rotates with the long lever arm that is the spine above the disc. During WEIGHT-BEARING FLEXION the long lever arm rotates around a fixed point to create a posteriorly directed compressive force or squeezing

75

pressure towards the posterior much like a fancy garlic press, nut-cracker, or claw hammer when the nail won't budge. Incredible amounts of force are brought to bear on a small surface area. If one can see how a foot-long claw hammer can generate enough force to tear off the top of a nail, certainly a three foot spine can squeeze a rubbery piece of cartilage through a 2-3 mm sheet of sinew. If the reader jumps ahead to the Section on AVOIDING WEIGHT-BEARING FLEXION, Figure 10 expands this diagram letting an obese clown show how these forces are magnified during lifting.

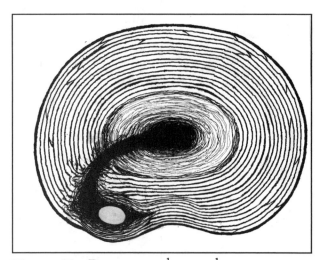

Figure 30 Disc material trapped in laminations of Annulus Fibrosus

As mentioned before, with age and its consequent desiccation (drying out) also comes a decreased elasticity of the annulus fibrosus making it less liquid in character and more solid, predisposing it to breakage. As this solidification progresses with age, trauma has more likely a capacity to result in fragmentation. As this degeneration occurs subsequent to repetitive trauma, larger areas of central disc material become cut-off from contiguous tissue upon which it relied for its nourishment. These fragments then become less vital, more brittle, and literally degenerate, hence the term "degenerative disc disease." As the solidified material of the nucleus pulposus is forced against the annulus fibrosus's laminations as in heavy lifting in a flexed position, a fall with the back flexed, or even prolonged flexion with just the weight of the upper body, these fibers break, creating widened radial tears or fissures, allowing the hard, normally centralized, disc material (either fragments of solidified nucleus pulposus or the larger disc-shaped solidified nucleus pulposus itself) to migrate into spaces previously occupied by flexible, more liquid, deformable material.

Once these hard inner disc materials or fragments push their way through bands of the annulus fibrosus, they can stay positioned off center. So long as force is continually applied by the weight of the body, it can remain off center, often effectively becoming trapped between the broken concentric bands of the annulus fibrosus (Figure 30). **These pieces of hard material can act as a fulcrum to create an effect that causes pain through mechanism described more fully later; but the more important consideration here is that it <u>can</u> cause pain even though it does not necessarily create an actual disc bulge that can be easily appreciated on imaging studies.** These imaging studies often are interpreted as though the disc cannot be the problem because no obvious distortion of the capsule can be seen. In reality, the displaced disc material still is the problem. It is only hidden from easy diagnosis due to its failure to show a bulge or herniation on an imaging study.

This hardened nucleus pulposus can also tear sufficiently through the annulus fibrosus to create a pressure bulge in the posterior or lateral ligaments on the periphery of the disc. This is what is known as a disc bulge, protrusion, or prolapse. When the hard, normally centralized disc material is pushed completely through the ligaments, this is said to constitute an extrusion. See Figure 27 showing various and progressive degrees of damage.

For a moment I need to digress so that the reader understands what physical reality is being represented by these definitions. By defining the different herniation terms statically, there is an implicit assumption that these descriptions constitute an either/or phenomena. When no disc bulge or simply a mild disc bulge is seen on an imaging study, it is often incorrectly assumed that it is only a mild protrusion, incapable of being consistent with the patient's described symptoms of pain, loss of function, or altered sensation. Such is not the case in nature where one is dealing with kinetic and flexible materials as well as reality wherein there is usually a spectrum of damage, at both the instant of injury as well as over time. Making an alternative assumption is a trap that sometimes taints the ability of individual medical doctors or research science in general to adequately portray or explain reality when applied to the individual. Often, the compulsive scientist is limited in his ultimate understanding by a need to rigidly and accurately define his terms so that there can be no confusion when attempts are made to reproduce the results. In the act of attempting to exactly define an entity that defies a static or rigid definition by virtue of its complexity and variability, errors in logic are the consequence. When applied in the context of practicing medicine, suffering usually results because these errors involve people.

For instance, if one were to do a study on the outcome of patients with protruded discs versus patients without protrusions, the protrusion definition and, hence, diagnosis must be fixed by some objective evidence. So, persons without evidence of protrusions on imaging studies are, by definition, eliminated from the study when, in reality, they may have suffered an extensive protrusion that has recoiled or spontaneously returned to a more centralized position by the time the diagnostic imaging is accomplished. **It is important to understand that these pieces move, and, at the time of the study, the "protrusion" may not be protruded. It may only protrude when flexion combined with weight bearing forces are placed on the disc**. The imaging studies might well have been done while the patient was in a reclining position with differing deformational pressures. So, for the purposes of the given study, this patient is not seen to have a protrusion and is likewise eliminated from the study's consideration; or, worse, relegated to the realm of a malingerer if the doctor cannot reconcile the imaging study with the described degree of pain or disability.

The reason why I engage in this seemingly tangential discourse, here, is because there is a tendency to rely too heavily upon and simply equate what is seen (or, better, not seen) on an imaging study with the reality of the damage. **If an imaging study has evidenced that a patient does not have a protrusion, that only means that at the precise instant the imaging study was accomplished, a protrusion was not seen.** It does not mean that the patient has not suffered a protrusion event, and it may well be that the disc material only intermittently protrudes and spontaneously returns to the center with random motions.

An example of this phenomenon was inexplicably expressed in a medical journal wherein a physician reported that his back pain resolved when he flew his plane upside down. Essentially, he was unconsciously performing a traction MANEUVER that moved the displaced disc material centrally by a mechanism described at the end of this chapter. Also, numerous inversion traction devices have been marketed which inadvertently capitalize upon this mechanism; however, it is very uncomfortable to hang upside down. Nevertheless, the limited success of these methods, intentional or otherwise, demonstrate that the disc system is not static.

Disc herniations can produce a changing spectrum of symptoms depending upon the actual position of the herniated disc material, explaining why occupationally debilitated patients can, from time to time, be nearly symptom-free and perform activities in which, logically, their described disability would seem to be irreconcilable with their other performance. This explains why a person disabled from his employment as a brick-layer can be filmed by an insurance company's private investigator playing basketball; yet still be legitimately disabled. Basketball can be played without much necessity for engaging in lumbar flexion, yet brick-laying requires it. Also, the disc material may be spontaneously centralized occasionally enough to engage in a non-flexing sport from time to time without significant pain. Yet, the instant that the patient goes back to his usual occupation, he flexes while carrying a weight, and the disc again decentralizes, returning him to pain.

Besides my own personal experience, to further support the reality of this phenomenon, I have seen at least two cases in which I have been able to closely examine the patients immediately after the injury (whereupon a clinical examination demonstrated that the nerve roots had been damaged at the instant of injury by compression against the vertebral bones due to a severe protrusion); yet the imaging studies (NMRI) portrayed only moderate disc bulges by the time they were actually done. Reconciling the clinical exams with the clinical outcomes forced me to conclude that they indeed have residual nerve damage; but, based upon the imaging studies, the protrusion did not involve the nerve at the time of the study. The erroneous conclusion was drawn that no nerve damage existed in the disability claim. The patient had definite nerve damage evidenced by atrophy of involved muscle groups; yet the back pain management "expert" physicians who evaluated this case relied nearly exclusively upon the imaging studies to determine that the patient was not truly disabled.

Not only does a kinetic spectrum of damage exist at the instant of injury; but it also exists over the lifetime of an individual. The manner in which successive damage occurs starts with any event that puts excessive forces on the disc. These forces, for the most part possessing a posteriorly directed vector, during flexion and weight-bearing, start by tearing small fissures in the innermost lining of the annulus fibrosus layers. This weakens that area and allows the nucleus pulposus to preferentially enter the space created. Successive traumatic pressure events then allow the radial tear to advance.

If the force is of sufficient magnitude, it can create large radial tears all at once; however, normally centralized elements of the nucleus pulposus, both liquid and solid, can also slowly continue to advance the radial tear over time and repeated small traumatic events. These tears can then dissect between laminations of the annulus fibrosus to create circumferential tears as laterally directed pressures likewise occur pushing the nucleus pulposus deeper into the separating layers of the annulus fibrosus. The mobilized elements of the nucleus pulposus can even be caused to move circumferentially between the laminations by a forceful, weight-bearing circumductional movement such as lifting while twisting (as mentioned above), even to the extent of becoming trapped by the bordering laminations of the annulus fibrosus (Figure 30). Once they are positioned to be able to do that, relatively small forces can dissect the laminations, widening the circumferential tears and allowing increasingly larger volumes of nucleus pulposus material to decentralize. This, then, predisposes the disc for a widening of the radial tears with the next weight-bearing, forced flexion event.

It is easy to visualize how this **decentralized disc material can create tracts or tunnels by fissuring through layers of the annulus fibrosus**, allowing the displaced disc material to move a number of ways either spontaneously or intentionally. **It can continue to advance away from the center, follow the same path directly back to the center, or it can move circumferentially requiring a more complex series of movements to get it to re-centralize.** This is when the problem is increased in complexity and much less likely to spontaneously resolve. In this instance, special consideration must be given to get it to re-centralize. **The MANEUVERS of** *The O'Connor Technique (tm)* **are designed to re-centralize this aberrantly positioned disc material intentionally so as to reduce symptoms as soon a possible rather than to wait for random activity to generate equivalent forces in the ideal sequence over a protracted period.** The method and means to accomplish this is discussed at length below.

This series of injuries can continue until the solidified nucleus pulposus actually leaves the confines of the capsule to become a sequestered or extruded disc fragment (See Figure 27F). Prior to this point, there is every reason to believe the mechanical problem can be managed and the damage prevented from advancing with *The O'Connor Technique (tm)*; however, after the disc material escapes the capsule it usually can only be managed with surgical intervention if it produces loss of sensation, paralysis, or pain.

The intent of this chapter and the essence of *The O'Connor Technique (tm)* **is to teach the back pain sufferer to understand the functional anatomy, forces acting upon, and the mechanics of the disc so as to be able to reproduce forces in an opposite direction to the original damaging forces and, thereby, re-establish the proper configuration of the disc relative to its containment structures. A person who masters this method can look forward to a future in which disc pain can be predicted, prevented, controlled, counteracted, and the spine protected from future injury and pain.**

Recall the oxtail described above. It provides a nearly identical, natural, representation of the actual anatomy of a disc. I would seriously encourage the reader to go to a supermarket and find a package. It cannot be frozen, the meat must be fresh and the oxtail must be large because the smaller ones don't adequately represent a disc approaching the size of a human disc. This is as close to a model of the human disc as is readily available since it represents the standard mammalian design. Of course, since the tail of the ox is not a weight-bearing structure there are small differences which must be overlooked. For this discussion, one is only interested in the anatomy and basic physical characteristics of the disc portion or the white, plastic-like, central portion.

Put your finger on the central white portion of the largest oxtail you can find. By continuously pressing down in the center with a finger and moving the hand in a circular motion one can often feel a central hardened area moving within gelatinous surroundings. This hardened center is equivalent to the central portion of the human disc system that hardens equivalently in the aged human condition. Now, if you imagine what would happen in the forced flexion position with downward pressure applied with the incredible gravitational forces that the back sustains, it's easy to see how that hardened piece of cartilage-like material could break through and penetrate the circular, softer, concentric rings that are designed to keep it in place.

Look closely at the oxtail's center and see those concentric rings of firm gelatinous tissue.

79

If you really want to get the picture, make some oxtail stew out of them and cook them well-enough that the meat is falling off the bone. By biting into this material, you can appreciate how tough it is; and how it is indeed constructed of circular rings of cartilaginous tissue. By conceptually enlarging it in your mind, you can see how successive events of forced, load-bearing flexion can cause the radial tears that allow for the central material of the disc to move laterally and eventually escape the disc unit all together, resulting in an extrusion.

By picturing in your mind what would happen if that hardened disc material were to be traumatically forced against the rings of cartilaginous material by 500 lbs of pressure, you can envision how **the layers would break and create a pathway (fissure) for the solid, central, disc material to traverse to the exterior leaving behind a canal of torn material. This is equivalent to a fissure (wide and long radial tear) in the human disc, and these are caused by a similar series of events wherein the central disc material (nucleus pulposus) is forced against layers of the annulus fibrosus breaking them to create a pathway through which the pieces of broken, hardened nucleus pulposus and fragmented disc material can freely travel.**

Most people with injury-induced back pain, especially first-timers, have the type of tear with herniation, as opposed to an obvious disc protrusion or bulge. These herniations are usually invisible to the majority of medical imaging modalities. Discography (an X-Ray technique wherein dye is injected into the disc space highlighting the fissures created when the central disc material tears channels in the annulus fibrosus) is the most accurate means to detect these earliest of degenerative changes--tears or fissures of the annulus. These are difficult to detect by NMRI but, nevertheless, must exist in anyone with discogenic pain. Several studies support this finding.[4] **Due to the difficulty these tears have in being seen with imaging studies, multitudes of people are mis-diagnosed as having back sprain, muscle pulls, or pinched nerves.** The presence of these fissures together with their herniated disc material can cause pain in any number of ways. This pain can be correlated and explained in terms of the mechanical anatomy.

CORRELATION OF MECHANICAL ANATOMY WITH DISC PAIN

Pain is an extremely interesting phenomenon, it can protect and teach while at the same time can intimidate and destroy nearly all enjoyment of life. Back pain is no different. Without adequate explanation or relevant education as to its source, mitigating factors, or potential duration, it can be interpreted as random, unpredictable, confusing, frightening, and apparently perpetual. When back pain strikes that can't be alleviated in the usual time frame in which one is accustomed to seeing pain resolve, it can transform one's life expectations into constant apprehension. Back pain is somewhat unique in the scope of body pains because it carries the added prospect of one's potentially becoming disabled. Add to it the fear of losing one's livelihood or the realistic potential for paraplegia and even a small injury can magnify any sensation to an inconceivably frightening level.

Psychologists tell us that **the stress induced by pain can be markedly better endured and tolerated so long as it is not perceived as random, it is made controllable, and predictable in both its onset and termination.** Any pain can be tolerated much more easily if the seeming randomness is explained and understood. The purpose of this section is to lift the "blindfold" on the most common form of spinal pain by defining its source as discogenic (originating in the disc), familiarizing the sufferer with its various manifestations, and, through education, make the unseen source of pain understandable, manageable, predictable, and ultimately preventable.

To remind the reader, it is well-established that the nucleus pulposus and the inner portion of the annulus fibrosus have no nerve supply.[5] Only the most outer portion of the disc unit, the ligamentous capsule and peripheral aspect of the Annulus Fibrosus, has sensory innervation. Some misuse this anatomical fact to assume that there should not be pain associated with either the tearing of a solidified nucleus pulposus through the laminar rings of the annulus fibrosus or the degenerative process in general. To a certain extent this is true and explains why people often relate that during the twisting or lifting event that they know initiated their pain, they just felt a pulling or a "pop." Only later did they gradually experience the sharp, debilitating pain. Also, people within hours of a whip lash injury describe the same experience. Immediately (minutes) after the trauma, they are a little sore, but the real grinding and immobilizing pain often comes hours later or the following morning when they wake up and try to move their neck. This is perhaps the most paradoxical aspect of spinal trauma. One would think that, if significant damage was occasioned, it would be immediately apparent and obvious at the scene of the trauma as in the case of a motor vehicle collision. After all, whenever someone pulls a muscle, breaks a bone, or sprains a ligament, the pain is apparent immediately.

One must consider, when trying to make sense out of the pain, that the entire disc system has very little tolerance for misplaced parts. Simply because one cannot feel the actual damage being done as the hardened components of the nucleus pulposus herniate through the annulus fibrosus doesn't mean that once they come to rest, placing direct pressure on the outer ligamentous bands of the annulus fibrosus or posterior longitudinal ligament, that they won't induce pain as the pain receptors within those ligaments are excited and the inflammation process begins.

DIRECT PRESSURE PAIN

First, tears of the annulus allow the de-centralized disc material to move towards the disc's periphery and put direct pressure on the ligamentous capsule that surrounds it. **Movements putting the affected part of the spine in forward flexion can be seen to actually squeeze the hardened nucleus pulposus or other pieces of disc material posteriorly to put direct mechanical pressure on the posterior aspects of the capsule (See Figure 31).** These capsular ligaments are very well-supplied with nerves and are quite capable of generating severe pain.

Also, the residual liquid component of the nucleus pulposus can participate in this pain scenario, especially when weight-bearing flexion causes the liquid component of the disc to exert hydraulic pressure on the posterior peripheral capsule. Considering what is occurring anatomically when trauma tears free the solidified nucleus pulposus and forces it through layers of the annulus fibrosus, there are areas of liquid nucleus pulposus that now have the capability of entering the fissure and hydraulically adding to the pressures that are felt on the posterior capsule. The hardened nucleus pulposus as well as its liquid counterpart are free to dissect through the fissure to reach the sensitive capsule to generate pain when the nerve-supplied ligaments are stretched.

81

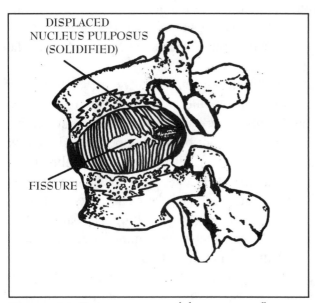

DISPLACED
NUCLEUS PULPOSUS
(SOLIDIFIED)

FISSURE

Figure 31 Cut-away view of disc unit in flexion showing a displaced nucleus pulposus

When flexing in the weight-bearing condition (WEIGHT-BEARING FLEXION) hydraulic pressure or mechanical pressure on the nucleus pulposus forces it (or fragments of desiccated cartilaginous material) into the outer bands of the annulus fibrosus and posterior longitudinal ligaments, and pain is the consequence (See Fig 31). This effect can occur instantaneously or over a prolonged period of time due to successive events of pressure. This type of pain can be looked upon as originating from direct pressure applied to the capsule's ligaments.

The pressure on and damage to the peripheral ligamentous component of the disc (the capsule) and the posterior longitudinal ligament are probably the most important contributors to pain in the disc system and are largely responsible for the majority of pain attributable to back pain in general. Others may argue pulled muscle, sprain, arthritis, or some other mechanism, but, since the time I have been able to manually reduce disc herniations or put "in" de-centralized disc material with *The O'Connor Technique (tm)*, my experience has shown me that the greatest component of spinal pain originates in the direct pressure placed on the exquisitely innervated joint capsule that surrounds the disc unit when decentralized disc material exerts pressure on those ligamentous structures. I "know" this because, once I have relieved this pressure through manipulation, the pain relief is usually instantaneous. In fact, it is very uncommon for me to have a back pain patient that I cannot prove has disc disease as the source of pain by virtue of my ability to relieve it. This leaves me with no other conclusion to draw.

As elaborated above, the peripheral ligamentous structures surrounding the disc, the joint "capsule," contains the sensory nerve fibers that tell where the upper body is in relation to the lower body. This innervation is the reason why you can stand upright and a baby (who is too young to have these pathways functional) falls over, even if only seated. It takes a high density of sensory fibers to be able to discriminate extremely subtle movements. When this same density of sensory receptors is applied to pain sensors, it implies that a little stimulation can go a long way in producing pain. That small amount of stimulation can come from a relatively small piece of displaced disc material pushing against the capsule or when, off-center, it creates a fulcrum effect in concert with the adjacent surfaces of the vertebral bodies.

These parts of the body rarely feel pressure or experience trauma during the youthful formative years of neurologic development due to their deep location in the body and their being surrounded by protective muscles that prevent their routinely experiencing painful stimuli. Therefore, when forces induce pain, it is registered by the brain as a novel phenomenon which usually translates to pain the severity of which has never been experienced by the average person any prior time in their life.

For this reason, annular tears can be very painful; yet patients with just these tears (in the absence of a bulge or protrusion) are often dismissed as having psychogenic pain motivated by secondary gain,[6] mostly because discography is not done to demonstrate the true pathology. However, doctors don't routinely order discography and for good reason. It is a dangerous and invasive procedure. Only highly trained and qualified physicians are willing to stick a needle into the disc because it is painful and risky. If the radiologist is only a couple of millimeters off, a nerve root could be injured leading to paralysis. Since it is so difficult to identify these tears with non-invasive methods like X-Rays, CAT, or NMRI scans, the most convenient but alternative, erroneous, diagnoses are usually made instead.

FULCRUM EFFECT PAIN

The other major contributor to mechanical discogenic pain can be appreciated by considering what happens when, over time, with successive small injuries, a major lifting injury, or a traumatic flexion event the central disc material breaks its way through the layers of the annulus fibrosus but doesn't necessarily reach the peripheral capsule. The broken fibers of the annulus can close like one-way doors behind it, trapping the normally centralized disc material in an off-center position. The hard disc material then acts as a fulcrum. The vertebral body and the portion of the disc above it acts as a lever with the weight of the body providing the moment arm's force during flexion.

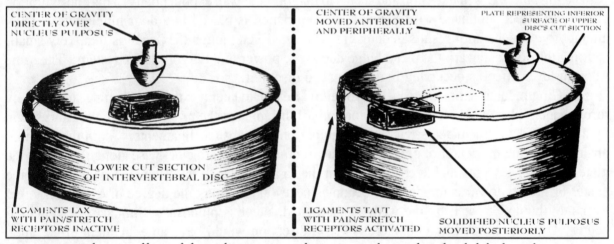

Figure 32 Fulcrum effect of disc when center of gravity is changed and solidified nucleus pulposus is displaced.

This phenomenon is not difficult to comprehend. Figure 32 schematically portrays a disc cut in horizontal cross-sections. The inferior surface of the superior section of the disc is shown as a transparent plate resting above the inferior component of the intervertebral disc. The displaced disc material or hardened nucleus pulposus is represented by a "brick" that rests between these virtual surfaces. The figure on the left describes the neutral (normal) situation where the center of gravity (fat arrow) is directly above the nucleus pulposus. In this configuration, the ligaments are relaxed and no pain is felt so long as the body is balanced directly above the center of the disc.

The figure on the right shows the condition in which some previous traumatic forward flexion event has displaced the hardened nucleus pulposus towards the posterior periphery. Then, the act of moving the center of gravity towards the periphery (as shown in the drawing on the right by the movement of the fat arrow), in this case equivalent to antero-lateral flexion, puts an inferiorly directed force on the "plate" causing it to teeter on the "brick" (the solidified nucleus pulposus) which stretches the "rope" (representing a ligament with pain/stretch receptors). When the force of the weight of the body acts with a fulcrum effect upon the component of the disc (the "plate") immediately above the hardened nucleus pulposus the forces stretching the ligaments become quite substantial. I term this FULCRUM EFFECT PAIN.

In the presence of a herniation, during my examination for diagnostic purposes, when I cause patients to change their center of gravity anteriorly (in a forward flexion directly away from the site of pain while standing, they easily agree that the **pain is stretching due to the mechanical or hydraulic pressure on the posterior capsule. This pain is the pain of direct pressure. However, they then agree the pain is wedge-like when I keep them bent and circumduct them until the point that the fulcrum effect stretches the capsular ligaments adjacent to the displaced disc material.** They recognize the pain as if something was physically wedged in their back when I then shift the center of gravity around to the other side of the herniation by circumducting them in the opposite direction. The slightest increases, beyond the point where pain begins, increases that tension and seems to magnify the pain exponentially. This configuration creates an effect similar to what happens when a pencil is placed in a door hinge wherein any attempt to close the door results in damaging forces. Even though the pencil is relatively small, shutting the door can warp the metal hinge due to the power of a fulcrum/lever system. The same fulcrum/lever effect is occurring in the damaged disc unit.

Circumduction moving from antero-lateral flexion to lateral extension (leaning successively through a circular, clockwise, range of motion) of the spine at the problem disc level causes pain by a fulcrum/lever mediated stretching of the peripheral capsular ligaments. As in the diagram analogy, moving the center of gravity along a circumferential path clockwise along the rim of the plate, successively puts and keeps tension on the ligaments such that, the closer one moves the center of gravity towards the brick, it becomes necessary to relax the degree of extension to get over the "hump" created by the wedged, hardened, nucleus pulposus. Similarly, moving the center of gravity around in a counterclockwise direction would have an equivalent effect upon other ligaments equivalently situated to the displaced disc material on the opposite side. The effect of this type of action is discussed in depth in the section on DIAGNOSTIC CIRCUMDUCTION wherein the pain and arrest in circumduction can be used to determine the position of the displaced disc material. Feel free to return to this drawing to understand that concept as well.

Just as the tiny pencil placed in a door hinge can stop the door from closing, so, too, can a small piece of cartilage-like material, when off-center, cause pain as the surrounding ligaments are stretched by a fulcrum effect. Attempts to force movement in spite of the misplaced disc are often met with excruciatingly sharp pain. The pain is often immobilizing because no matter what direction you turn or what position you assume other than balanced directly above the nucleus

84

pulposus, the pain increases.

These factors explain why, during an acutely painful back event, the sufferer can neither bend forward to any extent, move to wards the painful side, nor extend enough to stand up straight without increasing the pain to an intolerable level. In any of these movements, the hard, off-center disc material can serve as the fulcrum for any of a number of possible levers and moment arms created by the cartilaginous and bony surfaces contiguous with that disc and the displaced disc material. Depending upon which of the other sites on the adjacent surfaces of the vertebral bodies is farthest from the displaced disc material, it becomes the moment arm. The site with the shortest distance becomes the lever. The lever then can stretch peripheral ligamentous tissues with forces much stronger than would otherwise be generated without the lever/fulcrum effect.

For instance, let's assume that the solidified disc material is displaced off-center to the midline posterior in the neck not enough to cause a direct bulge or protrusion, however, enough to impede competent movement. When the patient tilts his head forward and to the right, the displaced disc material, now turned elevated fulcrum, causes the left posterior peripheral ligamentous elements to be stretched with far greater force than they ordinarily would be caused to be in the disease-free condition. This causes a stretching pain to be felt to the left of the displaced disc material. The same thing happens when the head is tilted to the left, only this time the stretching type pain is to the right of the herniated piece of disc material.

As above in, Figure 32, the forces acting on the disc's ligaments can be equated with a rope (about the length of the brick's height) tied to the edge of a circular shaped board and secured to a platform. If a brick were placed in the center of the board and someone were to stand on the end of the board farthest from the rope, the rope would probably not break because the end of the board where the weight was applied would hit the ground before that could happen. However, moving the brick closer and closer to the rope's site of attachment, the board (just as the displaced disc material moves closer to the peripheral ligaments as it is displaced posteriorly and peripherally) increases the fulcrum effect so that, when it is nearly touching the rope, even small amounts of force on the far end of the board can be seen to be capable of snapping the rope.

I have ascertained to my own satisfaction that this mechanism of pain is the predominate cause of a condition known as torticollis or "wry-neck syndrome." Usually it is seen more often in children; but is also seen frequently in adults; but their necks don't seem to go into as much of the uncontrolled spasm as is routinely seen in children. Rather, the adult is most of the time unable to look over the shoulder to the same side as the displaced disc material. However, it is not unusual for the condition to be chronic or even perpetual. The disc material is usually displaced more laterally than posteriorly, and it causes the sufferer to turn his face away (due to contraction of the sternocleidomastoid muscle) but bend his neck towards the side of the herniation (due to a combination of same-sided paracervical muscle spasm and an attempt by the individual to keep the weight of the head's center of gravity directly over the displaced central disc material. To anterior flex the neck to the opposite side as the displaced disc material creates pain so the head and neck are kept rigidly immobilized partly because of spasm and partly because nearly any movement off of the center of gravity causes extreme pain.

It appears to some that muscle spasms are the source of the problem. So much so that, recently, some doctors have reportedly improved the condition by injecting a muscle relaxant into

85

the sternocleidomastoid muscle; however, I fear this practice is too dangerous and ineffective because , technically, it only treats a symptom of the problem and not the origin. Alternatively, I have found it is the FULCRUM EFFECT of de-centralized disc material stretching the peripheral ligaments that initiates the spasm. The disc material displaced is most likely liquid nucleus pulposus in the child and/or solidified nucleus pulposus in the adult which has herniated off-center. This herniation, I have found, after careful history taking, to be usually due to a flexion injury, either in the immediate past or the remote past (that only has acutely re-herniated due to so much as sleeping in the wrong position).

On occasions too numerous to count, acting upon these assumptions by using *The O'Connor Technique (tm)* **I have been able to non-traumatically and immediately reduce the subluxation with manipulation rendering the patient free of pain and restore full range of motion**. This success is contrasted to reports in the literature of this condition lasting for years in the absence of definitive management. In fact, there are so many people in this country that have this untreated condition that they have formed a society.

Understand that the above described intervertebral disc fissure-facilitated mechanism of disc material displacement pain can occur over a long period of time with repeated nearly identical flexion injuries or instantaneously with a sufficiently powerful force. After repeated events that progressively damage the annulus fibrosus, even a seemingly small force can result in debilitating pain since the disc can be poised at any time to suddenly travel the same damaged route to reach the intervertebral ligaments. This explains why people can be doing something as apparently innocuous as taking out the trash early in the morning and "put out" their backs, resulting in a permanently painful back condition requiring surgery. Such is the case in many incidents which are usually not believed by the patient's doctor to be sufficiently traumatic to result in a disc protrusion or herniation.

You see, in cases like this, where someone comes into the doctor reporting that a sneeze or simply waking up and putting on shoes initiated a severe back pain event, the doctor reasonably assumes that no major damage could have occurred to ligamentous or bony structures because the forces applied were inconsistent with the ability to damage these characteristically tough structures. However, the original event, that predisposed to the presently painful one, may have been a fall as a teenager or an auto accident years prior that resulted in only moderate, transient pain. The disc material in the first injury never moved enough to become trapped; but it damaged the annulus enough to create a pathway for future advancing of the injury. **Few people realize that the cartilaginous material that comprises the annulus doesn't heal or repair itself over time. Once it is fractured, it doesn't even scar**. It remains perpetually broken and capable of allowing the central, hard disc material to repeatedly migrate along a previously created pathway. This helps explain why studies show that **40% to 85% of patients will have recurrences of back pain within a year after their initial episode**.[7],[8] and **nearly one third of patients with low back pain have a relapse within 3 years of the initial episode**.[9] Each event in which a radial tear is created makes it more likely for a fissure to be created and another, future, painful event to occur. As time goes on, cumulative injuries predispose to progressively severe disease.

This phenomenon also explains why "degenerative" lumbar disc disease is said "to progress as a series of pathophysiological events, beginning with asymptomatic fissuring and fragmentation within the disk."[10] It is not widely appreciated, difficult to accept as fact, and worth repeating here that **a significant radial tear can occur in the annulus fibrosus without inducing a reasonably commensurate amount of pain because these structures do not have nerves supplying them.** The age-solidified nucleus pulposus, gradually and eventually, through repetitive trauma, herniates through successive layers of the annulus fibrosus, followed by prolapse of this fibrocartilaginous material into the spinal canal or the neural foramen.[11] **The pain comes only when the surrounding ligamentous component of the disc sustains pressure, stretching, or inflammation whenever the irritation is sustained.**

There is also a combination type of pain that is experienced when the centralized disc material (the solidified nucleus pulposus, the broken fragments of the annulus, and/or the liquid component of the nucleus pulposus) bulges or protrudes to the rims of the adjacent vertebral bodies due to a herniation that causes the capsule to significantly deform and bulge posteriorly. In this case, the pain comes from the disc material causing both a fulcrum effect and direct pressure pain by its being trapped during the act of extension (See Figure 33). **The decentralized disc material is positioned so far peripherally that it is actually pinched or squeezed by the vertebral body's rims.** This, too, puts pressure on the capsule and results in pain.

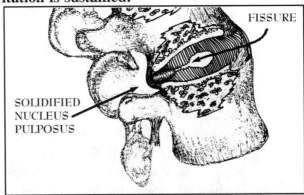

Figure 33 Herniated Nucleus Pulposus positioned to exert both a direct pressure and fulcrum effect

CRIMPING PAIN

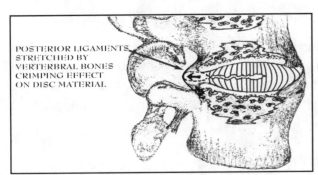

Figure 34 Cut-away view of disc showing crimping effect of vertebral body's rims coming together during extension on prolapsed piece of disc material.

When extending in the weight-bearing condition (WEIGHT-BEARING EXTENSION) extension is often only allowed until the fulcrum effect is experienced because pain stops the movement; however, another condition that is closely related to the pain of the fulcrum effect yet is more appropriately considered as a constant direct pressure pain is when the displaced disc material has protruded to the point where extension of that disc unit causes a crimping of the prolapsed disc material. **The crimping or pincer-like action happens when the disc material is pushed beyond the rim of the vertebral bodies and enough of it is outside of the circumference of the plateau portion at the rim of the vertebral bones to not allow it to move anteriorly in the presence of the body weight's compression**

forces (See Figure 34). Often, a fragment of displaced disc material is lodged in this prolapsed position; and the act of WEIGHT-BEARING EXTENSION traps and pinches it further posteriorly. This type of pain usually requires a protrusion or bulge-type herniation to be present, but one isn't absolutely necessary if the greater part of an ideally-sized piece of disc material is situated immediately peripheral to the point where the lips of the vertebral bones oppose each other such that their approximation when extension is occasioned creates a bulge.

RADICULAR PAIN

Radicular pain comes as a result of an extruding, protruding or prolapsed disc fragment coming into direct contact with a spinal nerve root (See Figure 35). **Since the sensory component of the nerve roots travel down to the areas to which they supply innervation, pressure on these large roots can cause pain to appear to be coming from the places where the nerve travels.** This type of pain is a searing, burning, or electric shock-like sensation that is often associated with a definite extremity weakness and loss of muscle strength because the spinal nerve contains fibers that carry, sensory, pain and motor (muscle movement) signals. Since this type of pain if persisting, signals a nerve root compression syndrome and most likely will result in immediate surgery to remove the piece of disc material that is compressing the

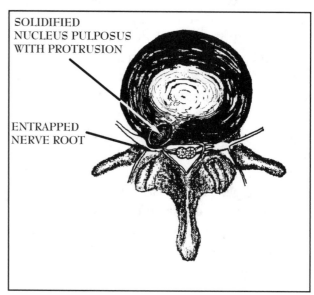

Figure 35 Protruding disc material causing direct entrapment and compression of a spinal nerve root.

nerve, it will not be focused upon too heavily here except to elaborate that there are definite nerve root impingement syndromes described to explain the consequent loss of sensation, pain and motor loss depending upon the particular nerve root that is damaged. If the reader experiences this type of pain, this book is not a wise solution until one has been rejected as a surgical candidate by a neurosurgeon.

REFERRED PAIN

None of these mechanisms thus far explains why the hip or leg hurts when the lower spine is supposed to be the problem or why the shoulder hurts when the cervical vertebrae's discs are supposedly the source of the pain when there is clearly not a protrusion seen on an imaging study.

The more commonly experienced **Referred Pain** reveals that the central nervous system isn't as smart as you think. In some ways, it is very unsophisticated, especially with novel events in which it has not been given time or capacity to become accommodated. By way of example, when a thorn is stuck in the leg while walking, initially, the brain recognizes that the leg hurts.

You cannot determine anything more specific than the right lower leg has pain. The next thing you do is attempt to localize the pain by feeling the area and reproducing the pain by touching the affected site to convince yourself that indeed, that specific point is where the pain originates.

Next time you have a small injury, think about the pain. Finger pain can seem like the whole hand hurts until focus is directed at the actual source to pin-point the site. Most times it is necessary to feel around at length to determine the exact site of a particular pain's origin. In order to localize and identify pain, it is usually necessary to bring in other modalities of the central nervous system such as sight, movement response, and touch in order to localize it. Well, when the actual source of the pain is hidden deep inside a part of the body that cannot be felt, seen, touched, or knowingly moved in such a manner to identify the true source of pain, the brain is forced to make, often incorrect, assumptions.

Take for instance a painful condition that most people have heard about. Heart pain is so rare to the central nervous system's experience that, when it occurs, it is often thought of and felt to be in the arm. This is explained because the nerves to the arm are embryologically developed from the same pathway as the heart's nerves. So, the mind, trying to determine the pain's origin, concludes that the pain must be coming from the arm because the nerves are being excited from the same general pathway as the arm. Since heart pain is so rare, the mind assumes that the pain must be coming from somewhere else more accustomed to receiving pain signals. After all, most heart pain suffers are older than forty years old. The central nervous system has been living that long without pain from that area and has good reason to not "believe" pain could be originating there. So, it is not unreasonable for the brain to make an alternative "assumption".

When it comes to spinal pain, the brain is equally confused. This was documented by a study in which subjects were injected with irritating solutions into the facet joints at various levels. They were unable to determine which level was being injected or whether the disk or facet joint was being injected.[12]

I am convinced that a similar pain pathway confusion frequently occurs when the nerves of the intervertebral disc's capsule are stimulated. Depending upon what level of inter-vertebral capsular ligaments are involved, take for instance L5-S1, the pain message emanating from this disc space is similarly accepted by the brain to have origination from the areas of the more customarily stimulated nerves' embryological distribution. The large spinal nerve root that exits the spinal column (that eventually supplies innervation to the muscles, skin, and joint of the hip) sends a small branch to the disc area, the Recurrent Sino-Vertebral Nerve (See Figure 10.) Both pain and proprioceptive impulses travel to the spinal cord and on to the brain through this nerve. When painful stimuli excite the small nerve from the disc's capsule, the impulse travels along with other fibers coming from other sites supplied by that particular, larger, spinal nerve. These pathways are so closely related that the mind frequently accepts the pain as having originated from the other sites which have been more accustomed to managing pain sensations throughout the life of the individual. Depending upon what spinal nerve is pertinent, the sensations, upon reaching the brain, are often accepted as having come from those areas of the body also innervated by that spinal nerve root in which the impulses from the disc also travel.

When the disc capsule's pain receptors are excited and pain impulses are produced, one can't very easily put one's finger on the actual site of pain at the L5-S1 disc level to convince the mind it is in error as in the thorn example given above; so, the central nervous system makes the incorrect "assumption" that the hip is what hurts and that site is from where the pain is mistakenly registered by the brain as having its origin. These areas correlated with the distribution patterns of spinal nerves are well-known and mapped out as sclerotomal, dermatomal, myotomal patterns corresponding to their respective spinal nerve levels. These patterns are delineated in more exhaustive textbooks for professionals and need not be reproduced here; but, ideally, by identifying what area the dull aching pain comes from at rest, one should be able to tell which disc is the source of pain. In reality, there is so much overlap of areas, the opportunity for further confusion is so rife, and that degree of exactitude is neither necessary or realistically achievable by the lay persons that I have elected to dispense with its discussion.

The O'Connor Technique (tm) makes such a pursuit academic. An individual can learn to correlate their own particular pain patterns with specific disc units simply by moving the spine and paying educated attention to where and when the pain is felt. Then, when that pain recurs, it can be assumed to be from the particular disc with the herniation. This will become more pertinent and apparent when, later, the reader is taught how to diagnose their own disc herniation because he/she will be able to specifically move their spine to find the actual discogenic source of pain regardless of where the pain radiates or refers.

Also, of note, something interesting about referred pain is that if you stimulate the area that appears to hurt, such as with a massage or rubbing, the pain temporarily disappears as if the mind, then, is saying: "Oh, the pain can't be coming from there because now I'm touching it and it is not being reproduced; therefore it has to be coming from someplace else." Then, the instant that the massage or stimulation stops, the pain recurs because the brain again returns to making an incorrect assumption like that elaborated above.

To better understand this type of pain, one should know that referred pain usually has limitations. It seldom travels beyond the elbow or knee. Rarely, in my experience, has referred pain gone below the knee in a lumbar disc problem or beyond the elbow in a cervical disc herniation when a nerve root is not involved. When it does, that can be a sign that the pain is radicular and caused by the actual pressure of a prolapsed disc on the nerve that passes through that segment of the spine. Radicular type of pain is usually described as "burning" whereas the referred pain is more often described as a "dull ache." Whenever pain seems to involve a strip that runs the entire length of the leg or arm, or is accompanied by actual weakness, that is a bad sign, made worse if it is accompanied by weakness of that same muscle area, and there should be no delay in seeking out a physician to determine if further studies or an operation is necessary to prevent destruction of the nerve.

A common source of not overtly obvious shoulder or leg pain is from an intervertebral disc referring the pain. Without other cues, the mind often cannot differentiate pain originating from the stimulation of a nerve at any point along the distribution of that nerve. The brain may register as the source of pain any site of stimulation whether it originates at the level of the nerve as it exits the spinal column, nerves that travel in the same bundle, or from the area innervated normally by the nerve.

As an experiment to demonstrate this phenomenon, the next time something hurts on your legs such as a bite, scratch, or any narrow area of trauma, without looking or touching, close your eyes and try to figure out exactly where the pain is coming from by just closing your eyes and focusing on the site. Your first impulse is to touch the area to determine the exact locality of the pain. You will probably realize, until this is done, you feel pain simply coming from a broad general area on the leg. In order to convince your mind where the exact location of the pain is, it is usually necessary to feel the area, actually reproduce the stimulation by pressing on the area of pain, and convince yourself that you have located the exact point of its origin.

Now, consider what happens when a disc or a nucleus pulposus puts pressure on the ligamentous bands on the periphery of the annulus fibrosus. There is no way that you can touch the disc with your hand to convince your mind that you have located the exact origin of the painful stimuli. Consequently, the mind must resort to guess work. The brain must assume the pain is coming from the nerves that innervate that area of the body to which the nerve being stimulated supplies nerve function.

In the case of the Lumbar region, the nerves are the same ones that go to the hips, buttocks, and legs. The pain is dull and no matter how much you touch the area that aches, you can't make it hurt more or reproduce the pain by touching areas from which the pain appears to come. If the pain were truly coming from the hip joint, moving just that joint should increase the pain, but it doesn't, neither does pressing on what seems to be the pain site. In fact, quite often, rubbing or massaging those areas stop the pain momentarily because the stimulation convinces the brain that that area cannot be the source. However, as soon as you stop, the pain returns.

As a pertinent aside, this paradoxical phenomenon can be explained by the Melzack and Wall gating theory of pain because sensory impulses travel faster than pain impulses and, when they beat the pain impulse to the spinal cord, they preferentially stimulate the nerves that travel to the brain by a gating mechanism. The brain receives the sensory input before it accepts the pain impulse.

Evolutionarily, this makes some sense since when running away from a predator, the organism is better served by a nervous system that physiologically ignores pain while allowing sensory input to have preference. It is apparently more a selection advantage to know where your feet are running than whether they hurt or not. Another model for this reality comes from the frequent experience of men in combat who describe no pain sensations while distracted by complex sensory input enabling them to continue functioning despite massive wounds.

The sensations of touch, temperature, stretching (so-called proprioceptive impulses), and vibration travel in very fast fibers. Consequently, these impulses arrive at the spinal cord's "gate" earlier and get through faster and more often than the pain impulses that travel in slow fibers. This explains why hot packs and ice packs both relieve pain. Unfortunately, they do very little to modify or heal the true source of the pain since neither heat or cold can reach the disc.

This information comes as scant consolation since one must first understand what is causing the pain to alleviate it. Towards this purpose, let us assume that a patient has hip pain on the right side. Many of my disc patients actually do not complain of low back pain per se, but describe it as predominately hip pain which accompanies the lumbar pain. This is also the case of the shoulder's relationship to the cervical spine.

They rarely have pain in the actual hip joint upon testing the range of motion of that joint so long as the back is prevented from moving during the testing. When traction is applied to remove pressure from the protruding disc, the first thing they notice is that the hip pain is relieved; and the spine becomes the site of pain. Only after having them do a DIAGNOSTIC CIRCUMDUCTION MANEUVER (to be explained later) in which they convincingly reproduce the pain and their movement is arrested, can I determine the position of the disc protrusion. Once the site of pain is identified, I put the disc back "in" with a centralizing MANEUVER. When they achieve relief of their hip pain, I can be certain that the disc was the source because that is the only area that was mechanically altered. Because I usually prove this is what is occurring by successfully putting the disc back "in" and the patient walks out without hip pain, I am forced to conclude that the pain relief would not have occurred unless the spine was the origin because that is the only area that had been mechanically altered.

I have also had a continuous opportunity to study this phenomenon on my own disc pain for years. This first-hand knowledge gives me a great deal of insight into my patient's experiences and the intricacies of spinal pain in general. When my disc is "out" the pain is more in the superior buttock than the spine. Upon completing a MANEUVER, the hip pain is likewise extinguished.

So, in evaluating your own low back pain, with *The O'Connor Technique (tm)* you can learn to recognize hip or buttock pain as originating from the disc material pressuring the nerve that refers pain to the hip. You can determine that the true source of the pain is coming from the spine by moving the spine in a very specific manner which will be discussed later in the description of the DIAGNOSTIC CIRCUMDUCTION or "THE O'CONNOR TEST." **When doing the diagnostic and therapeutic MANEUVERS described later in this book, be cognizant of what particular movement accentuates the pain and what particular therapeutic MANEUVER decreases it.** Usually, the DIAGNOSTIC CIRCUMDUCTION, when attempting to go to a full posterior extension, will be accompanied by arrested motion when the actual area of the displaced disc material interferes with the movement of that particular disc unit. Just as the point is reached where you feel as though, if you continued without letting up on the EXTENSION the pain would be unbearable, your extremity should start feeling the pain, and the sensation of something obstructing the movement should occur. This is the point where the surfaces of the vertebral bones interfacing with the discs are beginning to put pressure on the displaced disc material. It usually stops you from CIRCUMDUCTING further and gives the sensation that if you could just move the right way the pain would be relieved. It is often described as a "catch" in the back, like something is caught and prevented from moving further. That is the most characteristic component of disc pain that differentiates it from other types of pain. The following chapters go into much greater depth so don't stall here concerned that you have missed the point.

MUSCLE PAIN

Certainly, other sources of pain in the back do exist. People occasionally "pull" or "strain" the muscles in their back; but this is associated with a different type of pain. The pain of a "pulled" muscle (actually torn) in the erector spinae group is usually not associated with extremity pain or if it is, it is a pain that is reproducible and increased when the affected muscle is manipulated. Recall, the referred pain from the disc usually is made to feel better while being manipulated. The pain of a torn muscle is identified by tenderness (pain upon touching) of that specific muscle when it is palpated. When manual pressure is put on the torn muscle it becomes **immediately** more painful. So, with a backache, it is simple enough to test for actual muscle tenderness at the time of the injury, if it is present this gives reasonable evidence to conclude that the source of pain does not come from a disc. However, in my professional experience, a pulled muscle in the back is a rather uncommon event. However, **pain in the muscles is not necessarily that uncommon because muscle pain can come from secondary spasm due to a herniated disc.**

The pain of muscle spasm is sometimes hard to differentiate from pain due to a muscle tear because both are accompanied by a generalized hardening and swelling of the affected muscles. Spasm often follows a back injury in which a disc is herniated because that is the body's protective mechanism. The spasm can be expressed as an intermittent jerking with jolts of pain or continuous, depending upon whether or not the pain comes in short, rapid bursts (such as when a damaged ligament is stretched for an instant with movement) or sustained for long periods (such as when disc material is persistently deforming a ligament). By spasming, the segmented animal splints that area of the body so that injured midline structures are protected. Recall what happens when you pinch a worm, it curls towards the pinch. If you ever get the opportunity to handle an new born baby, place it face down with its stomach in the palm your hand so that its bare back faces you and its hips can move but each leg is straddling your arm. By running your finger down the back about one inch lateral to the spine you will see the Landau reflex. The baby will contract the erector spinae muscles automatically on the same side that the stimulus is applied. There is very little difference between this reaction and the reaction that occurs when a painful stimulus is applied to the spine later in life. The erector spinae muscles automatically and involuntarily contract towards the side of injury. When this contraction is sustained because the pain is continuous, the muscles go into a prolonged contraction or what is commonly referred to as spasm.

The best way of differentiating the pain of spasm from the pain of a pulled muscle is to feel the muscle itself. **Usually, the torn muscle will be tender at the site of the tear immediately after the injury.** The muscle that is painful due to prolonged spasm may become tender along its entire length but it does so only at a time distant to the injury and along the entire length of the involved muscle. The pain of both are increased when FLEXION away from the side of the pain is accomplished.

In order to differentiate between muscle pain versus disc pain, the job is much easier. When in extending to the side of the pain in the presence of muscular pain, the pain is reduced. Think about it, muscle pain from tearing is decreased when tension is taken off of the muscle and increased when tension is put on the muscle. So, when in a PASSIVE (without the activation of the muscles) EXTENSION position towards the herniation's side, a pinching of the disc should increase the pain. When passively extending to the side of pain, the erector spinae muscles will be relaxed to that side and result in less pain when the pain is due to a muscle tear. Additionally, there is usually no actual arrested motion in the presence of muscle spasm or tear. With a herniation, the displaced disc material physically stops the act of CIRCUMDUCTION. A torn or spasmed muscle might be painful to move, but it will not stop the spine from circumducting

INFLAMMATORY PAIN

A discussion about the sources of pain in the disc system would not be complete unless Inflammatory Pain were included. Whenever an anatomical structure in the body sustains trauma, especially constant or repetitive friction due to abnormal pressures placed upon a component, inflammation usually occurs. This inflammation results from chemicals produced by the white blood cells that migrate to an area to facilitate the repair of damaged tissue. When displaced disc material is mechanically impinging upon structures that have a blood supply, cellular damage is occasioned. As the disc material abuts against the ligamentous structures, inflammation is created. **Unfortunately, as long as the ligaments are being irritated by the continuous pressure of the displaced disc material, the inflammation will persist. It stands to reason that the pain of inflammation will also not resolve until the mechanical problem of the decentralized and aberrantly placed disc material is solved.** Later in the book, methods designed to remove the disc material from pressing against the ligaments will be elaborated. Once the friction is relieved, the inflammatory component can be managed successfully.

ADDITIONAL SOURCES OF PAIN

When a disc has severely degenerated for many years, the majority tissue that once constituted the actual disc can become simply a mass of non- or poorly functioning material that has lost its structural integrity, leaving the ligamentous capsule as the only anatomical structure joining the two vertebral bones. In this advanced disease, the vertebral bones can be caused to contact each other or slip relative to each other into abnormal and painful configurations of bone on bone or a combination of bone and disc material that stretches the capsule. Fortunately, this level of disease occurs only in a limited percentage of "old" bad backs; and the principles of *The O'Connor Technique (tm)* still pertain and can effectively be used to relieve pain. At this stage, though, sustained relief may only come with surgical fusion.

Finally, without question, back pain originates from and accompanies many other disease states. Spinal stenosis (narrowing of the spinal canal), ankylosing spondylitis, arthritis, spondylolisthesis, cancer, fracture, trauma, infections, etc.; however, in my personal medical and orthopedic experience, the **overwhelming majority of spinal pain originates in the disc and is due to some consequence of disc herniation**. Those orthopedists, chiropractors, and medical doctors are entitled to their opinion when they attribute acute (rapid onset) or recurrent back pain to pulled muscles, ligament sprain, lumbar strain, sciatica, sacro-ileitis, spasm, etc. because those events do occur but not nearly with the frequency of disc herniation. However, **they, more often than not, cannot make a convincing, logical argument with some form of objective proof to demonstrate the accuracy of their diagnosis because they seldom are required to design one. They are rarely held to the standard that their diagnoses be correct nor are they exposed to much of an untoward consequence if their diagnosis is erroneous. They simply make their best guess based upon what they assume to be fact, then rely upon Nature to remedy that which they cannot even adequately describe**. This may sound like an indictment or a criticism; however, it is not. It is simply a statement emanating from a realistic assessment of the widespread, contemporary, lack of understanding about discogenic pain.

Another means of differentiating whether the source of pain originates in a disc or from some other source is that **TRACTION can transiently relieve disc pain**. In muscle tears, "sprains," or inflammatory arthritis of a joint, the isolated act of traction, in and of itself, will induce pain. **TRACTION in the presence of a disc herniation will noticeably reduce the most severe component of the pain--the hydraulic or mechanical pressure induced component caused by the herniating or prolapsing material pushing against the ligamentous peripheral annulus, the capsule, or the posterior longitudinal ligament.**

In keeping with the balloon analogy used before to describe compressive forces, one needs to understand an equally important decompressive force that can act upon a disc. That force is mediated through TRACTION. One can imagine what would happen to a

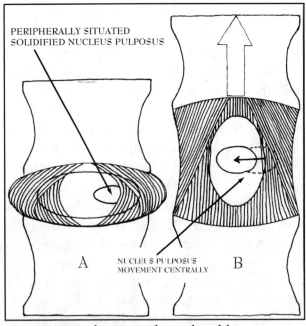

Figure 36 Tightening of peripheral ligaments and creation of negative pressure moving nucleus pulposus centrally due to TRACTION

liquid filled balloon that has been glued to the vertebral bodies similar to the manner in which the disc is anatomically secured in the natural condition. When the vertebral bones are separated along the vertical axis (or in other words, pulled apart along their longitudinal axis, superiorly and inferiorly), as would occur when a person hangs or is put in traction, the contents and periphery of the balloon would move centrally due to the negative pressure generated and the tension placed on the balloon's walls. Likewise, in the natural mechanics of the disc, when TRACTION is applied the disc contents are both drawn by central negative pressure from the relative vacuum created as well as pushed centrally by tension-generated inward directed pressure as the peripheral ligamentous structures are stretched and tightened. As the peripheral ligamentous structures are straightened, their circumferential configuration leaves no where else for internal disc material to move except towards the disc's center. Therefore, if the nucleus pulposus were previously in a more peripheralized configuration due to some prior event that has forced it there (Figure 36A), TRACTION would serve to move it centrally as seen in Figure 36B. **This is one of the more important concepts to understand because peripherally- displaced contents of the disc (principally the solidified nucleus pulposus or any internal disc material) can be <u>intentionally</u>, caused to move centrally by a combination of the negative pressure generated by TRACTION and the bow-string like forces generated by the stretching to full length of the ligamentous, laminated structures that surround the nucleus pulposus.** The separation of the vertebral bodies creates a relative vacuum in the empty spaces of the discs which were created by the displacement of the center's contents; and the straightening of the annulus fibrosus and capsule

95

creates a positive, inward directed, tension-mediated, force that physically pushes the displaced disc material centrally.

The capacity of the disc to perform this action is one of the principle reasons why *The O'Connor Technique (tm)* works. Of all the disc's bio-mechanical actions, this is arguably the most uniquely important in terms of the functional rationale and logic of *The O'Connor Technique (tm)*. When longitudinal (along the axis of the spine) TRACTION is applied at a disc unit, the peripheral ligaments are stretched to their full length. By this "MANEUVERING," the disc material encapsulated by them can be intentionally moved centrally regardless of where it is situated within the disc. **By adjusting the posture of the spine, different ligaments can be caused to be preferentially stretched and the disc material directed from the posterior to centrally, left to centrally or from the right to centrally depending upon how the TRACTION is applied in conjunction with FLEXION.** For instance, if the displaced disc material is posteriorly positioned in the disc near the periphery, TRACTION combined with FLEXION will selectively stretch the midline posterior ligamentous bands of the annulus fibrosus and capsule, causing the disc material (in concert with the negative pressure created by TRACTION itself) to be pushed anteriorly towards the center (See Figure 37).

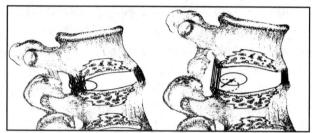

Figure 37 Cut-away disc unit with solidified nucleus pulposus decentralized to the posterior then moved anteriorly by tightening of peripheral posterior ligamentous structures with FLEXION IN TRACTION

Similarly, if the disc material is protruded to the left posterior, TRACTION combined with FLEXION to the right will selectively stretch the left posterior ligamentous bands of the capsule and annulus fibrosus periphery. This, in conjunction with the negative pressures created by the TRACTION, can cause the disc material to be moved to the right (centrally) and anteriorly thus re-centralizing it in the same fashion, only the direction of the forces are different..

With TRACTION, the central disc space volume (created by the nucleus pulposus' absence as it was displaced peripherally) is increased. This volume increase creates a relatively negative pressure, reducing the posteriorly directed pressure, removing the mechanical obstructions presented by the laminations of the annulus fibrosus, and allowing the disc material to migrate centrally as the peripheral ligaments assist to push it centrally when they tighten (See Figure 36). **This relief of pressure on the capsule and the posterior longitudinal ligament reduces pain, in many instances, instantaneously.** Usually some recognizable pain-relief is immediate as soon as the pressure acting upon the displaced disc material is relieved; however, relief is not sustained when the TRACTION force is removed,. Later in the book, a means to capitalize upon this mechanism will be presented to create and maintain a pain-free state by solving this mechanical problem. **Once the mechanical problem is solved, the inflammatory component is, theoretically, the only one left remaining to cause pain. Once the problem that is creating the inflammation is solved, competently dealing with the inflammation-chemical induced pain should, therefore, result in a pain-free state.** That process, too, is dealt with later in the book.

The dilemma arises, however, in that, before one can solve the mechanical problem, a means must be found to convincingly and precisely identify and define the pain as originating from a mechanical problem then devise a means to insure that the mechanical component of the pain is truly no longer acting. The following Chapter on **DIAGNOSING DISC DISEASE** deals with how that is accomplished.

1. Perey O: Fracture of vertebral end plates in the lumbar spine. An experimental biomechanical investigation. *Acta Orthop Scand* (Suppl) 25:10, 1957.

2. Nachemson AL: In vivo discometry in lumbar discs with irregular nucleograms. *Acta Orthop Scand* 36;426,1965.)

3. Borenstein DG, Wiesel SW, *LOW BACK PAIN Medical Diagnosis and Comprehensive Management*, 1989, W.B. Saunders Co, Philadelphia, London, etc., p.11.

4. Walsh TR, Weinstein JN, Spratt KF, et al. Lumbar discography in normal subjects: A controlled, prospective study. *J Bone Joint Surg.* 1990;72A:1081-1088.

5. Op.Cit., Endnote #3;p.14.

6. Sasso RC, Cotler HB, Guyer RD, Evaluating low back pain: The role of diagnostic imaging, *The Journal of Musculoskeletal Medicine*, May 1991:21-37.

7. Valkenburg HA, Haanen HCM. The epidemiology of low back pain, in White AAIII, Gordon SL (eds) American Academy of Orthopaedic Surgeons Symposium on Idiopathic Low Back Pain, St. Louis, CV Mosby Co, 1982:9-22.

8. Troup JD, Martin JW, Lloyd DC, Back pain in industry: A Prospective Survey, *Spine* (1981) 6:61-69.

9. Deyo RA, Back Pain Revisited: Newer Thinking on Diagnosis and Therapy, *Consultant*, February 1993: 88-100.

10. Vlok GJ, Hendrix MR. The lumbar disc: evaluating the cause of pain. *Orthopedics*, 1991; 14:419-25.

11. Deyo RA, Loeser JD, Bigos SJ. Herniated lumbar intervertebral disk. *Ann Intern Med*, 1990;112:598-603.

12. Mooney V, Robertson J. The facet syndrome. *Clin Orthop* 1976;115:149.

CHAPTER THREE: DIAGNOSING DISC DISEASE

DAMAGE/PAIN SCENARIO

At the time, that fall on your buttocks when you were roller skating as a teenager, the football injury where the guy landed on you while you were falling backwards into a sitting position, or the time your back snapped forward in an auto accident, all seemed to be relatively insignificant injuries. However, they were importantly detrimental physiological and anatomical events. Some may have hurt for so little time that you hardly remember them, yet they were nevertheless capable of setting you up for a *"Coup-de-Gras"* later in life which (sounding familiar to many) goes something like this:

As an ageing human *[your nucleus pulposus has solidified into a discus-shaped lump of cartilage]*, you wake up from a sound sleep in a soft bed *[your Lumbar disc has been in flexion for nearly the last 8 hours]* to recall that you forgot to take out the trash, and today is pick-up day. Unbeknownst to you, your desiccated nucleus pulposus has migrated to the end of the radial tear tunnel (fissure) that was created by past trauma to the spine and, as you raise your upper body off the bed to get up *[you induce weight-bearing flexion that exerts nearly 500 lbs of force]*, you feel a slight twinge that you discount as insignificant *[the disc material has just poised itself against the capsule]*. You hurriedly trundle outside in your pajamas as fast as you can so as not to be seen by your neighbors. You are caused to lean slightly forward because its the most comfortable position *[the disc material is exerting the fulcrum effect]*, and it is difficult to stand erect without slow adjustment which you don't have time for just now. Still half asleep with the majority of your muscles remaining relaxed from your slumber and, therefore, providing no protection, you bend over, lifting the can that turns out to be a little heavier than you expected. So, you jerk it up--WHAM! *[The last fibrous band of the annulus fibrosus ruptures, allowing the central disc material to be squeezed towards the edges of the vertebral bodies, pushing before it the thin ligamentous capsule with all its delicate nerve endings, herniating into and prolapsing the disc.]*

The pain takes your breath away, so you lean forward on the trash. The pain increases so rapidly that you can't bear the weight of your own body; and you find that lying in trash isn't so bad after all. You finally muster enough will power to try another attempt at erect posture. Now, the ground seems like the only site of solace. There, you can at least assume the fetal position and the grinding pain, like someone is using "the jaws of life" on the bones of your spine, is somewhat relieved just so long as you don't move *[any reduction in the load bearing on the disc reduces the hydraulic pressure on the peripheral ligamentous capsule]*. You feebly call out for help but no one can do anything because the slightest movement results in agony. All that you can think to do is seek out medical care and prepare for the economic hemorrhage that is soon to come.

Your doctor can't conceive of the possibility that you have herniated or prolapsed a disc because the lifting of a trash can in his mind isn't sufficient force; so, in the absence of neurological findings you are diagnosed as having a "back strain," given some pain pills, a few muscle relaxants, bed rest, some physical therapy, and told that it will get better. The only problem is that it doesn't; and you are then faced with the task of figuring out what is wrong because you aren't getting the answers you need and can't see yourself living with this kind of pain for the rest of your life.

One needs to understand that a herniated disc is a mechanical problem; and mechanical problems have mechanical solutions. In order to solve a mechanical problem, you first have to determine physically where and what constitutes the mechanical lesion. When a disc goes "out," it does so physically and, therefore, has a dimensional reality. It actually travels to another position that causes pain. **In order to determine the best method or MANEUVER to put the displaced disc material back "in" to the center where it belongs, the location of the out-of-place disc material must be identified.** The level of the vertebral column where the pain originates and the position of the fragment within the disc space must be fixed in the mind so that a mechanical strategy can be designed that will be both specific and effective. Before one can move a piece of matter, one must first know where the material exists in space.

There are expensive means of determining the location of a displaced piece of disc material; and there are self-administered, free, ways to accomplish the same task. The beginning of this section will briefly discuss the options available using standard, costly, diagnostic modalities ordered by licensed practitioners and the remainder will be dedicated to **teaching the reader how to accomplish a "do-it-yourself" diagnosis.** Taking the time to understand the options will assist the reader in making the best, most cost-effective decision. Without this understanding, the reader might end up spending thousands of dollars and getting nothing.

CONVENTIONAL DIAGNOSTIC METHODS

Understand at the outset, that medical science's understanding of the causes of back pain is so limited that there, to this day, is no agreed-upon method of diagnosing a structural abnormality of the spine despite two extensive reviews in the medical literature.[1],[2]

Nevertheless, when a patient presents with back pain to a chiropractor or physician, the most commonly ordered diagnostic imaging study is a spinal, plain film, X-Ray series. This usually amounts to long-axis side views, front to back views, and oblique views oftentimes focusing on the specific area of pain or the Lumbar region by virtue of its statistical probability of being the site of an abnormal finding. They cost Medicare $50; but, for everyone else, they can cost 2-3 times as much. Even more disconcerting is the amount of radiation to which the patient is exposed in light of how little they contribute to elaborating the cause of back pain.

People have a need to know how much radiation they will be exposed when "the routine X-Rays" are taken in an Emergency Room, the Chiropractor's office, or when ordered by a physician. Undergoing a three view lumbosacral spine study is equivalent to having a Chest X-Ray study done every day for at least three years![3] This is one of the major reasons why a person should think twice before allowing themselves to be X-irradiated. A lot of people dispense with the risk by saying that we are always being exposed to radiation from natural sources. That is true, but there is a "natural" rate of cancer, too. Not only are you being forced to take your risks of getting cancer simply by choosing to live on this planet; but now when some other people on the planet want to make money off of you by increasing the amount of radiation you are exposed to by hundreds of times higher doses, I tend to get infuriated. Add to that, the doses calculated were probably measured with reasonably new equipment. Many facilities have purchased the old machines without image enhancing capability; and the doses are much higher. Evidently, the fact of radiation-induced genetic damage and its ability to cause cancer has escaped the educations of those people who down-play the 400 mRads of radiation to the female gonads and bone marrow entailed in every medically unjustified study they accomplish.

True, the cells of the body have a capacity to repair the genetic damage induced by radiation, however, that capacity has been evolutionarily designed to deal with background levels of radiation, not the logarithmic excesses to which some would have them exposed. Justification for the use of X-Rays (including CAT scans) exists, but it is limited by a few considerations which are pertinent to a patients decision to consent to an X-Ray procedure. Swedish investigators concluded that **one might expect to find X-Ray evidence of a diagnosis not indicated by the physical exam in only one of every 2,500 adults under age 50 with low back pain**. Many X-Ray findings are unrelated to symptoms of back pain and are found just as often in asymptomatic individuals.

If the first back pain episode started when a patient is over 50 years old or as a teenage athlete with activities strenuous to the Lumbar spine (i.e. gymnastics, wrestling, etc.)[4] the yield of a plain film X-Ray study <u>may</u> justify the expense and radiation risk, especially if there has been a history of steroid use, a reasonable suspicion of ankylosing spondylosis, prior history of cancer, weight loss, bowel or bladder incontinence, a history of substance (drug or alcohol) abuse, significant trauma, **failure to improve with conservative therapy within 4-5 weeks** (*The O'Connor Technique* constitutes conservative therapy), or motor neuron deficits.[5]

A condition that usually first affects athletic young people causing them to seek medical attention is called *spondylolisthesis*, which is a often a congenital (present since birth) defect or traumatic fracture of vertebral pedicles (the *pars interarticularis*--the bridge-like bones that join the front portion of the vertebral bones with the back portion). When the segments are separated, it is called *spondylolysis*. Either can be painful or simply found incidentally during an X-Ray done for other reasons. That reality makes it a confusing problem to indict as the source of pain and also difficult to manage. This condition, however, is decidedly a statistical minority.

I mention this specific condition here because if you are one of the few people who have this condition I cannot be sure *The O'Connor Technique (tm)* will be helpful. I doubt that it would be harmful because, in that event, the pain would not be helped by the technique and those patients would reasonably stop practicing it. In the worst case scenario, it might increase the pain, and logic would dictate that you would stop doing what hurts before any serious damage could be done. For more information on this condition especially as it relates to sports, go to the SPORTS Section of this book.

Another situation in which an X-Ray examination may reveal the source of pain is in the presence of pain that is constant, not improved by lying down, or does not respond to bed rest. These findings suggest a systemic disease or cancer. By "constant" it is meant that the pain stays largely the same regardless of what one does to try to alleviate it. Discogenic pain usually is reduced by lying down and returns when a person tries to get back up. If the pain were caused by cancer, no matter what one does, the pain of the tumor encroaching upon a nerve will not reduce in severity.

The other two most common diagnostic modalities used in the evaluation of back pain are the CAT Scan (Computerized Axial Tomography a.k.a. CT Scan) and the NMRI (Nuclear Mass Resonance Imaging a.k.a. NMR).

The CAT Scan is basically an X-Ray machine hooked up to a computer that takes lots of X-Rays, pools the information into one picture and gives an X-Ray cross-sectional slice-through-the-body. Because different tissues of the body allow X-Rays to pass more freely, those tissues with major differences in density can be differentiated from each other and not just bones are outlined. Its two largest draw-backs are the amount of radiation to which the patient is exposed and the limited resolution--especially in the neck region. To get some idea of how old the technology is, it was developed by money from The Beatles rock group. Since there are a lot of the machines still around and they have been paid off already, they can sell the images cheaper. But not even The Beatles can solve the radiation problem--it is even worse than that of the standard spine series. The problems of both cost and radiation can be somewhat mitigated by asking the physician ordering the study to limit it to just the painful area. Unless there is a compelling reason to irradiate the entire Lumbar region, you may reasonably request that the study be limited to just the painful area (which you can demonstrate to the radiologist). This way, if the pain is localized to one or two disc units your probability of seeing what is wrong by just examining those discs stands to be much more productive with respect to cost and radiation exposure.

CAT scans were once the best means of seeing into the spinal anatomy; but the NMRI is its higher-resolution competitor. The most accurate picture of the spine, especially the intervertebral disc structures, and least dangerous, is the NMRI (Nuclear Mass Resonance Imaging). It is about twice as expensive as the CAT Scan, but the resolution is much better without exposure to radiation. It actually is an amazing device. Patients are placed in a large magnetic field, and the manner in which the atoms of the body vibrate in that magnetic field differs from tissue to tissue and the difference can be detected with sensors. So, one gets a picture of the internal muscles, bones, cartilage, and other soft tissues. Whereas the plain X-Ray only sees the bones, with an **NMRI device, the displaced disc material can actually be seen**; and the position of it relative to the vertebral bodies and, more important, the spinal nerves can be determined.

The draw back here is the cost. It is a relatively new technology and expensive. If you are paying for it, you are looking at upwards of a thousand dollar bill. That's a pretty hefty sum, and it is very difficult to get a doctor to order one because they are hassled and intimidated by HMO's, administrators, or third party payers' refusal to pay. Or worse, the managed-care doctor himself (when your health care dollars are paid to him and capitated in advance) can have become reluctant to spend his "own" money on you. The conflict of interest inherent in capitation warrants an entire book; but, suffice it to say, that, if you are in a capitated care plan, this book is probably the only way in which your back will be made to get better. **When anyone is getting paid more by delivering less care to your back, it will probably get better on its own before they do anything that can realistically be expected to alter the outcome.**

The most common justification they give for not ordering any expensive modality is that at any given time, probably 20% of "normal" thirty-year-olds who undergo an imaging study (CT, myelogram or NMRI) can be shown to have asymptomatic evidence of herniated discs.[6] This statistic is then often misused to justify a belief that the finding of an herniated disc on an imaging study is not equated with pain. I fervently disagree. **The presence of a herniated disc on an imaging study constitutes irrefutable evidence that the patient has suffered an injury to the disc system; and the burden of proof, then, rests upon the physician to prove that the disc is not responsible for the pain's origin.** Until that is done, the disc should be considered the most likely source until it is proven that such is not the case. Admittedly, this advice deviates markedly from the current approach to back pain management; yet I am convinced that, as the reader completes their understanding of *The O'Connor Technique (tm),* they will logically conclude that it exposes a fundamental inadequacy in the current "academic" approach to this human problem.

The finding that a substantial percentage of asymptomatic people are usually found with evidence of a herniated disc simply establishes the reality that far greater numbers of people (than currently believed) could be suffering from disc disease. These people simply may not have had the diagnosis made previously. That doesn't mean that they don't have disc herniations, it just means that they don't have symptoms at the time of the study. Any time a "scientific" study establishes the statistically significant presence of undiagnosed disease, it is equally probable that the explanation rests in a failure of the diagnosticians to have previously elaborated the disease through adequate histories and physical examinations.

Many patients may have unconsciously, unknowingly, or coincidentally accommodated to the problem by limiting their activity, become so accustomed to the pain and limitations of movement that they no longer accept or perceive it as abnormal, stopped complaining about it to themselves or their physician's, or the area has become scarred down and physiologically, spontaneously, stabilized. Denying the significance of a disc herniation does not, however, make it go away or provide assurance that it will not again become symptomatic later.

The event that caused the herniation also could be so distant in time that a recollection of the event is difficult; but it is these very types of patients who probably constitute the population of persons who (seemingly inexplicably) are immobilized by pain when the already herniated disc only requires a relatively small amount of force to push it into a painful configuration. These are the type of patients who give a history to their doctor that they were simply taking out the trash or sneezing when suddenly they were immobilized by pain. The doctor feels the area, finds muscle spasm and assuming that the force described could not have been sufficient to cause a herniation, then erroneously concludes that the source of the pain is a pulled muscle--which is now in spasm. They then conclude that no imaging study is necessary with that diagnosis and elect the cheapest and easiest strategy: "conservative management" (which is no more than what we physicians call "benign neglect") relying upon the assumption that within two months most of these patients will again be pain-free.

You may find it difficult to obtain an NMRI if your doctor's compensation is capitated by your insurance or health care program because the doctor is now spending <u>his</u> money. This whole movement in medicine called "managed care" is the worst of all systems from a quality point of view because an inescapable conflict of interest is designed into it. If your doctor is paid up front to take care of you, when it comes to ordering an expensive study or sending you to a specialist-- the money comes out of his pocket. As perverse as it may seem, human nature being what it is, don't expect your doctor under that type of system to do anything but the cheapest management possible unless he is a Saint. The most important factor influencing his decision appears to be how much risk he is willing to take with <u>your</u> well-being yet still not get sued.

This book is not the ideal forum to expose the particulars about how bad the basic philosophy of these HMO's, Kaiser-like plans, or capitated programs truly are because that's another entire book that belongs more in the horror stories section of the book store. But it is appropriate to address the motivations of those persons charged with the responsibility of your health because, when it comes to the costs relegated to back pain, those paying for the care do not want to spend any more money than is absolutely necessary. It seems that everyone is jumping on the "get-it-done-cheaper-at-any-cost-band-wagon" and, those that don't climb aboard of their own volition, are being economically drummed out of the practice of medicine by the administrators and business people who are reaping enormous profits from this scam (right now, their "take" averages 12% of the health care budget in any market they can capture). It is accurate to say here, that if the "bean-counters," whether at a governmental or corporate level, can persuade a doctor not to order an expensive test, they can take that money and give it to themselves. So, more often than ever before, beneficial (and even essential) diagnostic information is not obtained because someone along the line is willing to play the odds such that, by withholding any particular procedure or diagnostic test, they can stumble along without it (regardless of the excess pain and prolongation of ignorance that such a strategy entails) so long as they are willing to sustain the reality of your not getting better, staying in pain longer than necessary, or suing them.

An excellent example of this mentality is represented by a recent case known to me. JM is a physical laborer who sustained a fall and has never been able to alleviate the back pain subsequent to that trauma. Two years after the injury, he presented with obvious clinical symptoms of disc prolapse with possible spinal nerve root involvement at the clinic where I practice. I attempted and then taught him some self-administered extension MANEUVERS to see if he would benefit, but he not only achieved no obvious relief, but he had to stop doing them because they hurt more.

The degree of pain involved and the potential presence of nerve root impingement indicated that the safest and most prudent course would be to acquire an NMRI to make certain that he could mobilize the spine by without risking additional nerve damage. When I ordered the NMRI, a nurse with absolutely no knowledge of the specific patient or back pain in general refused the imaging study and insisted that he go to an orthopedist specialist for consultation. Because the local Medicaid managed-care organization refused to pay local orthopedists a reasonable compensation for their work, he was sent to the University where he was seen by a student doctor. Without knowing whether the patient had a partial extrusion that could reasonably be expected to be made worse by extension exercises (a risk I was unwilling to take in light of the fact that extension was so painful), he ordered physical therapy with extension exercises before determining the extent of the protruded disc material with an NMRI. This was done in the presence of the fact that in my consultation request I informed the doctor that previous extension-type physical therapy attempts had met with a worsening of the condition.

It seems now-a-days, that economics are the most influential determinant with regard to whether an NMRI is "necessary." An NMRI costs about $1,000.00. The physical therapy costs $60 a week. If he's hurt by the exercises, it helps convince a physician that the fellow has a real problem--the pain and neurological function gets worse. Then, only after his condition gets worse or no better will some other strategy be tried. The problem with this scenario is that JM unnecessarily must be put through weeks of pain before being "allowed" the imaging modality and risk suffering a permanent neurological deficit when treated by an exercise instructor who has no true knowledge of the injury's extent. In fact, even the doctor doesn't know it because he failed to obtain the "road map" NMRI. So, I was forced to stand by and watch this man's future ability to walk jeopardized because money wouldn't be spent by a nurse (who's job is to refuse services) and the doctors within this system were willing to proceed with a demonstrably dangerous plan from a perspective of elective ignorance. The frequency with which this occurs is so great that it defies description; however, I present it so that the reader will at least be forewarned about the current state of affairs in medical management decisions and be better prepared to deal with it.

My solution was to send a letter to his lawyer, outlining the problem, and to the doctor reminding him that extension exercises were already unsuccessfully attempted and persisting with them presented the potential for further harm. In that way, the entity that chooses not to do the proper imaging study will have a legal "sword of Damocles" hanging over its head (rather than mine). You see, when capitated health plans deny services, the legal liability for that decision still remains with the physician unless he makes a good-faith effort to protect the interests of his patient. I protected my patient while at the same time transferring liability away from myself. If the other physician is so arrogant as to persist with his plan to proceed blindly, he would be the one to end up in court explaining his methods to a jury. My ethics won't allow me to violate the trust engendered in the physician's precept *primum non noicere* (first do no harm) nor ignore the published guidelines that justify an imaging study if the patient has gone greater than six weeks without alleviation of symptoms. However, health plans are not governed by that creed and can choose to ignore any given M.D.'s orders. Their interest is in acquiring wealth regardless of patient's additional suffering or risk. The reality is that these machinations exist so far beyond the understanding of the patient that the administrators can get away with just about anything. They act upon the assumption that their decisions will not be legally questioned until it can be proven, afterwards, that they caused damage. Even in the presence of damage, it is very hard to prove that they actually caused the damage, so it behooves the patient to become sufficiently educated to manage their own back problem through the system, to prevent irrevocable damage. I designed this book for laypersons because they must be able to make their own diagnosis.

Don't mistake my loyalties, **most physicians I have met are hard-working, humanitarians with altruistic goals and genuine concern for the welfare of their patients**. However, as hard as it may be to believe, (because doctors are sometimes seen as "all-powerful") they are often victims of forces beyond their control. In that instance, few of them are martyrs enough to suffer in your stead. All too often, they, by their own experience with "the system" have become complacent and unwilling to stand up for their patients' well-being let alone their own.

Here's how it works. If a particular capitated program's cost-control officer looks at the statistics and sees a particular physician is ordering too many NMRI's, he will be either intimidated into ceasing this practice (by volumes of additional paperwork, "guideline" educational seminars, demands for specialty referrals, or "de-credentialed" if he persists. These capitated plans and HMO's usually have clauses in their contracts that allow them to remove a doctor from their provider lists "without cause." To even the best doctors, this can mean being put out of business. It is a modern form of corporate "Black-Listing;" and it especially happens to doctors who "cause trouble" when they protest decisions of the health care plan not to approve expensive procedures.   If you suspect you are suffering this situation, don't attack your doctor, write a certified letter to the healthcare plan demanding an alternative decision. By demanding that they put in writing the specific criteria they are using to deny you that service and indicating that any future pain, suffering, or disability resulting from a failure to adequately diagnose the problem, you intend to hold the persons making the decision liable for damages because, inherent in the act of refusing legitimate diagnostic or therapeutic modalities, they are practicing medicine without a license.

If your back pain is not getting better and, after practicing *The O'Connor Technique (tm)* enough to convince yourself that you have given it an adequate opportunity to work, you feel that having an anatomical image of the problem will make the definitive diagnosis, and you are paying for it yourself (or have a doctor that is paid up-front by your health care plan that refuses to order the study), there may be a compromise. You can reduce the cost by specifically asking your doctor to order just a limited study of the area in question. Usually, the painful area of the spine only involves a few segments and, after you have lived with the pain for a while, it is not too difficult to determine where the specific area of the spinal pain is located. It is unnecessary to image the entire spine when only a small area is actually affected by pain. So, if you want the best imaging study to determine if a disc is herniated, a limited NMRI may be the best option. By reading on, you will be given a means to localize the site of the problem if an NMRI or CAT Scan becomes necessary.

However, **the greater purpose of this book is to teach the reader how to make their own back better**. In large part, that must include figuring out, _for yourself_, without great expense, what is actually wrong. The following describes how you can do it yourself because, in fact, **you are the best person to do it**. No doctor known to me is aware of this method, nor is it, to my knowledge, described in the medical literature (and believe me, I am well-read in the field of back pain); so, up until now, patients have really been left to their own devices, anyway. So, at worst, the situation hasn't changed with the advent of this book. At best, the reader has every reason to believe that they, themselves, can be made competent enough to figure out if they have a disc problem and remedy it by a few simple movements.

SELF-DIAGNOSING YOUR DISC

I am convinced, through experience teaching *The O'Connor Technique (tm)*, that, for the average person with back pain, **it is possible for a patient of normal intelligence with no medical training to identify, without expensive modalities, the exact origin and site of the pain and thereby learn to make their own diagnosis. This is done by performing specific movements of the spine and focusing on what happens to the pain**. These movements can be categorized and technically defined as a **DIAGNOSTIC CIRCUMDUCTION** because the movements employed constitute what is known in anatomical or orthopedic parlance as "circumduction." Based upon a knowledgeable and logical deductive reasoning process, anyone properly educated can arrive at their own diagnosis by engaging in DIAGNOSTIC CIRCUMDUCTION and, thereafter, **identify the exact location of their displaced disc material**

so as to, later, be able to manipulate it back into the pain-free configuration.

This method of DIAGNOSTIC CIRCUMDUCTION to diagnose a disc condition is so successful for me in my practice that, many times, I get an NMRI (Nuclear Mass Resonance Image) or CT Scan simply to confirm my clinical diagnosis. I seldom find a major discrepancy between the image study and my clinical exam, except in the presence of spondylolisthesis.

Now, the reader may scour the existing medical literature on back pain in search of the clinical term--DIAGNOSTIC CIRCUMDUCTION. To my knowledge, it does not exist outside of this book, and I have been specifically exploring back pain literature for well over 15 years. Moreover, no mention of DIAGNOSTIC CIRCUMDUCTION is made in the newly published government guide to back pain management which, by virtue of its "definitive" auspices, should contain it or a similar test if it exists. Therefore, when DIAGNOSTIC CIRCUMDUCTION is used by professional clinicians to diagnose a disc herniation, in the absence of alternative nomenclature, it can best be referred to as **"THE O'CONNOR TEST."** If it can be shown that some other author described it prior to 1990, I would gladly re-title it; however, until such time, I will continue to represent it as my contribution to clinical medicine.

In developing this technique, I discovered that, **whenever a person with back pain attempts to circumductionally pivot (as in Figure 1) the spine at a particular vertebral level where disc material is herniated and significantly displaced, they almost invariably experience pain that has an arresting component to it.** That is, their **CIRCUMDUCTION is physically stopped by the obstruction caused by the displaced disc material.** As they CIRCUMDUCT through that particular arc where decentralized disc material is located (almost always in the extended configuration), they begin to trap, pinch or put pressure on the disc material that is off-center; and **a very specific pain is produced that is easily distinguishable from other types of pain.** This pain, as described in the previous chapter is due to the fulcrum effect. It is a pain that stops movement as though an actual object was physically obstructing the movement, not highly unlike a pencil had been put in a door hinge and the door attempted to be shut. One can't continue to force the door shut without breaking something. Similarly, **when one**

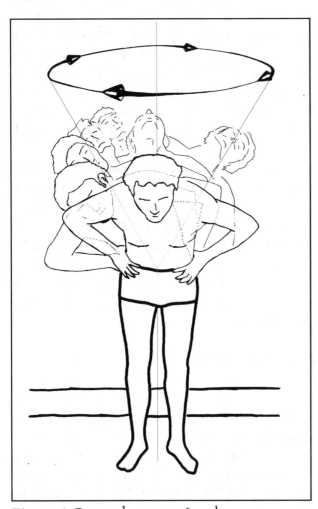

Figure 1 Circumduction at Lumbar spine

tries to gyrate through a point between two vertebrae where a piece of disc material is de-centralized, one cannot complete the CIRCUMDUCTIONAL movement while maintaining the same degree of lateral bending or extension. When this action is attempted, the person with a decentralized disc feels something like a wedge is stuck in the way. This is the sensation that frequently is described as a "catch," as if something were "stuck" in the back or something in the back "went out." **The sufferers almost uniformly feel as though, if they could just move in the right way, the pain would resolve or the back "go back in."**

The pain more often than not feels like an object is stuck in the spine at a fixed point. **Every time the person rotates the painful area of the spine through CIRCUMDUCTION and reaches the same area where the wedge is stuck, they have to stop or the pain becomes too great.** Either way they CIRCUMDUCT, (clockwise from left to right or counterclockwise from right to left) upon reaching approximately the same point where the disc material is herniated, they are arrested in their range of motion by pain. The person senses that if they persist in the CIRCUMDUCTION without reducing the degree of lateral bending or extension, the pain will become unbearable. So, in order to continue CIRCUMDUCTING, they have to relax the degree of extension (or leaning) over the site of the herniation by dropping the hip, bending the knee on the same side of the pain, or straightening up slightly to reduce the degree of lateral bending or extension. Once this is accomplished, the CIRCUMDUCTION can usually be continued unimpeded because by so doing, they are shifting the center of gravity at the problem disc to a configuration wherein the vertebral bones are no longer putting fulcrum-like forces on the displaced disc material.

After they adjust their center of gravity so that the increased pain is no longer present, the usual background pain may still be present; and, no matter how many times they try, the range of motion through that same part of the arc at the particular spinal level is repeatedly and reproducibly impaired. What is happening has been anatomically described in Chapter 2 as the FULCRUM EFFECT.

Often, when a person is CIRCUMDUCTING and they come to the point of restricted range of motion, they often will automatically bend the knee on the painful side so as to drop the hip and thereby reduce the degree of lateral bending. When I am examining a patient I sometimes move their upper body in such a way that maintains the degree of lateral bending and extension and doesn't allow them to try to return to the neutral position. This forces them to bend their knee or drop their hip to avoid the pain, and it is a sure sign that I have

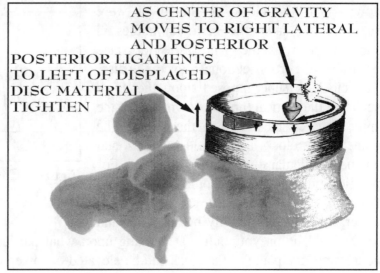

Figure 2 Fulcrum effect causing pain as CIRCUMDUCTION proceeds clockwise until arrested by displaced disc material.

identified the site of the disc displacement. The presence of an ARREST IN CIRCUMDUCTION might properly be termed a **"POSITIVE O'CONNOR TEST"** in medical parlance since, to my knowledge, this distinction has never been made before in the medical literature.

The pain is generated by the same type of forces that strain the hinge when an object prevents a door from closing. A long moment arm is acting on a very small fulcrum-to-object lever arm length. In the disc's case, the hard, displaced, disc material is acting as the fulcrum, the vertebral body and the adjacent disc component above and anterior to the displaced disc material is the long moment arm, and the ligaments that hold the vertebral bodies together are equivalent to the "objects" moved by a fulcrum when it operates. Just as a long pry-bar can lift a heavy stone, similar force applied to tighten such short ligaments results in pain. (See Figure 2)

In order to discover where the displaced disc material is actually located along your spine, you need to learn how to perform a DIAGNOSTIC CIRCUMDUCTION in which you attempt to CIRCUMDUCT in a leaning FLEXION that progresses clockwise or counterclockwise to an EXTENSION such that the body is pivoting at the disc unit level where the spine is most painful. This is done by first leaning forward slightly (flexing) such that the body is bending exactly at the site of spinal pain. Ideally, the area below the pain should stay immobilized as best as you can and only the vertebrae above it should be allowed to engage in CIRCUMDUCTIONAL motion.

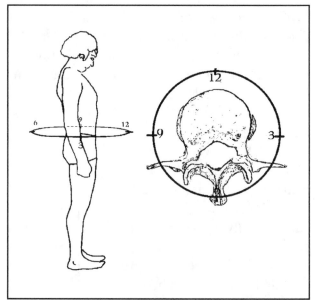

To understand how to perform a meaningful DIAGNOSTIC CIRCUMDUCTION on yourself as well as how the designation of clockwise and counterclockwise is used in this book, you need to view (in your mind's eye) a clock face from a perspective such that you are looking down upon the clock as though it were superimposed upon the vertebral bodies in such a manner that the plane of the clock face is parallel to a cross-sectional view of the disc. The clock is superimposed upon the spine such that the vertical (up and down) axis of the spine transects the center of the clock. The plane of the clock face should be horizontal and perpendicular to the axis of the spine. For practical purposes 12:00 should be directly in front of you. The 6:00 position would, understandably, be directly behind you, and

Figure 3 Clock face superimposed upon body and vertebral bone for orientation

9:00 would be on your left. Depending upon what particular disc unit of the spine you are addressing, the plane of the clock can be elevated or lowered in your imagination; but it should always be kept perpendicular to the plane of the spine. The intricacy of this designation is not important. What is important is that you develop some way of orienting yourself to some conventional diagram for the purposes of this discussion and future reference because, if properly aligned, the horizontal plane of the clock face is superimposed upon and parallel to the horizontal plane of the discs (See Figure 3). It is as if the problem disc now has clock face numbering system superimposed upon it so its reference points can be discussed and the reader can be directed without confusion.

Now, to perform a **DIAGNOSTIC CIRCUMDUCTION, start by facing towards the 12:00 position on the clock,** putting your hands on your hips for balance and support, and mildly lifting your upper body off of your lower body by pushing inferiorly with your arms (this takes some hydraulic pressure off of the disc and makes it easier to know which pain is acting); then **flex anteriorly** (flex approximately 15 to 20 degrees but no greater than 30 degrees forward off of an upright posture). If you flex forward too much, that will increase the prolapsing pressure and unnecessarily increase the pain. One way of knowing if you are flexing the right amount, flex forward (anteriorly) until a stretching pain comes to your back, then back off (reduce the amount of flexion) until that pain stops.

Leaving your feet firmly planted at about shoulder width, **begin smoothly leaning/CIRCUMDUCTING** (not twisting which is technically termed axial rotation) **only that portion of your body above the painful site in one direction or the other.** If the pain seems to give you more symptoms to one side or the other then start CIRCUMDUCTING towards that direction.

For this example, I choose to CIRCUMDUCT clockwise (to the right) first, pivoting at the level of a lower Lumbar disc. So, begin to tilt towards the 1:00 position (clockwise) while keeping the angle of the upper body at the same degree of flexion. The leaning is continued by a tilting of the body above the pivot site to this same side while eventually you will be moving from flexion to extension. You should be only allowing the spine superior to the site you are pivoting around to flex or extend, the segments below the site should be kept in neutral position. When you start CIRCUMDUCTING to the right, you lean more and more to the right; and, in a smooth continuous motion, you progressively CIRCUMDUCT in an arc, a little more each time by leaning more to the right and posteriorly until at the end of the movement, it is as though you were leaning backwards in full extension (as in Figure 4).

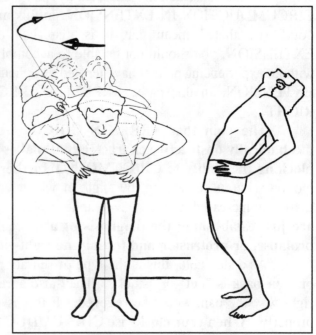

Figure 4 CIRCUMDUCTION to right (clockwise) ending in full extension

Since this may be difficult to understand, I will elaborate in other words. At the level of the spine where the pain is located, try to make your spine bend or lean enough to reproduce the same-sided pain you are usually experiencing with movement. About 15 to 30 degrees off the axis of a normal erect posture should be sufficient. While keeping this same degree of tilt, slowly and

109

carefully make a gyrating-like rotational movement (like a gyro-scope or a top when it begins to run out of energy and begins to carve out an inverted cone in space) so that, by the time you progressively CIRCUMDUCT to the 3:00 position, you are in effect leaning sideways to the right as much as you can without losing your balance. This DIAGNOSTIC CIRCUMDUCTION is not to be confused with twisting. You are not twisting the spine during this test. Continue this same movement towards the 4:00 position. You may at this point have to thrust your hips forward (like you were sticking out your belly-button) at this point to keep the center of gravity of the upper body over your legs. If your back pain usually gives you pain more on the right side of your body this means that the disc is herniated more to the right than directly in the posterior midline; so, somewhere between about 3:00 and 6:00 the pain should begin to increase so much as to prevent you from CIRCUMDUCTING further without straightening up slightly or dropping the right hip or bending the knee to allow the movement to proceed. **If your motion is arrested, what is arresting your motion is the off-center displaced disc material that has begun to act as a fulcrum**; and, as the peripheral portion of the vertebral bodies progressively compress from the 3:00 to 6:00 positions on the periphery of the disc, they begin to compress and pinch the displaced disc material, forcing it to act on the intervertebral ligaments with a fulcrum effect (review Figure 2 here and Figure 32 in Chapter 2) and creating increased pain to the point where you have to stop. The obstruction caused by the displaced disc material makes Continued CIRCUMDUCTION IN EXTENSION, in this manner, realistically impossible. If the disc is "out" (by that I mean that it is displaced enough to impede CIRCUMDUCTION IN EXTENSION, you should not be able to accomplish full extension over that point of herniation without experiencing pain. I have termed this phenomenon ARRESTED CIRCUMDUCTION IN EXTENSION, in this case, ARRESTED CIRCUMDUCTION IN EXTENSION TO THE RIGHT.

The pain that ARRESTS CIRCUMDUCTION IN EXTENSION should have a mechanically obstructive character that makes it feel as though something were physically blocking the ability to CIRCUMDUCT further. That is, you sense that if you continue the motion without decreasing the angle at which you are leaning or extending, the pain will be markedly increased, possibly even unbearable. When this happens, **don't force it further, you are just establishing the diagnosis of a de-centralized piece of disc material, herniation, prolapse, or protrusion and testing the right-sided margin of the disc bulge at this point.**

As a side note, this is the type of sensation that patients routinely describe as a "catch," or their back is "out" or "stuck." They also agree that it feels like if they could just move the right way the pain would be relieved. If this is the sensation you feel, you are doing the test properly. **When your clockwise CIRCUMDUCTION is halted by this obstructing pain, you have just identified the position of the right margin of the displaced disc material.**

In most cases, you will be stopped in your movement to the right (or clockwise) before reaching the region of the posterior midline. Then, you continue THE O'CONNOR TEST by repeating the movement to the left (or counterclockwise) by starting from the front again and, only this time, successively perform the flexion, abduction, extension, and adduction in sequence to the left which similarly brings you around leaning progressively more posteriorly until finally you are leaning backwards. To do this, go back to the 12:00 position and repeat a similar leaning/gyration-like movement in the opposite direction as before. This time, move to the left (counterclockwise) by continuously leaning/CIRCUMDUCTING to the 11:00 position then on to 10:00 position, and so on. As you did before, continue to smoothly CIRCUMDUCT and thrust your hips gently forward when you get to the 9:00 position if necessary. **As you go from 9:00 on towards 6:00 and the back begins to assume an extended posture, the pain should be elicited at some point in the CIRCUMDUCTION before reaching the posterior midline if the disc material is herniated predominately to the left.** Similarly when you moved in a clock-wise direction, your movement should be arrested by pain when you reach the point where the pressure created by the two vertebral body's edges begin to apply force to the herniated disc material. **The point that now stops you defines the left margin of the displaced disc material.**

If your pain is predominately one sided, (and for the purpose of this example I will assume that it is more to the right) one should notice that the movement counterclockwise is not arrested until CIRCUMDUCTING somewhere well beyond the 9:00 position. It will usually become arrested again at least when one approaches the 6:00 position (the posterior midline) from a counterclockwise direction because the vertebral body's peripheral margins will be compressing the other side of the herniated material as the DIAGNOSTIC CIRCUMDUCTION proceeds to this point. Of course, the actual site of the arrest is largely dependent upon the actual position of the displaced disc material. The more lateral the obstructing disc fragment, the more lateral the range of ARRESTED CIRCUMDUCTION. Unless you have two discs out simultaneously, one on one side and another on the other (this would be unlikely if this is the first episode of severe back pain, but not unusual if you have had several traumatic flexion injuries) your motion should be arrested predominately to one side. If only one piece of disc material is to blame it usually is apparent which side the herniation is on because the pain will be mostly on that same side. As you repeat these DIAGNOSTIC CIRCUMDUCTIONS alternately clockwise then counterclockwise, the places where your motion is arrested identifies for you the borders of the displaced disc material.

As a procedural consideration, if your pain is predominately right-sided, then start with a clockwise CIRCUMDUCTION because that should get you to identify the most anterior aspect of the prolapsed disc first. Then, to locate the other side of the disc bulge you next CIRCUMDUCT in the counterclockwise direction. Keep doing this until you have fixed in your mind the position of the aberrant disc material.

This is much like being given the task of finding the position of a brick placed between two barrels with your eyes closed. You do it simply by progressively rocking the top barrel in a circular/gyrating fashion until you can figure out where the most force is necessary to roll the barrel over the hump that the brick creates. As you "CIRCUMDUCT" the top barrel, the closer the rim gets to the brick, the more energy it takes to force it over the hump. The barrel would be analogous to the barrel-like component of the vertebral bones adjacent to the herniated disc and the herniated disc material would be the brick. I doubt that anyone would have trouble describing the position of a brick between two barrels with their eyes closed, so one needn't make finding a disc herniation any harder than that. You just have to picture the vertebral bone gyrating above a piece of hard material resting on another similar barrel surface, unmoving below it.

Now, if the disc is herniated directly to the posterior (in the posterior midline) and it is a wide bulge, arrest can occur as early as the 9:00 position CIRCUMDUCTING counterclockwise and again at the 3:00 position while CIRCUMDUCTING clockwise. This is not unheard of, so when this happens one can assume that the disc bulge is directly in the mid-line, extremely wide based, and herniated directly to the posterior. When this is the case, usually the back pain doesn't seem to be directed or radiating to one side or the other but stays centrally in the posterior midline or gives pain to both sides more or less equally. In my experience, the centralized disc bulges usually only occur in the lower Lumbar region. I believe this is owing to the extra anatomical strength afforded by the posterior longitudinal ligament as it ascends to the superior reaches of the vertebral column making midline posterior prolapses less likely as one ascends the spinal column. When it enters the lower Lumbar region, the wideness of the vertebral bodies causes the posterior longitudinal ligament to be spread thinner, thus predisposing to posterior midline disc bulging. Also, this area usually sustains the greatest forces when flexion injuries occur, and most people flex directly forward when they lift.

It is so unusual for discs to herniate anteriorly except under extreme traumatic stress such as in an automobile accident or major fall in which the spine is violently hyperextended that I do not feel a discussion of that condition is appropriate here; but if the pain is indicative of an arrest in motion when CIRCUMDUCTING through the 9:00 to 12:00 to 3:00 positions, then suspect an anteriorly prolapsed disc.

In the approximately ten years of treating disc herniations, I have seen only a single anterior herniation. Of course, in the event of a major traumatic injury such as mentioned above, an examination by a qualified medical doctor is in order, and an appropriate imaging study might just as easily and safely demonstrate the lesion. Nevertheless, repeated DIAGNOSTIC CIRCUMDUCTIONS around from one side to the other should allow you to fix in your mind the approximate direction and position of the disc bulge.

The level (i.e.: L5-S1, C5-C6, etc.) of the spine where the pain is elicited and at which you should be pivoting tells you the level of the disc segment that is herniated, bulging or prolapsed. For instance, if you lean your torso and center your pivot at the area right where the spine meets the hips and an arrest in motion occurs, your protrusion is probably at the L5-S1 disc space level. If you only need to lean your head to one side and rotate it (as if looking over your shoulder) and the motion is arrested, it is at the C2-C4 level. Depending upon how much you have to lean that portion of your body superior to the area of pain away from the mid-line tells you how far down the putative segment is located. This is understandable because the more away from the midline you have to lean your upper body to get to the painful segment, the lower the portion of the spine that will be required to bend in order to allow for the movement. As that segment bends in the direction of the herniation, bulge or prolapse, the wedge-like, painful sensation is elicited as the bulge is squeezed and the peripheral intervertebral ligaments containing the bulge are stretched.

So, **once you have fixed in your mind the borders of the disc bulge** as described above, you can **carefully aim a leaning extension directly over the center of where the herniation should be**. The onset of the pinching, wedge-like, pain (immediately upon the degree of the leaning extension being sufficient to put pressure on it) should confirm the exact center of the disc herniation, bulge, or prolapse. Strictly speaking, when you are compressing the disc directly over its herniation, the pain you feel is mostly due to the hydraulic, direct mechanical, or pincer-like pressure exerted by the displaced disc material pushing against and deforming the posterior component of the capsule (depending upon the displaced disc material's position relative to the disc's center). The instant you move off of that point directly over the displaced disc material, the fulcrum pain comes in as adjacent capsular ligaments are stretched.

If there is no arrested motion or pain during this test, either your pain is not due to a disc or you are not leaning far enough off the vertical axis to ideally effect the spinal segment with the herniation. It may sound obvious, but if you are attempting to CIRCUMDUCT by pivoting at the lower Thoracic region, you are probably not going to illicit sufficient discomfort to diagnose a herniation at a low Lumbar lesion and visa versa. To insure such is not the case, you can do some experimental testing by increasing the degree of off-center leaning to find the location of the problematic disc unit.

DIAGNOSTIC CIRCUMDUCTION can be used at any level of the spine to determine whether a particular disc is herniated. In the Cervical region, CIRCUMDUCTING the head at the neck such that you pivot around the lowest vertebral segment that is painful will give the best determination of the level of the herniated disc material. The Thoracic spine is somewhat more difficult due to its inherent lack of mobility; however cocking the shoulders to effect a leaning gyrating CIRCUMDUCTION and focusing your pivotal point slightly below the area of discomfort usually will reveal what segment of the spine is involved. For the Lumbar region, pivoting at the hips usually is enough to confirm where the pain precisely stops your motion. Regardless of the spinal region, the more you increase the angle of the spine superior to the area of concern, the more you activate the disc segment in question. If you keep the spine superior and inferior to the site of pain and the disc unit you are testing relatively straight. That way you can be certain that you are testing only a single disc unit.

You may note, leaning or flexing anteriorly too much towards the opposite side relative to the disc herniation during this test can sometimes elicit a stretching type of pain near the site of the disc herniation because the degree of leaning is so great as to stretch the peripheral intervertebral ligaments affected by the disc herniation or due to the hydraulic-type pressure exerted by a bulging disc material (depending upon the actual type of herniation and degree of off-centered position of the herniation). This means that you are over-doing the degree of anterior flexion or leaning; however, this pain can usually be distinguished from the range of motion, obstructing-type, pain or disc-bulge, pinching, sensation. **The pain of too much flexion is more of a stretching type pain and different from the pain induced by trapping and squeezing a herniated piece of disc material that comes while CIRCUMDUCTING IN EXTENSION. Also, the stretching type of pain, although brought on by the movements, doesn't arrest CIRCUMDUCTION anteriorly so much as it is so painful that you don't want to continue to flex forward. Too, straightening up from this pain sometimes produces pain actually greater than the pain you induced by flexion.** You should also feel the discomfort on the posterior side opposite to the side towards which you are anteriorly flexing. **This is the pain caused by weight-bearing flexion on a herniated disc** (to be covered in greater depth later). This is a consequence of the de-centralized disc material being pushed further posteriorly, but I don't want to confuse the reader anymore by focusing on it, except to say if it occurs, straighten up until it is relieved before it causes the disc to prolapse more and potentially compress a nerve root.

As I indicated above, there are other ligaments, inflamed tendons, and torn or spasmed muscles all possibly present concurrently, any one of which is capable of generating back pain; and, therefore, capable of confusing the picture, especially just after an injury. Since standing and CIRCUMDUCTING while weight-bearing involves the activation of these structures, it can be difficult to distinguish between these sources of pain when trying to determine if de-centralized disc material is the source or if a major contributing component is due to the activation of damaged muscles or tendons. In reality, one can expect these other types of pain, especially spasm, to participate in the total back pain experience especially when in close proximity (both anatomically and near in time) to an injury. In that event, wait a few days or, if necessary, as much as a week or two to let these other structures calm down. They will heal, the disc's structural tears will not. One can be reasonably certain that if the disc is involved, it will stay broken and eventually it will become apparent that such is the case.

If the DIAGNOSTIC CIRCUMDUCTION test described above is not obviously and convincingly successful in distinguishing whether pain is from a piece of decentralized disc material or some other source while weight-bearing, you can try lying down and reproducing the same test in a reclining position. Simply put pillows in such a manner that you can roll or change your position successively to reproduce the same configurations as achieved when leaning and extending from an upright posture. For instance, for the neck area, the obstructive component of the pain can be identified without interference of any other active muscular motions by simply relaxing and propping the head up on a pillow then log-rolling the entire body. In effect, the angle formed by the neck with reference to the axis of the body doesn't change as the neck is fixed in its orientation and the body moves through space. This moves the selected disc unit through its range of CIRCUMDUCTION motion equivalently to the manner which is accomplished while standing only, in this case, it is on a horizontal axis and the body below the disc is doing the moving.

In the reclining scenario, the previously described "O'CONNOR DIAGNOSTIC CIRCUMDUCTION TEST" would be referred to as "**PASSIVE**" and can be differentiated from the standing test which would be conversely designated as "**ACTIVE**." In the upright posture, the body is actively moving and contracting muscles, activating other potentially inflamed soft tissues, and stretching those structures necessary to balance the body; but, in the reclining case, the body is more passively determining the site of the lesion because the disc unit is only moving as a consequence of the body rolling and the non-disc structures are exempted from fighting gravity.

For Thoracic spinal pain, similarly propping the upper torso on pillows or any suitably comfortable structure will suffice. For the Lumbar region, especially while in acute pain, lying on a soft mattress is an excellent vehicle. You will probably be doing that anyway, so you might as well "make hay while the sun shines." As the body sinks into the mattress while a pillow or the elbows raise the prone torso up, the Lumbar spine passively assumes an extended posture. Rolling through the same pattern as above can reveal the same information. Instead of leaning and gyrating, you only need to roll from side to side to localize the site of the de-centralized disc material. The principle is the same, only the passive positioning eliminates the likelihood that spasm and inflamed tendons or muscles are being activated to cause the pain.

After becoming very familiar with these methods, through repeated experience, the reader can expect to instantly identify when the disc material has become de-centralized and instigating the pain from any position. Once familiar with the feeling (especially if your disc material repeatedly is prone to de-centralization), every time it goes "out" you can immediately tell if it is "out" by gently CIRCUMDUCTING from even a seated position. It isn't necessary to make a big project out of CIRCUMDUCTING after you conceptualize the mechanics and become adept at the movement. After awhile, simply rolling the neck or shoulders around from almost any position will reveal the presence and position of Cervical or Thoracic decentralized material, and gyrating the hips without so much as changing your seated position can be expected, eventually, to be all that is required for the "expert" you can become at your own back pain diagnosis.

I've become so adept at doing it, when I suspect (due to the onset of discomfort) the disc material has migrated, I only need to lean towards the place where it usually displaces and feel the characteristic "wedge-like" pain to confirm whether it is truly "out" or not. I don't necessarily have to go through the entire DIAGNOSTIC CIRCUMDUCTION process I described above. Don't think that just because I described it in such exacting detail that you need to obsessively adhere to the entire rigmarole forever. Even while driving, I can shift my hips in a leaning posture and feel the "wedge" or "lump." I then can do the appropriate MANEUVER (to be described later) and relieve the pain. There is no reason why anyone else who comprehends the mechanical principle of this test cannot do likewise. Reading on, the MANEUVER will be taught so that once the displaced disc material is identified, it can be re-centralized with equal ease.

In the absence of DIAGNOSTIC CIRCUMDUCTIONAL ARREST throughout the full range of posterior extension, it is harder to evoke a decentralized disc as the origin of the pain. If nothing stops or limits you when making these gyratory movements, the pain is possibly not from herniated, protruding, or de-centralized disc material's effect upon the capsular intervertebral ligaments and the re-centralizing MANEUVERS described later will have a lower probability of helping your type of back pain. However, I have known patients who involuntarily splint the affected segment and despite attempts to CIRCUMDUCT at the affected segment; instead, unconsciously they CIRCUMDUCT only at the segments above or below it. Therefore, **simply because you do not get a pain that arrests your movement does not mean that the MANEUVERS outlined in this book will not help you.** I have had several patients who are helped by my method yet never had an arrested motion that I could identify. In one case, I was able to conclude that the person was so flexible and had accommodated to the pain for so long that other segments of the spine performed all the circumductatory movements without necessitating the activation of the involved segment or she was so accustomed to the pain that she unconsciously avoided the use of that segment. The MANEUVERS worked very well in this patient, ending her years of neck pain.

Consequently, I would suggest that the readers attempt the MANEUVERS described later in the book, regardless of whether or not they have a rotational CIRCUMDUCTION ARREST or if they understand how to diagnose their own disc. **Anyone with back pain has nothing to lose and everything to gain by trying *The O'Connor Technique (tm)* MANEUVERS.** Sometimes, when I see that patients are not arresting in their own CIRCUMDUCTION attempts even though I have instructed them in what to do, I can usually properly guide their movements so as to insure that the affected segment is being loaded or stressed. This usually proves to me that, indeed, they have an arresting component due to a disc problem; and I can locate it even though they cannot without physical, individualized, and personal guidance. However, it is impossible for me to examine everyone of this book's readers who have herniations but are unable to properly perform a DIAGNOSTIC CIRCUMDUCTION. This series of movements is designed so that you can do it yourself; and, thereby, identify the site, direction, and position of the displaced disc material. If that cannot be accomplished, no big deal, continue reading; and, after the method becomes known to you, you can come back and try it again to see if you can succeed. In other words, don't get frustrated, disappointed, or give up just yet because the foregoing appears to be too complex or difficult.

Of note here, even though I'm getting ahead of myself, **when the MANEUVERS described later in the book are successfully accomplished, one can expect this "wedge"-like pain that arrests your movement and the obstructive component of the pain to be instantly resolved.** As the disc material is re-centralized, it no longer impedes the normal circumductatory and gyrational actions of the spine. When the displaced disc material goes back into its central location, it does so usually with dramatic relief because it no longer obstructs the normal circumductatory capacity of the spine. If the MANEUVERS are accomplished and no dramatic relief is achieved, then probably either a disc is not the problem or the corrective MANEUVERS are not being accomplished properly and, therefore, not yet successful in replacing the misplaced disc material.

Repeating this "test" but treating it as a component of a MANEUVER while unweighting the superior part of the body above the lesion at the end of one of the MANEUVERS that are described later in this book also can re-seat a displaced disc that is not very much off-center. I often see people with mild back symptoms performing this type of movement (especially after getting out and stretching after long drives) because it gives those with minimally displaced disc material relief from the "stiffness" they experience due to the prolonged WEIGHT-BEARING FLEXION of driving.

Often, the MANEUVERS I describe later in the book are able to move the disc material almost completely, but a little extra nudge is necessary to get them to seat completely. Simply doing a mild weight-bearing THERAPEUTIC CIRCUMDUCTION nearly identical to the "O'Connor Test" frequently accomplishes the "coup-de-Grace" and provides the final effort necessary to completely re-seat the disc, but more about this aspect later.

Another reasonable rule of thumb to be guided by is that, if there is no arrested motion on weight-bearing DIAGNOSTIC CIRCUMDUCTION, the disc material (or fragments of same) are probably not decentralized. An interesting problem sometimes prevents the immediately successful resolution of all components of the back pain. The disc material can have been returned to the proper centralized position, yet a residual pain may still be present. When it seems that even though you are doing everything as you are supposed to do and recreating the same sequences of MANEUVERS (as will be described later) that were successful in the past, yet still nothing seems to totally stop the residual pain, it often is the case that the disc fragment has been putting pressure on the capsule's ligaments so long that an inflammatory focus has been created. In this case, there may be pain associated with flexion or extension; yet no actual arrested motion.

In that event, using anti-inflammatory medications and rest to prevent repetitive irritation of the inflammatory focus is the best policy to relieve residual pain. More on that subject follows later in the section on medicines and strategy for pain relief; but inflammatory pain is of a dull

116

aching or warm (like heat generating) character, continuous, and present regardless of the position. Then, it probably originates from an arthritis-like inflammation of the joints, ligaments, or tendons acting on some nearby spinal segments. Especially, the accessory articulations of the vertebral bones (the facet joints) can also become inflamed. **Facet pain is usually distinguishable from the pain of a herniated disc because facet joint arthritis pain has no physically arresting component, hurts when standing, and relieved by sitting (the opposite of disc pain.)** In this case, drugs like acetaminophen, aspirin, Ibuprofen (Advil, Motrin, Nuprin, etc.) or other non-steroidal anti-inflammatory drugs are indicated. These drugs are often helpful for pain of disc origin, also; but, usually, they don't offer much relief if the disc material is still "out." After the disc has been re-centralized, the anti-inflammatory medicines are especially helpful in reducing the pain caused by the disc material rubbing against the ligaments or the inflammatory arthritic pain caused by the vertebral bodies rubbing together when discs degenerate to the point that the disc space has collapsed.

The key to this consideration, of course, is the understanding that if the disc is decentralized, the "wedge"-like pain that stops your movement will be present while leaning and CIRCUMDUCTING IN EXTENSION. If you have completed a successful MANEUVER that frees up the circumductatory capacity of the involved spinal segment such that there is no longer the arrest in DIAGNOSTIC CIRCUMDUCTION that there was before completing the MANEUVER yet there still is pain coming from that area, this is probably a residual soreness or inflammatory-type pain. Understandably, if a disc has been protruding and tearing the adjacent ligamentous structures, they will have been damaged or at least irritated. Be aware that once an inflammatory focus is set up after prolonged pressure due to protruding disc material, it is reasonable to assume it will take some time and anti-inflammatory medication to achieve total relief.

Many times, I have "fixed" a person's back to the extent that they no longer have arrested motion; but they continue to describe pain for a short time afterwards. Usually, the pain is of such reduced severity and so closely related to the MANEUVER done to them that they acknowledge the relief came from my method. Most patients recognize that the majority of the pain is gone the following day, attributing my application of *The O'Connor Technique (tm)* as the point when their recovery began.

DOCUMENTING YOUR DISC

Back pain episodes are frequently separated by long intervals between painful events. For that reason, it is easy to forget the site of the displaced disc material or, more importantly, the particular MANEUVER or sequence of movements that successfully alleviated that unique pain. So as to give your back its best chance for the earliest recovery, take notes to document the major components of the pain. By identifying the areas of pain for future reference, any particular pain pattern can be reasonably assumed to be originating from the same disc in the same position when it recurs. Therefore, **if a particular site is identified and a unique MANEUVER (the MANEUVERS are to be described later) is successful, you can document both the level and direction of the displaced material as well as the movements that were most successful in alleviating that pain.** Then, when an identical pain recurs at some time in the distant future, that

MANEUVER or sequence can be immediately employed to occasion relief without relying solely on the memory or trial-and-error.

It is best to characterize the pain in a systematic fashion. **First, locate it by level of the spine where the pain is greatest.** Certainly, you wouldn't be expected to be successful doing the same corrective MANEUVER for a problem centered at the high Thoracic level on the left that you would do for a pain originating at the Low Lumbar region on the right. So, it makes sense to keep track of where the problem is physically located so that the proper MANEUVER can be chosen later. Next, on a diagram like the one provided here (Figure 5), cross hatch the exact region (level) of the particular spinal pain where it seems to be centered and to where it radiates. Note where the sharpest pain is the most severe and any movements or positions which increase the pain.

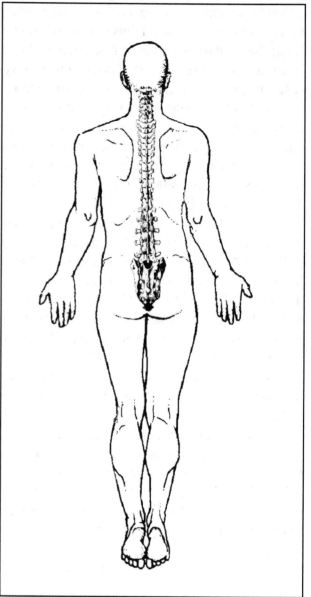

Figure 5 Posterior view of back with spine superimposed.

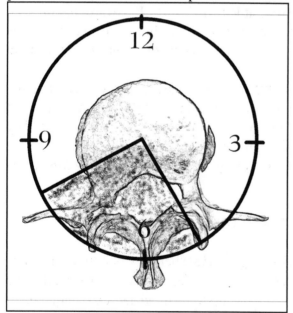

Figure 6 "Pie Chart" superimposed upon a disc showing arrested range of motion area.

After that, on a view that looks down upon the disc, draw a triangular "piece of pie" over the area which brings on the sharp pain during the DIAGNOSTIC CIRCUMDUCTIONAL motions described above in "SELF-DIAGNOSING YOUR DISC". It matters little whether you choose a format like a clock or a 360 degree circle to diagram the wedge shaped area of arrested motion so long as it is in some way recognized, understood, and documented. I find it advantageous to draw a diagram like a pie chart so that the areas with pain-free range of motion are distinguished from the areas where range of motion is arrested and pain is elicited (Figure 6).

Keeping such documentation helps to recall the exact location of the de-centralized disc material so one needn't repeat the testing every time. You will appreciate the necessity for documenting or fixing in your mind the exact location of the displaced disc material, later, as the MANEUVERS are described because you will also (later in the book) be asked to document the exact MANEUVER that gets you out of pain; and you will want to reference a particular drawing to a particular MANEUVER. The diagrams provided in this book (Figures 3 and 5) can be copied and drawn on to serve that purpose. Like writing down the description and combination to a safe, this becomes especially helpful and necessary if you have multi-level disc problems or if the disc is particularly difficult to re-centralize.

Documentation becomes especially important whenever there are complex cases in which the pain appears to move from side to midline, side to side, or from midline to the side during a WEIGHTED CIRCUMDUCTIONAL movement. This can mean that you have a mobile piece of disc material moving laterally through a concentric tear or a piece of disc material moving within a space between the laminations of the annulus fibrosus or between the capsule (the ligamentous peripheral layer of the disc) and the annulus fibrosus (as portrayed in Figure 7).

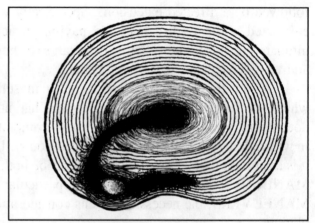

Figure 7 Disc material trapped between layers of annulus fibrosus

In that event, a recollection of where the original pain started and where it went to during any particular MANEUVER may give a clue as to the location of the disc material. Sometimes such a method can elaborate the original tract through which the disc material traveled. The eventual goal is, then, to design or describe a means by which you can work the material back to the center of the disc as though you were playing a "BB in a maze" game.

If the degree of disc degeneration is extensive and the product of multiple traumatic events the goal becomes not highly unlike moving a BB through a circular type maze game. In order to get the BB to the center you have to move the BB centrally at precisely the right instant where a gap in the walls will allow its movement to proceed centrally. In order to get to that gap, the BB has to be caused to move circumferentially by progressive application of forces directed to allow its movement to proceed in the ideal direction. In this analogy, the walls of the maze are the laminar array of the fractured annulus fibrosus laminations contained within the intervertebral capsule ligaments and the BB is the solidified central disc material that once was the liquid nucleus pulposus. Unfortunately, you cannot see the BB to know when it is in the ideal position to move centrally. This causes you to rely upon trial and error. **When you are successful, it probably is in your best interests to document what you did to succeed so as to reproduce that same**

119

series of movements the next time.

This is a potentially important distinction to be made and documented because if one has a disc like that seen in Figure 7, a DIAGNOSTIC CIRCUMDUCTION in a counter clockwise direction can result in the pain changing from the left posterior to the right posterior. You should take note of this type of reaction when documenting your disc pain. The significance of this will become apparent in later reading on MANEUVERS.

Don't get frustrated by reading this because of its apparent complexity and not knowing yet what constitutes a MANEUVER. Statistically speaking, you probably don't have a disc of this configuration; but, if you do, and the simple efforts don't seem to work, you may have to resort to a more complex strategy. In that case, the first effort would be made to return the disc fragment to the site where the pain originated, then find the tract through which it traveled so it can be moved back to the center. This may require a gentle WEIGHT-BEARING CIRCUMDUCTIONAL movement before an unweighted flexion in a certain position then followed by a directed extension. Specifically writing down the exact sequence of movements correlated with the disc map and paying particular attention to the successful positions that ultimately result in the relief of pain can save hours of ineffective movements being repeated if and when your back goes "out" again.

Even though I'm getting ahead of myself by discussing MANEUVERS, the nature of which are still obscure to the reader who has not yet read Chapter 5, a discussion describing documentation of a "puzzle" would not be complete without including a recommendation to retain in writing the solution to the puzzle, or if you will, the combination to your "safe". In summary, it is important to take a few notes to describe both the pain pattern and the directions for the ideal MANEUVER that gets you out of that particular pain pattern. Later, as you are exposed to the MANEUVERS, the necessity for this consideration and the means to accomplish it will become obvious.

1. Leblan K, et al. Report of the Quebec task force on spinal disorders. *Spine*. 1987;12:S1-S8.

2. Op.Cit. Chapter One, Endnote #2;AHCRP publication 95-0643.

3. Helms CA, Pearson DO, Neck and Spine, *Patient Care*, (1996) Sept. 30: 55-74

4. Sward L, Hellstrom M, Jacobsson B, et al, Gothenburg University, Gothenburg, Sweden, and King Faisal Specialist Hospital and Research Center, Riyadh, Saudi Arabia. *Back pain and radiologic changes in the thoraco-lumbar spine of athletes*, Spine. Feb 1990;15:124-129.

5. Deyo R, Diehl AK, quoted in Lower Back Pain: When do you order X-Rays?, *Emergency Medicine*; October 30, 1989:63-66.

6. Bowden SD, Davis DO, Dina TS, et al. Abnormal magnetic resonance scans of lumbar spine in asymptomatic subjects. *J Bone Joint Surg*. 1990; 72:403.

CHAPTER FOUR: PRINCIPLES

The preceding sections should have created a fundamental, basic, foundation of knowledge about the spine, discs, and the origination of discogenic pain. The following sections, preceding the actual instructions on how to accomplish the MANEUVERS unique to *The O'Connor Technique (tm)*, describe principles, concepts, and elements common to nearly all of the subsequent understandings essential to the prevention and management of back pain. **These principles are important to comprehend because they are pertinent to the understanding of the MANEUVERS one can (and most probably will) learn to use to relieve discogenic pain.** Treating them repeatedly during a description of every MANEUVER would be redundant; and, if their descriptions were only incorporated into the instructions for a particular MANEUVER, it might give the impression that they pertained largely or singularly to that particular MANEUVER. They are treated here as a prelude to the directions on how to accomplish the MANEUVERS so that the reader can become familiar enough with them, in advance, so as to be more able to focus, later, on the specific MANEUVERS rather than having to deal with the distraction of learning the associated devices and theory common to nearly all MANEUVERS.

Whenever appropriate, I have endeavored repeatedly to refresh the reader's memory as to these concepts during the descriptions of the MANEUVERS. The reader should plan on referring to the following sections wherever and whenever it becomes necessary to fully comprehend the reasons and justification for any particular given movement instruction.

Since certain concepts rely upon a foundation of prior understanding, it was necessary to assemble the principles in a conceptual sequence to facilitate the learning process. Therefore, the order chosen to assemble the principles should not be interpreted as to reflect their relative importance. **The two major concepts, AVOIDING WEIGHT-BEARING FLEXION and MAINTAINING EXTENSION are, by far and away, the most important general concepts applicable to the prevention and management of the overwhelming majority of discogenic back pain.** So, they should predominate in the reader's armamentarium regardless of their distanced and non-sequential placement in the text.

AVOIDING WEIGHT-BEARING FLEXION

The avoidance of WEIGHT-BEARING FLEXION is probably one of the two most important concepts comprising application of the total *The O'Connor Technique (tm)*. Once this understanding is cognitively internalized, it will inevitably alter the way in which a back pain sufferer moves for the remainder of his or her life. This concept centers upon the advantages of **judiciously avoiding WEIGHT-BEARING FLEXION of the spine at all times and at all spinal levels to prevent disc damage and pain.**

Current studies suggest that activities such as lifting, pulling, or pushing objects and awkward working postures such as bending forward or twisting account for 28% to 50% of Low back problems in the adult population; and the most dangerous jobs with respect to back pain are those 10% of jobs that involve activities requiring rapid lifting of heavy objects combined with bending or twisting.[1],[2] The common element that unifies these sources of back pain is **the act of WEIGHT-BEARING FLEXION which, if avoided, can reasonably be expected to prevent the attendant disc damage**. This is especially relevant at the site of previously damaged discs because WEIGHT-BEARING FLEXION at those discs has a higher probability of causing additional damage that will result in pain when compared to an intact disc.

First, the principle of avoiding WEIGHT-BEARING FLEXION needs to be viewed as being comprised of two negative components: WEIGHT-BEARING <u>and</u> FLEXION. In any event where WEIGHT-BEARING FLEXION occurs or can occur, it can be mitigated or reduced in its propensity to induce damage and pain whenever either component can be favorably modified. That is, if you must flex, then don't bear weight. If you have to bear weight, then make every effort to not flex while so doing. These simple caveats, if adhered to judiciously in all aspects of your activities of daily living, will prevent untold numbers of pain events and avoid immeasurable damage to the discs.

If you don't believe this, simply wait until the next time you go from the pain-free situation to the point when you notice that your back pain is present (or if your back pain is always present, what you seem to be doing when it increases). **You will undoubtedly find that the onset of back pain is almost uniformly preceded by a WEIGHT-BEARING FLEXION posture.** After you have paid attention to this detail enough times to convince yourself of its reality, you must then **program yourself to avoid this situation by choosing alternative postures and positions that do not require WEIGHT-BEARING FLEXION**.

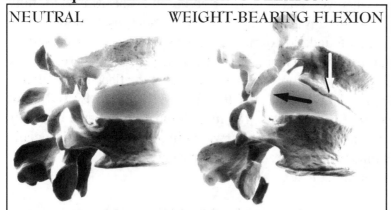

Figure 1 Disc unit in WEIGHT-BEARING FLEXION showing pressure directed posteriorly

Far from being a theoretical pontification, this understanding comes from an obvious yet articulate comprehension of anatomy, physiology, and physics. **When a spinal unit accomplishes flexion with a weight on the vertebral bodies, the pressure generated tends to force the contents of the disc posteriorly (See Figure 1).** Most back pain and disc disease originates when the disc material's neutral anatomy is disturbed by such flexion forces. The earlier sections on COMPRESSION FORCES and the CORRELATION OF MECHANICAL ANATOMY WITH DISC PAIN cursorily discussed this; so, it is unnecessary to repeat the bulk of it here. However, in the earlier chapter, it focused predominately on flexion forces as the origin of acute pain and damage to the disc. WEIGHT-BEARING FLEXION must also be accepted as a source for chronic pain, the re-exacerbation of quiescent pain, and the magnification of existing pain as well as damage.

Flexion, of course, is the process of anteriorly bending the spine. The use of the term throughout the book usually refers to forward bending whether there is a lateral component to it or not. Bending strictly to one side or the other would be properly termed "lateral flexion." Certainly, the definition of flexion also includes bending to one side or the other, but by flexion in this context, I am specifically referring to the act of anterior flexion. Anterior flexion is a bending at the spine that usually assumes that the part of the body above the reference disc (joint) is moved in an anterior direction. This includes the understanding that, if one is in extension, flexion has to be used to return to the neutral position.

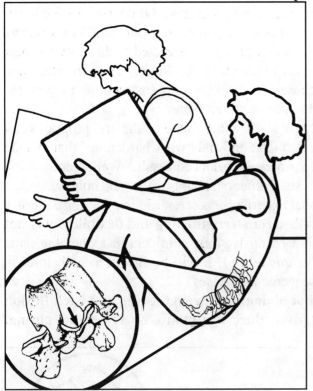

Figure 2 Fall in flexion can result in a disc herniation

The distinction I further make, that WEIGHT-BEARING FLEXION must be avoided, applies to any load-bearing on a disc unit. The weight about which I speak is not limited to the carrying of excess weight, it also pertains to the actual weight of the body above the disc unit in question. This consideration is inclusive of conscious as well as unconscious, unintended, acts. Falling upon your buttocks while the back is flexed is a form (albeit violent) of WEIGHT-BEARING FLEXION, as is the simple act of bending over to pick up a pencil off of the ground. It may appear exceedingly difficult to avoid these sorts of activities; but once you are convinced that such actions can result in disc damage or pain, it actually becomes quite simple to prevent.

This concept is one of the simplest yet all-inclusive innovations of *The O'Connor Technique (tm),* **advancing beyond the previously advocated "wisdom," since most, if not all, current and past back pain management programs employ exercise with almost equal advocacy of flexion as extension, with no recognition of the damage that WEIGHT-BEARING FLEXION can inflict.**

To my admittedly inexact calculation, this obligates the back pain patient engaged in those programs to at least a 50% disadvantage at any given time. By that, I mean, any deviation from the neutral position has to involve either flexion or extension. Since no pre-existing program applies traction or even a non-weight bearing consideration, the back pain sufferer has previously had only two choices when exercising the back--flexion or extension. So, in a fifty/fifty proposition, when they elect flexion, they are selecting the one worst choice out of two alternative possibilities. Therefore, the bulk of the limited success that previous back pain programs achieved can be explained largely due to a vagary of chance--equivalent to the flipping of a coin.

Consider that in nearly every exercise decision, a person has an equal probability of performing a movement that will hurt as one that will help. Any patients helped by previously advocated programs probably only got better because there is an inherent probability bias contained in the element of pain that prevents WEIGHT-BEARING FLEXION such that they would preferentially engage predominately in extension rather than flexion regardless of their exercise prescriptions. Any betterment in their back conditions must be attributed to something besides rational directives since any gains made by the neutral position or EXTENSION are counteracted by an equivalent or greater harm when WEIGHT-BEARING FLEXION is advocated or allowed. It has to be luck for anyone to get better when forced to subsist with the existing lack of insight in the currently advocated back pain management programs. Of course, for the lucky ones, common sense combined with the natural propensity for people to avoid painful movements keeps them from flexing in weight-bearing even though they are instructed to do so by the best intended clinicians and physical therapists. From my perspective, the "lucky" ones, in better than half of their choices, had to have routinely chosen to disobey their instructions to perform WEIGHT-BEARING FLEXION or they would not have gotten better.

Now, some may consider this heresy because all the other "state-of-the-art" programs and exercise books have major components of "back stabilization" and "work hardening" that include heavy doses of flexion exercises in an attempt to produce a balanced result. Well, I don't think their success rates give them bragging rights; so, I understandably differ in opinion. This difference of opinion is based as much on personal experience as scientific inquiry since **studies show that traditional exercise programs prescribed for strengthening and flexibility may not be helpful in restoring low back function**.[3],[4],[5] Contrarily, I am confident that when the same inquiry criteria are applied to *The O'Connor Technique (tm)*, it will be shown to be helpful in restoring low back function in a majority of discogenic pain cases.

Moreover, **clinical trials have shown that abdominal strengthening and back flexion exercises do not actually help patients get over their symptoms or return to normal activities**.[6] Further, such exercises are poorly tolerated, having a patient attrition rate that averages 50%.[7],[8] As explained above, I suspect that the patients more than likely stop doing these exercises because they very soon learn that flexion exercises while weight-bearing do not succeed in reducing pain. It doesn't take a psychology degree to recognize that when no reward or pain is

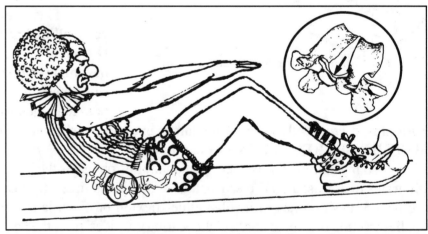

Figure 3 Sit-up exemplifying the posteriorly directed pressure on the disc material during WEIGHT-BEARING FLEXION.

forthcoming after a particular behavior, the study subjects fail to perform that behavior.

Others may interpret these findings in such a manner to conclude differently; however, I guess that is what makes this a free country and me thankful for freedom of the press. I can demonstrate that the weighted flexion that they employ such as in a sit-up is not only "not helpful" but actually harmful (Figures 3 & 4).

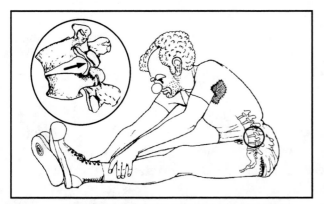

Figure 4 WEIGHT-BEARING FLEXION
putting especially painful posteriorly directed
forces on the disc

One of the main reasons I stress this principle as unique when compared to other methods is because many current "therapeutic" regimens demand repetitious and forceful sit-up type exercises. It is impossible to do any type of sit-up without committing some area of the spine to WEIGHT-BEARING FLEXION. Even the partial sit-up ignores the reality that the Thoracic and Cervical portions of the spine are capable of undergoing disc degeneration and protrusions. In my experience, the incidence of persons with Lumbar disc disease and concurrent disc disease in other regions of the spine is too great to attribute to coincidence. Rather, I have concluded that persons with the same intrinsic weaknesses at one part of the spine leading to disease are more apt to have a similar disc problem at other levels. I am not certain, but it seems to me to be a combination of genetics and trauma. Those with congenitally more flexible joints appear to have a higher incidence of back pain problems and certainly those with histories of flexion injuries usually have damage to the spine at more than one level. It is because the force engendered in a flexion injury usually occurs when more than one area of the spine is simultaneously in a relatively high degree of flexion, and the damage, likewise, occurs at these areas in the greatest amount of anterior flexion. For those with disc disease at one level, WEIGHT-BEARING FLEXION recommendations can easily be seen to cause the currently painful disc unit, as well as other segments, to become symptomatic. This other level otherwise would not have become painful had the patient not been convinced to purposefully engage in repetitive WEIGHT-BEARING FLEXION exercises.

For those who hold the opinion that WEIGHT-BEARING FLEXION is harmless for the Thoracic spine due to its rigidity, I would argue that the Thoracic spine is no stranger to this phenomenon despite its relative inflexibility. Up to 1.5 % of disc herniations occur at the Thoracic level[9]. I have found that the lack of flexibility has less to do with the incidence of Thoracic back pain and more to do with the difficulty in treating it. Such is the two-edged sword of life. In actual practice, despite the comparatively low incidence of actual operative herniations, I have found disc disease of the Thoracic vertebrae common enough to not allow any type of sit-up exercise in my list of recommendations. In fact, one of the worst places a person can apply WEIGHT-BEARING FLEXION is to the Low Cervical and High Thoracic region because it is so easy to damage and difficult to treat. Therefore, *The O'Connor Technique (tm)* insists upon intentionally avoiding sit-ups at all levels, symptomatic or not.

A back pain patient could accomplish very limited and controlled sit-ups so long as they have never had Thoracic pain by insuring that the neck was protected by the hands and Lumbar spine was protected with the support offered by a towel or pillow that maintains the Lumbar spine in EXTENSION so that all levels are is kept in EXTENSION. However, the same abdominal

125

muscle-toning effect can be achieved with leg-lifts that don't endanger the remainder of the spine.

In this book, I have taken the liberty of extracting from recent medical periodicals the actual drawings of back pain exercise recommendations (designed to educate physicians) and modified them with the most appropriate clown outfits I could fashion to simultaneously pay both homage to their imprudence and avoid any allegations of copyright infringement. I also had to find a way to demonstrate these bad examples yet make it clear to the careless readers that I was definitely not advocating them. Therefore, "Bozos" have been drafted to demonstrate these non-productive and self-defeating exercises.

The sit-up is particularly dangerous because the entire weight of the body above the level of the Lumbar spine is being applied to a Lumbar vertebrae while in maximum flexion. This generates a force on the Lumbar vertebrae nearly twice the weight of the body and predisposes the disc material to posterior migration.

Some attempts to hold onto the belief that sit-ups are still necessary to increase or maintain abdominal tone, even if they are shown to hurt the patient, have been instigated to substitute a partial sit-up for a full sit-up (Figure 5). **This may allow a few more clowns to perform it, but it neglects the reality that most people with low back problems have the same underlying weaknesses or prior injuries that predispose other segments of their spine to the same disc disease as the Lumbar region.** People doing exercises that do not insure protection of the

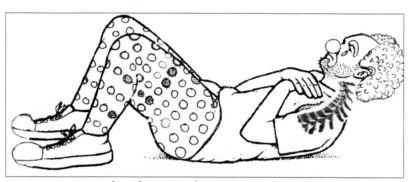

Thoracic and Cervical vertebrae, yet force these discs into sustained and repeated WEIGHT-BEARING FLEXION, can rely on these segments to become painful with time. One must remember that regardless of which segment goes into flexion, the movement of disc material to the posterior periphery is increased by a function of the weight above the segment in question. By

Figure 5 Cervical and upper Thoracic vertebrae exposed to posteriorly directed disc material de-centralizing forces

some calculus-described mathematical/mechanical physics, the degree to which that weight translates to a measure of pressure on the hydraulic system of the disc could probably be calculated; however, the proof is in the pudding. Even doing a halfway sit-up puts enough pressure on the neck and thorax to generate pain in a susceptible disc. I know this from personal experience as well as countless patient examinations in which pain is induced by the sit-up or its equivalent. **It is so reliable as an indicator of disc disease, that pain during directed sit-ups can be used as a test to substantiate a disc herniation diagnosis.**

If a back pain patient absolutely feels that they have to get abdominal muscular tone increased, the same effect produced by sit-ups can be safely accomplished by a structural and procedural modification to the exercise that AVOIDS WEIGHT-BEARING FLEXION. First, don't risk doing sit-ups at all if you have a chronic history of neck or thorax pain or a history of "whip-lash" injury. Second, support the low back with some Lumbar support and then do leg-lifts to tone the abdomen rather than lifting the upper torso. If the neck is ever caused to flex, in order to participate, make sure the Cervical spine is kept in slight EXTENSION by using the palms of the hands in a prisoner of war surrender-like position; and only go so far as this will allow you to flex without discomfort. That is, if any spinal elements are caused to go into painful flexion by sit-ups (either at the outset or later in close proximity to the time you started them), they should be deleted from any exercise repertoire.

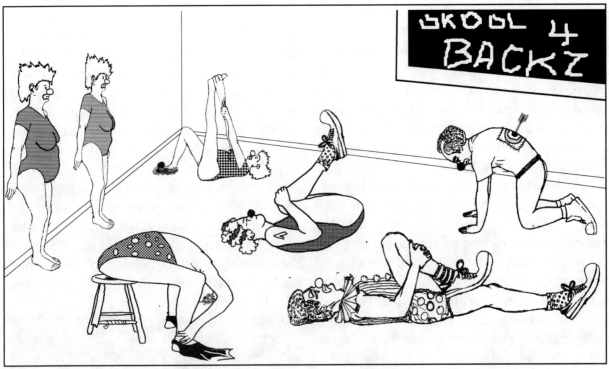

Figure 6 Traditional back school exercises engaging WEIGHT-BEARING FLEXION

In Figure 6, I have irreverently created a "Back School for Bozos." Each of these exercise depictions were reproduced from actual back pain exercise directions printed in medical literature and relied upon by the traditional "back schools" as a source of inspiration for those who are trying to help patients with their painful backs. Now, don't instantly jump to the conclusion that I am inconsistent when you are directed to use related postures advocated later in this book in the MANEUVER sections. A principle difference is that these clowns are doing non-sequential, random, exercises (routine muscular excursions) which are supposed to make them better but take no consideration in the mechanical consequences of the forces employed in the presence of disc herniations. There is a major contrast between committing a controlled, specific, action for the purpose of intentionally and beneficially moving disc material and unintentionally moving disc material into a painful configuration through an ill-advised exercise program. I have, on too many occasions, interviewed patients who have been through these physical therapy torture chambers, to not know of what I speak.

Each exercise I have bozo-depicted involves a contra-indicated WEIGHT-BEARING

127

FLEXION movement that can be seen, in some fashion, to induce the disc material to migrate to the posterior periphery. Even if that flexion is slight, such as when "flattening" the Lumbar curve against the wall while the patient is standing (the so-called "pelvic tilt"as portrayed by the patients against the wall to the left, still, WEIGHT-BEARING FLEXION is being encouraged. This puts a measurable pressure (at least half the weight of the body, mostly directed posteriorly) on the discs while in relative flexion, since **straightening the neutral Lumbar curve constitutes flexion**. Performing the same MANEUVER while reclining and flattening the Lumbar spine by pulling on a cloth wrapped around the foot results in similarly significant pressures and aggravating pain, as practiced by the lady in the corner.

Most of the "Back School for Bozos" is directly related to the Lumbar spine; however, the Cervical region is no stranger to bad advice. The diagrams seen in Figure 7 are excerpted from a patient education handout which directs neck pain sufferers in exercises which supposedly are designed to alleviate pain. Not that I am a cynic, however, it was published by a pharmaceutical company who stands to gain if people are kept in pain. I have selected several of their instructions which, from my point of view and experience, are typical and can only lead to increased pain for the majority of patients with herniated discs as their underlying malady, which, to my assessment, also constitutes a majority.

The directions associated with Figure 7, #2 recommend that the neck pain patient "push chin downwards, trying to touch it to your chest...Repeat 5 times," then goes on to advocate the same effort directed towards the sides of the neck. Figure 7,#4 convinces that the addition of a twisting motion adds some advantage, but you only need to repeat this three times. Later, in Figure 7,#7, the reader is directed to swing a 1-2 pound weight in a circular direction for one minute in each direction. Figure 7, #9 advocates flexing the neck with restraining force applied by the hand; then, later, tells one to do the same thing to the side.

I could wax poetic about the innumerable other instructions that are contraindicated, pointless, or have no basis in mechanical or scientific reasoning; however, the one consistently problematic component that evokes my criticism for current neck programs equivalently as for low back pain is the repeated and erroneous advocacy of WEIGHT-BEARING FLEXION. In addition to "not helping" (which, in surgeon's vernacular, is the equivalent of saying "we have only induced pain without apparent gain"), it must be repeatedly stressed that any FLEXION exercises cause needless pain, advance damage, and defeat the body's meager natural healing mechanism whereby scars contract to join tissue edges. **Every time a scar fiber forms or a ligament tightens, it is again stretched to the full**

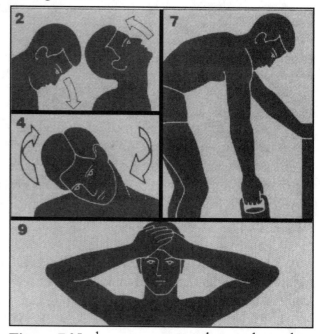

Figure 7 Neck pain exercises advocated in other spine pain literature

128

length position from the pressures exerted by the herniated or prolapsed disc material putting pressure on it during **WEIGHT-BEARING FLEXION.** In the case of the posterior peripheral ligamentous structures, this only serves to weaken the fibrous wall that retains the disc fragments within the capsule. Repetitiously and forcefully stretching previously torn ligaments only causes the scar to thin. Other paraspinous ligaments and tendons that would otherwise undergo a contraction during the healing process, are prevented from so doing by repeated, misguided, INTENTIONAL WEIGHT-BEARING FLEXION events.

Later in the book, a flexion action is advocated; but the principle difference is that **it is not WEIGHT-BEARING**; and, therefore, there is little or no posterior-directed pressures placed upon the disc unit. In fact, traction is applied during flexion. This leaves ample space in the central region of the disc for disc material to migrate into, rather than giving it only the posterior route to follow towards the periphery. **If any benefit at all comes of traditional flexion exercises, it is by an inadvertent mechanism equivalent to the ligament recruitment MANEUVERS experienced in FLEXION IN TRACTION (to be described later) and certainly should never be attempted while the spine is weight-bearing.**

The foregoing should not be interpreted as a condemnation of **all** the exercises routinely or traditionally prescribed for back pain. They are not all useless or harmful. On the contrary, some traditional exercises give some measure of relief to persons with minor disc herniations by advocating the same use of EXTENSIONS as *The O'Connor Technique (tm)*. Unfortunately, they are usually recommended in the semi-weight bearing condition and without any preparatory measures taken in advance, which limits their helpfulness to those patients who do not have severe herniations. In any case, their level of success is, again, largely due to the vagaries of probability and chance; and not due to reasoned intellect and applied bio-mechanical theory.

I presume promoting a belief that exercise might be detrimental in an era where exercise is currently in vogue and promoted as the cure-all for everything from heart disease to hypertension runs the risk of criticism. However, the body has a mechanism wherein it takes up the slack of any joint/muscle system by tightening the muscles with fibrous tissue formation to accommodate to the limited range of motion. If the posterior musculature is not stretched by forward flexion, these soft tissues have a better probability of contracting down to a position that maintains extension and limits flexion. Just as a bow-string keeps the bow bent, the degree to which the posterior musculature of the back develops a contracture-like configuration or even a relative HYPERTROPHY (strengthening to increase the size of a muscle) is the degree to which the back is kept preferentially in mild, sustained, EXTENSION .

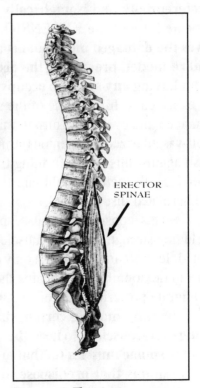

ERECTOR SPINAE

Figure 8 Figurative illustration depicting hypertrophy of erector spinae keeping Lumbar spine in EXTENSION

129

I can foresee no harm in practicing *The O'Connor Technique's (tm)* flexion avoidance to help effect the body's compensatory mechanism to limit flexion movements of the spine. For all intents and purposes, it is probably unreasonable to expect anyone to completely avoid flexion to the extent that the opposing ligaments, tendons, and muscle groups (the extensors) would become weakened or contracture to a detrimentally excessive degree. It should be easy to understand by looking at Figure 8 that if the erector spinae muscle were made stronger and tighter by not allowing the spine to flex, the curvature of the Lumbar spine would be more likely to remain concave to the posterior. Conversely, if the erector spinae were easily stretched to full length, the Lumbar spine can be expected to spend more time in counter-productive flexion.

The degree to which the Lumbar spine (by avoiding the stretching effect of flexion and the deleterious effect of strengthening the abdominal flexors on the erector spinae system) is made less likely to go into flexion defines the extent to which the posterior intervertebral spaces are kept closed. Keeping the posterior intervertebral spaces closed reduces the probability of the disc material escaping posteriorly during the resting state. This principle applies to the Cervical and Thoracic region as well and is further elaborated later under the heading of PREFERENTIAL STRENGTHENING/SELECTIVE HYPERTROPHY OF EXTENSOR MUSCULATURE.

The policy of avoiding flexion assists the effort of constantly maintaining an EXTENSION posture to protect the spine from posterior disc material migration. Preferentially and isometrically contracting the erector spinae musculature, as is done in repeated use of the EXTENSION MANEUVERS or a properly designed exercise regimen, gives the damaged interspinous and disc-associated ligaments the opportunity to scar down and re-model, preventing the disc material that would have otherwise migrated posteriority from having any space to occupy. Also, healing types of tissue known as granulation tissue can be expected to fill in some of the space created by the torn annulus fibrosus when the capsule is damaged and eventually turn to thickened scar, especially when injury tears the most peripheral, well-vascularized ligamentous structures. If the displaced disc fragments are allowed to constantly push against this newly forming tissue, as would be caused by WEIGHT-BEARING FLEXION exercises, the action would interfere with its confined growth and closure of the tears caused by the herniated disc material.

This consideration also speaks contrary to the belief that random exercise (especially including strengthening the muscles of abdominal flexion) is beneficial, since strengthening of the spinal flexors can accomplish only one foreseeable end--the increased likelihood of spending more time in flexion, thereby opening the posterior intervertebral spaces which allows the disc material to migrate posteriorly if done while the hydraulic pressure of weight-bearing is present.

So, by making certain that the spine is rarely flexed at the site of damage or pain, being ever-conscious to keep the spine in EXTENSION , and preferentially strengthening the erector spinae muscles (in that order), one can reasonably be sure that the mechanical forces and positions that predispose to posterior migration of disc material are not acting. This knowledge should give the back pain sufferer good reason to avoid positions in which the spine is continually, if inadvertently, flexed. Even **sitting in a chair in a slouched position puts a stretching force on the posterior connective tissue structures that gives the displacing disc material a space to occupy that it otherwise would not have.** Stretching the posterior muscles, ligaments, and tendons defeats the physiological mechanism designed to reduce this laxity.

Keeping the ligaments tight through an AVOIDANCE OF WEIGHT-BEARING FLEXION functions to deny the disc material a place into which it can protrude or displace.

In order to put into practice the principle of AVOIDING WEIGHT-BEARING FLEXION, by way of example, consider the "sit-up" most people execute while getting up from any supine position such as rising from bed. If sit-ups are pain inducing, this movement should be contra-indicated since it is mechanically equivalent to an exercise despite its usually only being done once a day in the morning. However, it is particularly more pain inducing for a person with a disc herniation problem because the prior sleep-induced muscular relaxation leaves the spine without its defensive waking muscle tone. This absence of tone puts the discs at a higher probability of displacing disc material posteriorly during the WEIGHT-BEARING FLEXION event most people commit as their first act of the day.

If you want to prevent WEIGHT-BEARING FLEXION at the onset of every day, you must consciously program yourself to dismount from a bed in a different manner. Later in the book, MANEUVERS are described to accomplish this in a therapeutic manner. However, one easy way to leave a bed and keep the low back in EXTENSION is to lock it in slight EXTENSION; then flex the outside knee while raising the thigh to just about the 90 degree angle formed by it and the surface of the bed (See Figure 9A). Bending the knee and using the hip to do the flexing allows you to lock and keep your Lumbar, Thoracic, and Cervical spine in slight EXTENSION while accomplishing this. If the knee is straight, you cannot bend at the hip and then the Lumbar spine is forced to experience a stretching and WEIGHT-BEARING FLEXION tension, and that tension allows or commits the Lumbar spine to flattening (or relative flexion) compared to an ideal slight EXTENSION .

In order to rapidly get your body to the erect position without using a flexed spine, the flexed thigh (preferably on the painful side and pre-arranged to be the side closest to the edge of the bed) is raised enough for the same side hand to grab the middle of the thigh underneath its posterior aspect. While the wrist is locked to hold the thigh, the leg is thrust downward off the side of the bed towards the floor. When the weight of the leg is being felt by the hand, the same arm that is holding the thigh rigidly flexes at the elbow like a weight-lifter's "curl." The combined action of the arm's muscles, the gravity assisted counter weight of the leg falling, and a tightening of the abdominal muscles without flexing the spine, brings the torso above the pelvis to the upright position (Figure 9B).

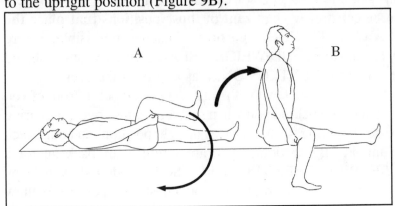

Figure 9 Bed dismount to avoid flexion

Quickly extending at the knee as the leg starts to fall adds thrust to the leg's fall assisting to give that added counter-weight to the teeter-totter effect that raises the torso. This gets the torso up without flexion at the spine. Your free arm can be pushed into the bed to assist your complete movement to the upright while the entire spine stays in EXTENSION .

Alternatively, if you don't mind rolling over on to your stomach and sliding to your knees each time you get out of bed or you feel that your back is painful enough to warrant daily using the MORNING EXTENSIONS described later in the MANEUVER chapters, you can always get up with those methods. Sometimes they are inconvenient and sometimes seems to take more energy and time than is necessary. However, during acute episodes of severe back pain, the methods described later in the book may be the best ways to get out of bed or any raised, flat, surface to AVOID WEIGHT-BEARING FLEXION.

Getting out of any supine posture in the usual and customary sit-up manner, unless assisted, requires an intermediary position wherein a WEIGHT-BEARING FLEXION ensues. Unless you can figure another way to raise the upper body to the erect position without suffering a flexion posture, I would suggest that you practice this technique for starters. Then, you won't join the ranks of the countless patients who have complained to me that they can be pain-free until they start to get out of bed--then the pain hits them. Some people, during back pain episodes, manage this pain-inducing activity by getting out of bed, letting their prone feet, legs and abdomen fall over the edge, in that order, while remaining in the face-down configuration. Then, they use their arms to bring them to the fully upright position. Very complicated, but I have used this myself on occasion. As I began to understand the mechanics, I arrived at the "MORNING EXTENSIONS/CASCADE MANEUVER" described in the MANEUVERS chapter of the book, then eventually graduated to the thigh grab technique described above; however, now, I rarely require any specific method except carefully extending my Lumbar spine and keeping it that way until I get to my feet.

If I am on the ground in a supine position and need to get up, I do so by rolling to a face down position, let my Lumbar spine assume a mild EXTENSION by raising myself up with my arms like the cobra yoga position shown in Chapter One, then, while keeping my back in that default EXTENSION posture, get on all fours before raising myself to standing. Regardless of the situation, I still hold the caveat to AVOID WEIGHT-BEARING FLEXION; and I can get up from just about any position without putting my back "out."

Although not so obvious, sitting upright on the floor with the legs in front is an exceptionally bad position due to the WEIGHT-BEARING FLEXION engendered. Leaning forward in a chair while sitting with the feet propped up is also dangerous for a bad back. It is impossible to describe every flexion event in which a person can engage; however, it is sufficient to caution the back pain sufferer to **be constantly cognizant of those positions that place the painful disc into a WEIGHT-BEARING FLEXION posture**. Whenever possible, before committing one's self to a FLEXION action (especially WEIGHT-BEARING) the position should be intentionally altered by changing to a spinal EXTENSION so as to protect the back.

For instance, let's say you are sitting on the lawn with your feet spread out in front of you resting back on your arms which form a tripod behind you when someone comes over, preparing to hand you a baby. Your first impulse is to bring the torso to the upright position, and outstretch the arms, preparing to accept the infant. By so doing, you are setting your back up for a tremendously stressful WEIGHT-BEARING FLEXION event. So, armed with your new knowledge of back protection, you ask the person to wait, and you adjust your posture to allow for the carriage of this weight by bringing your legs under you, you put your back in EXTENSION, and make them bring the baby to your torso rather than reaching out for it by keeping your arms close to your body.

With the advent of their children, innumerable women suffer from avoidable back pain unknowingly due to mechanically disadvantageous lifting and carrying techniques. It takes little or no extra effort to be alert to the necessity of AVOIDING WEIGHT-BEARING FLEXION. Instead of leaning over the crib and pulling the baby out like a crane, one simply need only put the rail down and roll the baby out. While keeping the Lumbar spine in EXTENSION, the baby would then be brought close to the center of gravity of the body and carried away without flexion. Although these two examples use babies as the object, any weighted object pertains.

AVOIDING FLEXION is closely allied to the MAINTENANCE OF EXTENSION, because they ultimately achieve one and the same goal and can appear (without further elaboration) to be nearly the same process because if you tell someone to keep their back bent backwards they, by simple logic, shouldn't be bending it forward. It is, by definition, impossible to flex a disc unit while maintaining it in EXTENSION; so, almost, it is as if you cannot do one if you are doing the other. If someone follows an instruction to MAINTAIN EXTENSION, they can't very well spend much time in flexion. Even though outwardly they seem to be the same effort, the difference is more than semantic.

It stands to reason, one shouldn't be flexing if they are supposed to be extending; however, there is a distinction to be drawn because **one can be in the neutral position while still AVOIDING FLEXION.** One doesn't have to be extending to avoid flexion. For instance, consider the seated position in a chair. By adopting a slouching posture, one places the Lumbar spine in WEIGHT-BEARING FLEXION. That is bad. Bringing one's self to the neutral position would result in just that--an anatomically neutral configuration. This position might theoretically seem comfortable enough and is the position which is advocated in nearly all the recommendations made by other back pain literature when they command to "keep the back straight, directly over the hips"; however, to do so requires energy to sustain that posture. Inevitably, the musculature tires and defaults into a WEIGHT-BEARING FLEXION slouch again. It is far superior to keep the spine supported in EXTENSION while seated, which constitutes a measure beyond simply AVOIDING WEIGHT-BEARING FLEXION. **If there is anything close to a caveat in this book: When sitting, reclining, or sleeping in the supine position, a pillow or some other back support cushion should <u>always</u> be employed to MAINTAIN EXTENSION.**

Many programs give their patients instructions on how to lift properly or hand them a brochure which is equally insufficient. **It is not enough to just say: "lift with your back straight". A straight back is insufficient for someone with disc disease who wants to prevent future back pain. What they more properly should be instructing is not only to AVOID WEIGHT-BEARING FLEXION but to take the additional initiative when required to lift so as to arrange one's stance so that the herniated disc unit is kept in a comfortable degree of EXTENSION.** This intentional alteration of posture to remain in EXTENSION most of the time is better treated separately under the MAINTENANCE OF EXTENSION heading. That will come later, here the discussion still surrounds its second cousin--AVOIDING WEIGHT-BEARING FLEXION.

It is equally important to appreciate what constitutes the "<u>weight-bearing</u>" of WEIGHT-BEARING FLEXION. It largely consists of the force of gravity acting on a disc unit in flexion at any point along the vertebral column; however, it can be expanded to include any axial force which acts to compress a disc. This is pertinent to both the herniated disc as well as any other disc; however, those discs with herniations will punish the violation more severely with pain. By bearing weight, I include the weight of the body above the level of the flexed spinal segment, any additional weight bearing on the spine, and any other weight that serves to deform the spine into flexion such as the abdomen's weight on the Lumbar region. Recall from Chapter Two, Figure 15, that even the reclining posture is attended by a measurable pressure on the disc contents due to the weight of the body (principally the abdomen). For a person who weighs 200 pounds, 25% of the standing force is not to be considered negligible.

Under the heading of WEIGHT-BEARING FLEXION is included the consideration of the weight of the body (especially of the abdomen) that is placed on the Lumbar disc units when in the reclining position. The simple flattening of Lumbar spine when exercising with hip thrusts is essentially a WEIGHT-BEARING FLEXION only the weight is supplied by the abdomen which causes the Lumbar curvature to flatten. If you think about it, **going from the relative extension that exists in the normal, neutral, lordotic, spinal curvatures of the Cervical and Lumbar regions to a flattened or straight configuration is, in essence, a flexion.**

Those exercise regimens that place a person against a flat surface and instruct them to flatten the Lumbar or Cervical curvatures in a hip thrust or neck straightening exercise are really causing the patient to undertake a WEIGHT-BEARING FLEXION usually at the site of a disc herniation (See ladies against the wall in Back School for Bozos above Figure 6). **It is impossible to go from an anatomically extended curve to a straight spine without engaging in flexion.** Even in this seemingly innocuous context, the flexion is counter-productive and serves to open the posterior aspect of the disc space between vertebral bones, allowing for migration of disc material posteriorly. Such a consideration may seem minor because the actual degree of flexion is so inconspicuous; however, when this movement is incorporated into daily, repetitive exercises, positions, or movements that are consciously undertaken to try to help the painful spine yet are only accomplishing additional pain from decentralization, they must be looked upon as contraindicated and avoided.

The amount of weight applied by the abdomen to the Lumbar region in the recline may seem paltry when one views the slim, perfectly proportioned models used for making the exercise brochures. It might make good copy, but it doesn't adequately represent the multitudes of obese abdomens that exist in the world of painful backs. An obese abdomen's weight can contribute substantially to the pressure exerted upon a given disc. Too, people with back pain are often given to lying on the floor flat on their backs to play with children, work on automobiles, and exercise. All of these types of activities can put a posteriorly directed weight on the Lumbar spine deforming it by flexion to the flattened, straight, configuration, because straightening the normal concave curvature of the Lumbar or Cervical spine nevertheless constitutes flexion.

BODY WEIGHT CONTRIBUTION TO BACK PAIN

It is essential to understand that AVOIDING WEIGHT-BEARING FLEXION includes not only the weights of objects that a person lifts but is combined with the actual weight of the body acting on the area of pain, as well as the length of time a person remains in flexion while bearing the weight. All of these variables function in the generation of disc damage and pain.

It is almost laughable to read the written disability criteria which attempt to quantify how much a person can lift safely on the job if they are preparing to return to work after a back injury. Speciously "scientific" numbers are generated within a framework of misunderstanding that fails to consider that how much one lifts is equally as important as how long one sustains the lifting. Compounding this assessment is how much the person weighs, the extent of their disc herniation, and the manner in which they lift.

The longer a deleterious WEIGHT-BEARING FLEXION position is held, the more time the disc has to migrate posteriorly to the point where the pain begins. A person such as an obese woman with two twenty pound weights (breasts) held at a foot from her spine bending over a low sink for a twenty seconds emptying a large pot filled with water puts much more combined pressure on a given disc unit than doing the same activity for only a few seconds. So, in this scenario, simply attempting to sustain the apparently minor weight of the pot waiting for it to empty in addition to the weight of her own body in flexion creates forces capable of putting her back "out." The action may have been otherwise sustainable for a couple of seconds, or if she were to alter her position to accomplish the same task, a longer period.

Anyone with back pain can relate to the time-dependence of this phenomenon because, without exception, leaning forward on a herniated disc for a long period makes it harder to straighten up again compared to flexion being engaged for only an instant. **The time it takes for the mobile disc material to move from a painless central location to a painful posterior location accounts for this observation. This leads to a simple conclusion: The more time one spends in WEIGHT-BEARING FLEXION, the more pain one can expect.**

The same time-dependent movement of disc material in the opposite direction explains why one can't straighten up too fast after forward-lifting (anterior WEIGHT-BEARING FLEXION) because the disc material takes time to re-centralize and pain is induced while extending to the upright posture until it does.

However, it may not be so readily obvious to most people how important it is to **judiciously avoid the generation of WEIGHT-BEARING FLEXION forces by actively avoiding the carriage of weight while in flexion in one's day-to-day, minute-to-minute activities.** In the scenario described above, the woman could have simply altered the forces acting on her spine by supporting the pan on the edge of the sink while it poured (instead of holding it up), backing away from the sink with her legs, and putting her Lumbar and Thoracic spine in EXTENSION by supporting her weight on her elbows. Outside of the obvious necessity to lose weight, it's little points like this that can turn a "good" day into a painfully "bad" one.

Even though it is impossible to totally eliminate the weight of the body above the painful segments; it is possible to eliminate some of it. For that reason, **weight loss is an essential component of making a bad back feel better**. If you don't believe this, pick up a twenty pound sack of potatoes in the grocery store and walk around with it while shopping. Every time you bend over to pick up something on a bottom shelf, keep holding it. You will soon discover how the extra 20, 40, 60, or 80 pounds above your ideal body weight becomes an important, yet sometimes inconspicuous, factor in your degree of back discomfort.

I frequently meet with some patients weighing 230 pounds or more, and I suggest to them that a major part of their problem is their weight. I usually get a sneering angry response and a comment referencing the fact that it couldn't be their weight because they were "this heavy for years and never had a back problem." Despite my contradictions, they usually persist in this defensive rationalization, and I become just another critic of their body image of which they have, as a denizen of the 90's, now become indignantly proud. It's obvious to me that the amount of WEIGHT-BEARING FLEXION to which they have been exposed has finally met the maximum ability of the spine to sustain that weight. In most cases, it is futile to try to convince them otherwise.

Imagine the stress placed upon the back during WEIGHT-BEARING FLEXION if the back pain sufferer is obese. Having upwards of one hundred pounds to be lifted about three feet every time they so much as get out of a chair. Recall the forces placed upon the back described in Chapter Two Figure 14, these were measured on an average 150 lb man. Those values are magnified by some enormous multiplicand when the center of gravity of the mass is moved away from the axis of the spine thereby increasing the moment arm's force of a fulcrum system (Figure 10) acting upon a disc.

To appreciate how immense the forces are, assume that half of a five-foot four-inch obese woman's weight is above the level of the Lumbar vertebrae, and she weighs 230 pounds, putting her almost 100 lbs over her ideal body weight of 130 pounds. If one accepts that greater than 115 pounds is attached above the Lumbar spine, it can be assumed that the forces generated while moving this person's body parts are equivalent to those forces placed upon any structure roughly equivalent to the spine.

Now, in your mind's eye, take a physical equivalent of that weight, a bar-bell type weight would be ideal, and secure it on the top of a three foot tall vertical broom stick with the bottom secured so as not to be able lift or slide out. Then, let the broom stick tilt off the vertical towards the horizontal. It will bend but probably won't break until about 20-30 degrees off of the vertical axis. As the angle advances, watch the broomstick snap like a match stick. The equivalent forces are acting upon the spine when an obese person so much as attempts to pick up an object off of the floor.

Figure 10 demonstrates schematically the multiplicity of forces acting when an obese person tries to take out the trash. (Employing a clown model, here, should not be construed, as above, to imply that the medical literature recommends that obese back pain patients carry trash cans at a distance from their center of gravity; rather, it merely gives philosophical substance to the absurdity of the human condition.) The numerous forces of gravity acting through long moment arms put extraordinary compressive forces on the discs.

The muscles, ligaments, and tendons that originate and insert on the vertebral bones' posterior elements (such the spinous and transverse processes) limit the extent to which the spine will flex. When they reach their maximum range of stretching motion, they anchor the posterior aspects of the bony structures. Then, when the normal weight of the body, the weight of the lifted object, and the excess weight of the abdomen act on the "lever" that is the rest of the spine above the point of flexion, the compressive forces squeeze the disc like a nutcracker or a fancy garlic press. The physiological consequences of this amount of force acting on such a small area is that herniations of the nucleus pulposus occur in the previously intact discs or disc material made mobile by prior injury is forced posteriorly.

Of course, all these mechanical forces act, albeit to a lesser degree, upon the non-obese spine as well; however, the obese condition provides an excellent opportunity to demonstrate how the simple act of picking up a trash can is capable of resulting in a disc herniation, protrusion, and paradoxically severe pain. It is this phenomenon that explains why, when an obese person gets a job that requires physical lifting like construction, nursing, or making beds in a hotel, the next employment-related event is that they apply for disability. It is no mystery why these types of occupations have such high disability rates and why the archetypal young jolly fat person usually becomes temperamental and not-so-jolly in middle age. They are usually in constant pain. An understanding, acceptance and application of the AVOIDING WEIGHT-BEARING FLEXION concept stands to substantially reduce those probabilities.

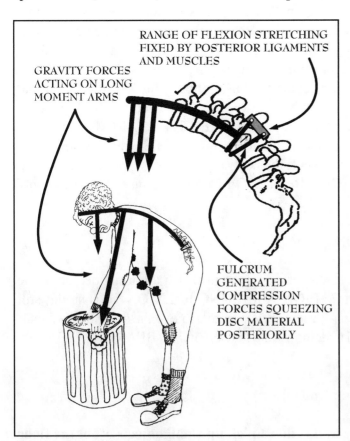

Figure 10 WEIGHT-BEARING FLEXION'S forces acting upon the Lumbar spine during a seemingly innocuous action

Regardless of whether or not you are obese, or if you have neck, thorax or Lumbar pain, one has to intentionally and continuously make a conscious effort to AVOID WEIGHT-BEARING FLEXION positions for all areas of the spine with pain. Because it is such a natural function, it is difficult to accept that it is harmful, especially to a person without a previous injury--but it is! If you have had a previous flexion injury, this is a concept you have to accept and incorporate into your daily activities in order to make your life less painful. Once convinced of the absolute necessity, it may seem overtly simple to follow a recommendation to avoid WEIGHT-BEARING FLEXION. In reality, it is impossible to totally avoid it, but you will discover, when your attention is focused upon it, just how often it occurs and how difficult it is to avoid. It takes vigilance and effort, but **you must program yourself to be constantly cognizant of situations that cause you to adopt it.** Its hard to recognize the absence of pain, so there is not much of a stimulus/reward mechanism to help you. However, the more of it you can avoid, the less back pain you will suffer.

Also, once you become aware of WEIGHT-BEARING FLEXION as the "enemy" you will notice that when you recognize the onset of back pain and you check your posture or position, or immediately recall the position you were in just prior to the onset of pain, it will be more than likely due to WEIGHT-BEARING FLEXION at the putative disc site.

Therefore, it becomes absolutely and literally necessary to **re-train yourself to prevent WEIGHT-BEARING FLEXION**. It is not as simple as telling yourself to do it and then figuratively sitting back to let it not happen. You have to **continuously monitor your posture** to guard against it. The easiest way to succeed in this pursuit is to convince yourself how important it is to avoid WEIGHT-BEARING FLEXIONS. Then you will be operating in your own self-interest. Pain is such a good teacher. Start by monitoring every onset of pain in which there has been none immediately prior. That is, every time you feel spinal pain, stop and consider in what position your spine was in immediately preceding the onset of the pain. You will find that almost exclusively a WEIGHT-BEARING FLEXION preceded the pain. Mentally back-tracking to figure out what particular movement or position put you into WEIGHT-BEARING FLEXION can tell you what movement or position you need to avoid in the future. After you have identified the particular WEIGHT-BEARING FLEXION event, the next step is to find a way to accomplish the same tasks without entering into the WEIGHT-BEARING FLEXION stance. Then, and only then, will you be able to avoid pain.

APPLICATION IN DAILY LIVING

It is impossible to describe and delineate every instance in which a normal person in the conduct of every day-to-day activity commits WEIGHT-BEARING FLEXION. It is harder still to describe an alternative movement that doesn't require flexion to achieve the same desired end; but here are a few examples I have developed to demonstrate that WEIGHT-BEARING FLEXION can, and must, be avoided.

Picking Up Objects

For instance, as in the left side of Figure 11, **don't pick up small objects off of the floor by using flexion of the Lumbar spine** if you have a low back disc problem. One way usually recommended in other books on back pain is to keep the spine "straight" and bend at the knees or the hips; but that requires the energy to raise your entire upper body weight back up to its former level (using the muscles of the legs or back) after letting it go down to near the floor.

A better manner in which to accomplish this task is to **put all your weight on one leg, flexing at the hip of the weighted leg you let your upper body "fall" forward while the other leg's hip and knee is fixed in a straight alignment. As the torso falls, the unweighted leg raises up as it acts as a counter-weight to the torso.** It is usually necessary to hold onto a fixed structure with the hand you are not using to pick up the object or place it on your knee for balance to insure that you do not fall. The

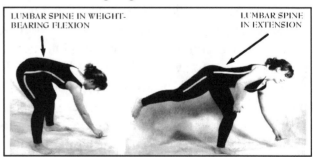

Figure 11 Leg raised method of picking up objects off of floor

raised leg gives balance which allows you to use it as a counter-weight to the upper torso when you bring yourself to the erect position again. **By locking the back into EXTENSION and using the weight of the leg falling as a counter balance, you can let the leg's weight lift the torso**

138

to the erect position again without ever causing the spine go into flexion.

When working on or manipulating objects below the waist such that flexion becomes necessary from a standing position, **spread your legs as far apart as comfortably possible and flex at the hip joints while keeping the back out of flexion and locked in EXTENSION .** This may take some practice to get into a "sway-backed" configuration; however, for efforts that would otherwise require prolonged flexed positioning , **it is most essential to insure that the back is kept in EXTENSION** because the longer you are flexed, the more time the disc material has to move posteriorly.

I frequently watched Southeast Asians planting rice for hours bent over in the rice paddies. I couldn't imagine a job more painful and intolerable. Revisiting this phenomenon, I concluded that people who perform this task comfortably are actually flexing at the hips, and their Lumbar spines are kept hanging in a nearly neutral position. For an older back pain patient who was not raised planting rice, it is unreasonable to expect instantaneous flexibility. It helps to keep the legs wide-spread during such attempts and, if you feel it is worth the extra effort, gradually increase the flexibility by stretching a little more each day to accomplish this. Exercises and practice mobilizing the hip joints to increase their ability to flex are reasonable, especially if your occupation or activities frequently involve reaching the ground from a standing position, such as house cleaning, working with objects on the ground, or gardening. Understand that this type of exercise, as is often recommended in other literature, does not directly function to make the back better; rather, **you are exercising for the purpose of increasing the ability of the hips to function in WEIGHT-BEARING FLEXION instead of the Lumbar spine.**

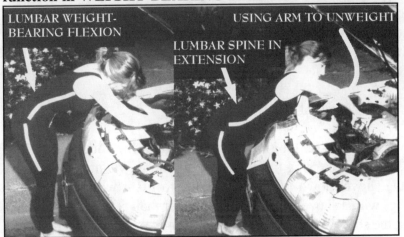

Figure 12 Incorrect (left) and improved means of working while leaning forward over an object

Any time you can take **some of the weight off of the body above the level of a damaged disc, you should attempt to do so. Where and whenever possible, try to find stable platforms upon which to rest the weight of the upper body with the arms.** If you find yourself flexing, use the arms for muscle power as a means of bringing one's upper torso to the erect position when raising the torso up from a plane lower than the region of back pain. If you are leaning over something such as the fender of a car, don't use your back to raise yourself up or lift parts out . Instead, plant one arm with the elbow bearing the weight of the upper body. Then with the Lumbar spine locked in EXTENSION use the other arm to do the lifting (See Figure 12).

Incrementally lift heavy objects only high enough to a place upon which they can rest long enough to give yourself an opportunity to re-position yourself with your back in EXTENSION to complete the task of moving the object. Don't try to "horse" objects up by leaning over and attempting to lift them with your spinal muscles. An especially damaging activity is leaning over the trunk of a car to lift something out. Injuries occur easily in this manner when the muscular forces of jerking the object upwards are added to its weight while the spine is flexed (see also Chapter 6, TRAVELLING WITH A BAD BACK).

Always remember, even if you are not actually stressing the previously damaged and painful segment of your spine, **you must continue to protect the remainder of the spine from minor, yet repeated flexion injuries as well. Guarding or making rigid only the painfully involved spinal segment is not sufficient because the forces are communicated to the adjacent segments.**

People who have had surgical fusion of a disc unit, assume that they shouldn't have problems with their backs ever again because it has become one, solid, piece of bone; yet they frequently do. So much so that at the ten year point, over-all, the surgical group are no better off than those who didn't have surgery. I explain this phenomenon due to the fact that they continue to make the same errors in committing WEIGHT-BEARING FLEXION post-surgically. Adjacent disc units undergo identical degenerative disc destruction due to the equivalently destructive WEIGHT-BEARING FLEXION forces which they continue to sustain; but, as the studies indicate, they do go through a symptom-free "grace" period before they are back into the same trouble. It just takes them several years to destroy their "new" backs. **An understanding of the necessity to AVOID WEIGHT-BEARING FLEXION should be communicated to every patient who has had disc surgery as a routine component of their recovery education or else they will be committed to making the same destructive errors the remainder of their lives.**

One must make every effort to avoid WEIGHT-BEARING FLEXION for the majority of the weight-loaded spinal segments. **This means taking a close look at every activity in which you usually participate or action you take, and find a means of doing it with a minimal amount of WEIGHT-BEARING FLEXION.**

Physical Labor

When you engage in physical labor, let long tools do your work for you. With a long tool, you needn't go into flexion. If you are trying to lift a rock, put the shovel under it and pry it up by pushing the handle of the shovel down rather than trying to lift it with your back in flexion. You can move many things with a shovel while standing rather than bending over to pick them up and throw them. Kicking the shovel while it abuts against a rock to move it, as if playing hockey, prevents you from having to flex in weight-bearing.

Think about this concept when you are gardening. You will find that using a small, cute little shovel or hoe is more painful than using a long handled one. When you pick-up something off of the ground, **use the long-handled tool like a support staff to help you get down and up by letting it, and your arms, support the weight of your upper body**. The only difference in the work being accomplished is that it should be done without as much WEIGHT-BEARING FLEXION. **If you flex, your weight should be on the shovel and not on your back.**

As you squat down to do anything close to the ground, realize that you are going into an unnecessary WEIGHT-BEARING FLEXION position. You would be better suited by getting down on all fours, putting your weight on your elbows and working with the arms, wrists, and hands. You would be even more comfortable if you allowed your back to "sway" while you worked by using a support device (See Figure 13). By that, I mean let your abdomen hang as low to the ground as possible like a "sway-backed" horse, rather than flexing it like a scared Halloween cat. Using some device to pad your knees, either an independent pad or those that attach to your knees like roofers and carpenters use makes you less likely to squat because one usually squats to prevent getting down on all fours. If you have a back condition, it is ultimately less painful to get down on all fours.

Whenever feasible, one should use the hands, arms, elbows, solid objects, or appurtenances (such as canes, staffs, or crutches) to take the weight off of the spine, especially during those times when pain is present.

Nurses and people employed to take care of the disabled, too, have some of the highest disability rates due to their constant flexion postures while they lean over people while trying to lift or adjust them. The nurses could eliminate many of their back injuries if they would use one outstretched arm (the non-dominant one) locked in EXTENSION at the elbow on the bed to support their weight, look up to insure that their spines are not in flexion while lifting, and use only the muscles of the other arm to lift or move their patients.

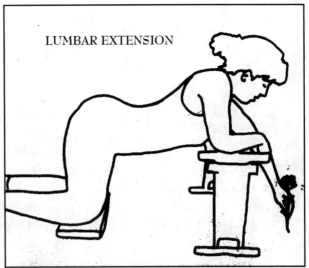

Figure 13 Working on ground with devices while avoiding WEIGHT-BEARING FLEXION

Usually, what they do is lean way over a bed and, with both arms, attempt to jerk the patient while lifting to get the mass moving. In that one movement, they put not only the weight of the patient on their spine but the weight of their upper body magnified by the contraction of the erector spinae while they lift with their back muscles. They usually can't continue this for long, because their backs give out and they become occupationally disabled.

In "the good old days" before hospital administrators figured out they could pay themselves higher salaries by eliminating the numbers of "orderlies," there usually were strong males coursing the halls of hospitals capable of helping lift patients whenever necessary. Now, the same administrators keep the wards perpetually understaffed so a nurse either hurts her back trying to support a patient, or the patient careens to the floor. My advice to nurses is to refuse to lift patients without help if it cannot be done safely. If there are not sufficient staff to perform that function, insist upon them being hired. It is either refuse to lift weights you were not designed to lift or end up with an early retirement of relative poverty and pain.

Driving

The act of driving or sitting in an automobile usually places one in a flexed, weight-bearing posture. If you could freeze the average person in the position in which they drive and,

141

without altering the configuration of the spine, place them on their feet, you would find that the person is stooped over into a very awkward flexion posture when standing (See Figure 14). This is the principle reason why truck drivers, fork-lift operators, and farmers who drive tractors all day have such a high prevalence of back problems.

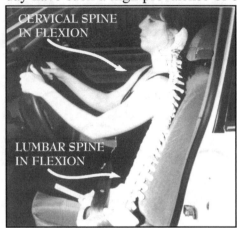

Figure 14 Cervical and Lumbar spine (especially L5-S1) in WEIGHT-BEARING FLEXION of driving.

I have read back pain literature that attributes this phenomenon to vibration exposure. The fact is that vibration is not the independent or primary precipitator of pain. Constant vibration when applied to nerves classically results in anesthetic neuropathies (numbness). **The largest contributor is not so much vibration inasmuch as it is from the repetitive WEIGHT-BEARING FLEXION events caused by up and down decelerations due to the rough road surfaces, as well as forward motion decelerations due to repeated braking's action on the disc.** These occupations' continuous flexion posture combined with the jarring of the vehicle causes a gradual, unrelenting, posterior displacement of the disc material. **This damage and pain can be prevented by placing a support in their seat to keep the Lumbar vertebrae in slight EXTENSION and driving with their Cervical and Upper Thoracic vertebrae kept in slight EXTENSION with a similar pillow strapped to the seat back (Figure 15).**

Another error is committed when people (especially professionals like truck drivers) leave the seated driving position to

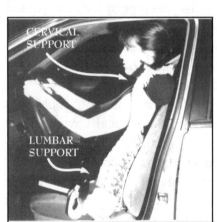

Figure 15 Using Cervical and Lumbar support while driving

get out of their vehicles. They usually commit another forceful and exaggerated WEIGHT-BEARING FLEXION (Figure 16) after hours of letting the disc material migrate posteriorly which sets them up for injury.

Ideally, they should dismount with an UNWEIGHTED EXTENSION MANEUVER similar to that described in the MORNING EXTENSION section of this book. By grabbing onto some part of the door frame of a car or a handle on the side of the truck, they can unweight while doing a few THERAPEUTIC CIRCUMDUCTIONS (Hula-like gyrations with

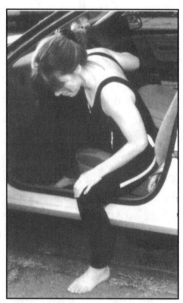

Figure 16 Neck and low back in bad WEIGHT-BEARING FLEXION upon exiting vehicle

the hips) before weight-bearing again in EXTENSION . Instead, they are usually seen getting out of their trucks in flexion then jumping to the ground only to land in flexion with the full weight of their upper body crashing down upon a flexed Lumbar spine with the posterior elements open, the disc material has been allowed to previously migrate to the limit of its posterior displacement and is just waiting for a worse herniation or protrusion when the right amount of force is applied.

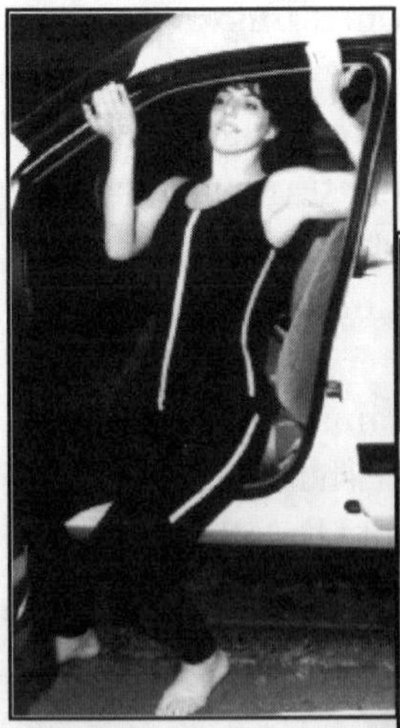

Figure 17 Neck and low back in EXTENSION upon exiting vehicle

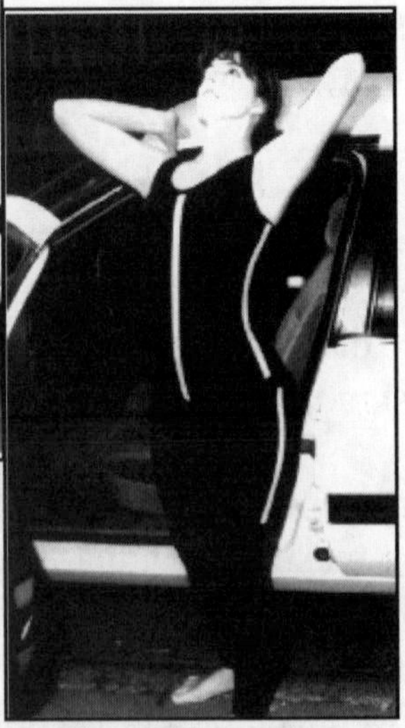

Figure 18 Spine in EXTENSION when re-weight-bearing

Applying the same principle of AVOIDING WEIGHT-BEARING FLEXION to getting out of a vehicle after a long drive can prevent a lot of unnecessary agony. Looking at Figures 17 & 18 which show how this is done, you will note that the model is laughing while exiting the car using a convenient means of applying UNWEIGHTED EXTENSION without having to go to your knees. The photographer at this point was ridiculing the absurdity of this practice. My reply was: "You don't have a bad back, do you? Someday you may not find this so funny." His retort was that nobody is going to do that." My final statement was: "They will when they discover how it eliminates pain."

Certainly, I don't always have to get out of cars like this; but, during those times in which I get out of a car when my back has been bothering me and I feel my back has been in flexion long enough to have caused a migration of the disc material, I simply perform this MANEUVER to stop the discomfort before it advances to pain when weight-bearing occurs.

Later in the book you will learn to do specific MANEUVERS similar to this and incorporate them into your daily activities as a choice. This is a preliminary exposure to that concept. The back pain sufferer can choose to leave a car in NON-WEIGHT-BEARING EXTENSION instead of WEIGHT-BEARING FLEXION and simultaneously perform an action which will serve to move the displaced disc material back to the center of the disc. Were I to get out with the usual WEIGHT-BEARING FLEXION (Figure 16), experience tells me I may pay for it with pain, so I make the choice to incorporate a back pain relieving MANEUVER into an action I have to take any way. The choice element is only that I choose to exit a vehicle in a different manner--that's all. If people without bad backs see this as ridiculous, that's their choice. They do not have to live with my back pain.

Coughing

Speaking of sick situations, I have noticed in my patient population that during colds and viral infections, more people complain of back pain. Also, I have had several patients come to me, with convincing complaints, who claimed that their back pain started when they caught a cold

143

or was significantly worsened during the cold. When I test whether this phenomenon is disc-related, it usually can be shown to be due to a herniation.

The consideration for AVOIDING WEIGHT-BEARING FLEXION is operant here as well. **A viral cold, allergies, or a smoking habit can make your back worse**. Why? Well, consider that most people lie in bed for hours, propped up with pillows, and their entire spine is configured in a long, sloping flexion. Since they still have the weight of their body pushing them into the bed, they are, in reality, weight-bearing; but they also are doing something every few minutes that is capable of putting a back "out." They are violently, uncontrollably, and paroxysmally contracting their anterior trunk musculature while taking deep breaths and bearing down on their abdomen and chest with forces sufficient to raise their entire chest off the surface of the bed--sometimes to the point of raising their legs off of the bed at the same time. What are they doing that you are probably telling yourself that you don't do, so this part of the book doesn't pertain to you?--They are coughing and sneezing!

Coughing and sneezing during a period when you usually have been maintaining sustained WEIGHT-BEARING FLEXION for hours at a time is extremely dangerous when viewed from a discogenic back pain perspective. Some of my patients say that they were told by other doctors that a cough or a sneeze was insufficient to cause a disc protrusion. However, a back pain sufferer knows differently and must excuse them their ignorance. A cold can bring out the worse in a bad back.

To prevent this, just before you are preparing to cough or sneeze, make sure you are in EXTENSION, as non-weight-bearing as possible, and make certain that you maintain this until the coughing fit is over. Try when you are lying in bed, especially under the influence of anti-histamines (which act as mild tranquilizers to relax the muscles because they keep you sleepy) to use pillows and positioning to support the Lumbar as well as the Cervical spine, especially. Re-structure your cough posture so that you don't bend forward. Straightening your airway by tilting the head back and putting the chin up actually improves the dynamics of coughing, actually making it more effective in removing secretions. Also, during coughing fits, hang your head over the edge of the bed so that you are no longer in WEIGHT-BEARING IN FLEXION. This will allow gravity to help you remove your secretions, and it will remove at least one factor in the generation of back pain. Taking the weight off of the segment of the spine that is most often flexed during a cough may necessarily allow flexion to occur but it doesn't make it a WEIGHT-BEARING FLEXION event. Therefore, it is made much less damaging.

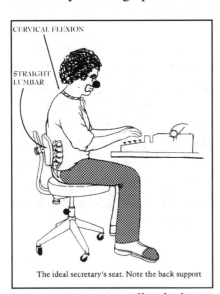

The ideal secretary's seat. Note the back support

Figure 19 Purportedly ideal position for prolonged seated work

Seated at Work

I could probably go on *ad nauseam* describing numerous situations in which **office workers position themselves in WEIGHT-BEARING FLEXION and remain so for nearly eight hours a day**. Even seated at a desk using

144

a computer lends itself to prolonged flexion and back pain by the end of the day. Sure, every book you ever read shows the ideal upright posture with the spine "straight" and the person seated as the clown in Figure 19. This drawing was extracted from a contemporary back pain book purporting to demonstrate the ideal office worker's posture. Unfortunately, this posture is unrealistic to maintain because the eyes must look down at the work; and, as they do, the neck goes into flexion to accommodate the eye's tendency to want to gaze at subject matter straight in front of them. Also, as the day wears on and the muscles necessary to support that posture begin to tire, the body slips into a flexion position at the neck and Lumbar spine. Then, the pain and stiffness sets in. **I advocate that everyone who is caused to sit at a computer or desk for prolonged periods re-arrange their work station so that they are sitting comfortably like in an astronaut's chair with their Lumbar and Cervical spines protected from flexion with tailored supports**. An astronaut's seat was designed to give maximum protection against the massive gravitational effects ("G" forces). The same forces are acting upon the spine at all times, albeit of lesser intensity. However, there is not much difference in total force sustained between experiencing four times the force of gravity for ten minutes while accelerating into orbit or facing the routine force of gravity for forty minutes.

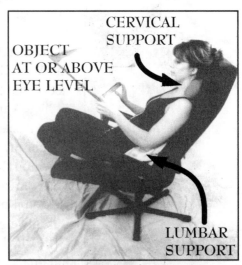

Figure 20 Ideal position for prolonged seated work keeping Lumbar and Cervical regions in EXTENSION

Either one will cause pain without support of the spine to prevent its unphysiological flexion. So, if it is warranted for astronauts, it is equally warranted for those stuck in chairs eight hours a day.

This support can be accomplished with "lazy-boy" type chairs that allow the feet to come off the ground and rest on a foot stool type support and with simple pillows in the Lumbar and Cervical areas. If a computer is used, the screen should be placed and angled such that a person can see it while comfortably lying back with the neck and low back in a neutral or slightly extended position (See Figure 20). This usually requires that the object being viewed be positioned at or above the level of the eyes. It is imperative to note that **repetitive flexion at the Cervical spine (by trying to look at some other object to the side or lower) or at the Lumbar spine (by raising the upper torso up off of the chair's surface or reaching repeatedly) constitutes repetitive WEIGHT-BEARING FLEXION. Such actions can negate this supported posture's benefits and should be consciously avoided.** Smokers have a statistically higher incidence of back problems, most probably because they repeatedly reach for cigarettes while seated and cough while in flexion.

Getting up from a seated position is perhaps the most common activity in which a person engages where AVOIDING WEIGHT-BEARING FLEXION is essential. The natural propensity is to plant your feet, put your arms forward, lean the torso anteriorly while falling into flexion (See Figure 21), and jerk yourself to the erect position. This is an ideal means of putting a disc out because usually the activity is preceded and initiated with a WEIGHT-BEARING FLEXION

145

due to previous slouching.

The act of getting out of a chair is also prone to WEIGHT-BEARING FLEXION pain. Most people move their upper body forward, flexing the Lumbar and Cervical spine, so that they can shift their center of gravity off of the chair. They then launch forward in WEIGHT-BEARING FLEXION. After sitting in prolonged flexion with a slouch, this is detrimental because the posterior intervertebral spaces have been maximally opened and are poised for a posterior migration of disc material when the WEIGHT-BEARING FLEXION is increased rapidly during the act of standing up from a sitting position.

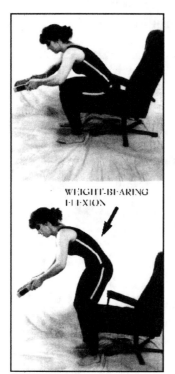

Figure 21 Rising from sitting incorrectly

A more ideal means of getting up from a seated position is to first take the weight off the Lumbar spine by pushing down on the seat or arms of the chair so you can adjust your spine out of any flexion it may have defaulted into. Once it is unweighted, a mild THERAPEUTIC CIRCUMDUCTION (gently make a hula-dance like action at the hips) can free-up any migrated disc material so that when weight bearing finally comes, you will be in EXTENSION and no disc material will be peripheralized to induce pain (See Figure 22). You then keep the spine in EXTENSION by contracting the posterior back muscles. Hold them contracted and slide your buttock to the edge of the chair until you are fully erect, usually by getting your feet underneath your center of gravity by moving in the most convenient manner at your disposal.

If you are in a lot of pain, you may have to slide to your knees and get up from the ground; but usually just using the chair itself as a launching platform for your arms, you can get yourself to the standing position with just extending your knees because you can lift your torso high enough with your hands on the chair to keep you unweighted.

Alternatively, at the point when your buttocks are on the edge of the chair, you can use your hands on your knees, lean forward and crawl them up your thighs to the erect position. The arms on the legs then can keep the Lumbar spine unweighted until standing. This is how old people routinely get up from sitting; and, for good reason, their backs are usually shot by that point in life. Nevertheless, they are able to take the weight off of the Lumbar spine long enough to get their back into an erect configuration so as to stand up after it has been in WEIGHT-BEARING

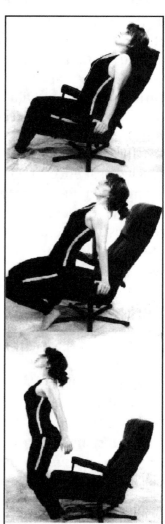

Figure 22 Rising from sitting ideally in EXTENSION

146

FLEXION for a prolonged period while sitting.

Squatting

In the spirit of avoiding WEIGHT-BEARING FLEXION, I need also to address the act of squatting. **When squatting, even without the intent to lift something off of the ground, the Lumbar spine naturally assumes a flexed position. It is nearly impossible to squat and not place the Lumbar spine in WEIGHT-BEARING FLEXION unless you consciously avoid it.** It is practically impossible to occupy a squatting posture and lift something off the ground without assuming a WEIGHT-BEARING FLEXION at the Lumbar spine.

Try it yourself. Squat down and then extend the Lumbar spine. Most probably you will fall backwards unless you are so obese that your abdomen keeps you balanced anteriorly. Even if you extend your Lumbar spine completely and then lower yourself to a squatting position, you will find that this position is very unstable because without flexing the Lumbar spine you will fall backwards.

For these reasons as well as personal experience, I have concluded that squatting is one of the most under-recognized pain-inducing and dangerous positions for anyone with a Lumbar back pain problem. Squatting while lifting cannot be underemphasized as a posture to consciously program yourself to avoid if you have a back pain problem.

The wearing of a tight belt or clothing with a tight-fitting waistline magnifies the problem because the pants, tightening in the squat, pull the constricting material superior to the hips inferiorly, aggravating the opening of the posterior aspect of the lower Lumbar disc units. This predisposes the discs to protrusion, especially in the act of getting up, because one is essentially caused to lean forward as the arms are extended forward for balance and jerk the upper body superiorly to regain the erect position. Squatting is one of the least recognized yet most pain-inducing postures I have identified. Usually, a person with Lumbar disc disease, including myself, can occasionally lift, lightly flex, and laterally bend in their activities of daily living so long as their back is not "out"; however, allowing myself the luxury of squatting, can usually be expected to result in a long period of pain before I can be rid of it by doing MANEUVERS. It took me literally years to figure out the destructive capacity of the squat.

Too, when people prepare to lift an object off of the floor, a squat is the position usually attempted. Not only because it seems the most natural way to do it; but if they have read the back pain literature, they recall distinctly the commandment to "keep your back straight and lift with the knees, not the back." This naturally brings one to the squatting posture shown in the clown on the Left in Figure 23. (Again, I have taken the liberty of excerpting an exact drawing from the "expert" back pain literature and clowned it up to

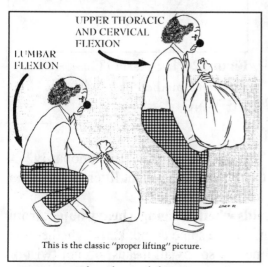

Figure 23 The classic lifting instructions given to back pain suffers (clown notations and clown attire mine)

147

display its obviously erroneous distinction from *The O'Connor Technique (tm)* ideal). In actuality, unless one intentionally attempts to AVOID WEIGHT-BEARING FLEXION by MAINTAINING EXTENSION during the lifting process, one naturally flexes at the Lumbar spine while lifting no matter how much they attempt to keep the back "straight." This happens because humans cannot elongate their arms at will. In order to reach the center of gravity and bottom lifting surface of a large object on the ground, something has to give. Usually it is the Lumbar region that is induced into an unintentional flexion by the squat position; therefore, I advocate avoiding squatting whenever possible.

Lifting Heavy Objects

However, I am a realist enough to know that it is nearly impossible to go through life without lifting heavy objects from the ground and, in order to accomplish this task, one has to assume a position that physically approaches a squat to do so. Therefore, in order to safely accomplish the task, one has to alter the pure squatting position into one that avoids WEIGHT-BEARING FLEXION.

The best way to accomplish the lifting of a heavy object from the ground is to start by looking up towards the sky before you even bend your knees to get the upper body closer to the ground. This locks the Cervical, Thoracic, and Lumbar spine in EXTENSION to prevent flexion. Then, snuggle up as close to the object as possible, use one knee to touch the ground for balance if necessary until you can grasp the object and use its weight to counter-balance the tendency to fall backwards when the back is extended and the knees are bent. Keeping the hands inside the knees whenever possible, you then look upwards with your face towards the sky during the act of lifting (See Figure 24). This forces the spine to assume a non-flexed and slightly extended configuration closely akin to a weight-lifter's stance. Weight lifters do not adopt their lifting posture because it is "cool" or stylish but because that is the physiologically, mechanically, evolutionarily, and

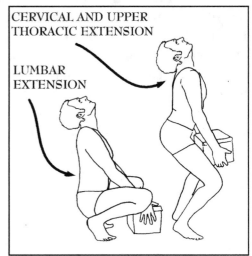

Figure 24 The ideal *O'Connor Technique* method of FACE-UP LIFTING

anatomically most advantageous position to adopt to protect the spine. "Evolutionarily" is figuratively used in this sense to discriminate between those "extinct" weight lifters who didn't lift that way and now are no longer lifting weights due to spinal damage.

The necessity to remain in EXTENSION also holds when bringing a heavy object from a high to low position on the ground. The forces acting on the spine do not know whether you are lifting or putting something down-- they stay the same. Also, by all means, do not twist or lift off-center or even allow yourself to lift heavy objects when there is a chance that you may lose your balance and be caused to twist or be caught with the weight off-center during the act of supporting a heavy weight.

148

Actually, lifting heavy weights can be accomplished safely (so long as your disc is "in" at the time) by holding to the principle of avoiding WEIGHT-BEARING FLEXION, even if you have a "bad" back. Most books will tell you simplistically to lift with your legs. Well, that is not bad advice, but many times you really cannot do so because you need the stability of a wide based gait, as in lifting furniture. You can still do things like this carefully and infrequently, by properly preparing yourself, using your legs as much as possible by bending at the knees first, getting as close to the weight to be lifted as possible, then, before you start to lift, look straight up above your head. This forces the spine into an extended posture similar to a weight lifter's stance. In fact, that is how they are able to perform such feats of human endurance without rupturing a disc. When they lift, they follow all the rules I have outlined here. They keep the weight as close to the body as possible, using the knees and arms as much as they can. It may look like they do, but they do not really squat in flexion. Their backs are in extension throughout the entire lift.

You will also observe how they cleverly avoid using the Lumbar spine muscles at all and do all sorts of careful alternatives to prevent WEIGHT-BEARING FLEXION. They use their knees to lift the weight to their waist; then, they use their arms and simultaneously re-bend the knees while lowering their body, to get their ideally extended, rigid Lumbar spine underneath the weight when they jerk. For a split second, they let the weight fall so that it becomes essentially weight-less so they can avoid WEIGHT-BEARING FLEXION.

The next time the Olympics are on TV, pay attention where the weight-lifters are looking when they bring the weight up to their waist. They may not always look up, but they rarely look down while lifting because that would allow the spine to slip into flexion and hurt them. Then, the next time you are asked to help move a sofa, during the lifting phase, try it with and without looking up. Also, after you have lifted a heavy object and are preparing to walk with it, be certain to aim your face towards the horizon so as to look where you are going because once you have raised the object to waist level, it is not as essential to keep your face looking up, just so long as your Lumbar spine stays locked in EXTENSION .

I mentioned above that lifting could be done if the disc was "in"; and one should prepare one's spine to insure that such is the case before lifting. By this, I mean, before lifting or carrying a weight, one should be certain that all the discs are in their proper alignment and all displaced disc material is centralized with an UNWEIGHTING EXTENSION MANEUVER quite similar to those described in the MANEUVERS sections. I'm getting a little ahead of myself here by advocating MANEUVERS which haven't been yet taught; however, this may be no more complicated than putting the hands on the hips then pushing down with the arms to unweight the Lumbar and Thoracic spine so that an unweighted DIAGNOSTIC and THERAPEUTIC CIRCUMDUCTION and EXTENSION can be accomplished. Once you have done this, you can be reasonably certain that no disc is "out" that will be further extruded when lifting increases the fulcrum-generated hydraulic pressure on the discs. "Seating" the discs in this manner insures that none are on the verge of being "out" and, therefore, are much less prone to injury while lifting.

Another device you will see weight-lifters use towards this end is to let the weight fall rather than cause themselves to go into flexion while putting the weight down. If you think about it, **the same forces on the discs are present when you are slowly putting down a weight as when you are lifting it.** The spine is loaded identically. So, when you are putting the furniture

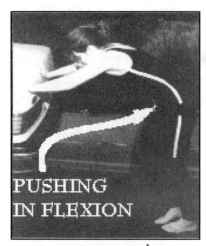

Figure 25 Incorrect choice in pushing car due to FLEXION

you are carrying down, you must insure that you do not go into flexion as well. A lot of people forget this and hurt themselves because they didn't consider that putting something down is equivalent to lifting it as far as the back is concerned. Putting something down is not exactly as dangerous as lifting it because you already have experienced the weight and you are not fighting gravity so much by letting it go to the ground; but, remember, **a lot of unbreakable things can be dropped if for some reason your back is accidentally forced to go into flexion**, you lose your footing, or pain starts. Its better to let a replaceable object unceremoniously hit the ground rather than risk your back. It may even be cheaper to let a couch fall if suddenly an unexpected move causes you to go into flexion at the Lumbar spine. So what if the leg on a couch breaks, you can go out and buy a new one--try buying a new Lumbar disc. Of course, if you do this too much your "friends" might not ask you to help them move their households.

Towards this end, you might consider thinking in advance of your preparing to lift something heavy or ungainly as to whether it is capable of being dropped or slid down the legs in the event that something happens whereupon you are forced to decide to hold onto it if you trip or lose your balance. Guiding a piece of junk to the ground so as to not let it make a noise at the expense of your back may not be a fair trade. Sometimes it is better to let even a valuable object fall and figure that you have just saved the lost income of two to four days of bed rest. It seems like it's unnecessary to monitor your condition so much; however, when the cost of not doing it can mean the rest of your life with pain, you might be convinced that such attention to detail is worth the effort. Unfortunately, most people make this assessment after they are in permanent pain and are retrospectively reviewing their actions to see what they could have done differently. By then, it is too late and simply an exercise in hindsight.

If pain occurs while lifting, no effort should be made to straighten up; but, rather, the weight should be abandoned and an attempt should be made to immediately find something to grab onto or support the upper body to take the weight off of the effected segment. If no support object can be reached, carefully lowering yourself to the floor on hands and knees to make the painful segment immediately NON-WEIGHT-BEARING is the best response. Then, letting the effected segment slowly move into an EXTENSION IN TRACTION posture before resuming WEIGHT-BEARING is essential. How you accomplish that is up to you, but a HIP-HANGING EXTENSION on the nearest piece of furniture is probably the best response. During these protective movements, the spine should be guarded so as to insure no motion is allowed that increases the pain.

Whenever possible, carry or move heavy objects behind you instead of in front of you or drag them behind you rather than push them in front of you. When carrying them behind you, you have a higher probability of weight-bearing in EXTENSION rather than flexion. As you walk, the forces are such that the disc material is not predisposed to a posterior migration. When pushing, you are unthinkingly forced into WEIGHT-BEARING FLEXION. The act of pushing places loads on the spine similarly to lifting. The harder you push the more the spine is loaded.

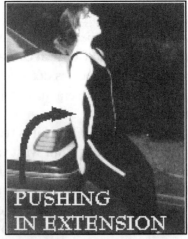

If you were to have to physically move a car, the low height of the car seemingly demands flexion (See Figures 25 & 26). The strength with which you push determines the degree of spinal loading. You will be able to exert much more force by facing in the opposite direction and pushing with the back in EXTENSION while you walk backwards. You would be surprised how much more efficient and safe doing it that way is.

Figure 26 Correct choice in pushing car in EXTENSION

Don't let your ego prevent you from asking for help or refusing to lift a heavy weight. Asking someone to help you get the heavy weight, you both plan to carry, up to the waist level until you can turn around so as to carry it behind you, still gets the job done; but you don't put your back at as much risk. If you aren't in pain and you wish to stay that way, don't be afraid to say: "Sorry, I can't do it, my back won't let me." It's better to let your ego take a hit rather than your disc. You can get over the embarrassment of revealing a "disability" in a millisecond. It may take months to get out of back pain.

All of this may seem like too much to remember or too great an imposition on your lifestyle; but, if you remember to practice the simple principle of avoiding WEIGHT-BEARING FLEXION in everything you do, as much as you realistically can, you will find that you can continue to enjoy most activities that you otherwise probably would have had to abandon because they brought on back pain.

I would hope everyone, especially those people without bad backs, could apply the principle of AVOIDING WEIGHT-BEARING FLEXION and adhere to these practices in their daily lives without having to go through the trauma of a disc herniation to convince them of the necessity. However, in reality, an ounce of prevention may be worth a pound of cure, but society would rather pour out billions of pounds of money treating back disease rather than preventively educating employees in back protection. I hope this book serves the purpose of stimulating employers and insurers to do something along these lines now that there exists a rational vehicle to effect that change via *The O'Connor Technique (tm)*.

TRACTION

"Traction" as it is used in spinal pain referenced orthopedic parlance consists of the process of stretching the vertebral column for prolonged periods of time with complicated weights, ropes, and hardware. In most instances, its past use has been relegated to a medieval apparatus with a corset-like device attached to the hips while a system of pulleys, ropes and weights are used to generate the traction employing the force of gravity or a motorized force. If one envisions the mechanical effect of putting the spine in traction as conventionally defined, two major consequences predominate. One, the entire spinal column as a whole is straightened and, two, the disc spaces between the vertebral bones are widened. The effect of the former is to straighten the Lumbar and Cervical curvatures, and the latter opens or widens the disc spaces. Both of these actions can be seen as detrimental to both the natural or damaged condition because no beneficial disc material movement can be expected using the current methodology of classic orthopedic traction.

TRACTION as it is treated and utilized by *The O'Connor Technique (tm)* **has a similar physiological basis but with vastly different mechanical and anatomic consequences. Without complicated apparatus, relying upon an enlightened use of body positioning, and capitalizing upon gravity's actions on body parts, displaced disc material can be favorably moved with TRACTION.** One of the major contributions to this technique's success rests in the ability of the back pain sufferer to learn how to effectively put the body in various positions to effect a site-specific traction at only the precise area of a damaged disc so as to widen the intervertebral space and give the displaced disc material a space into which it may re-centralize.

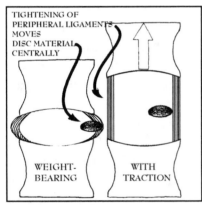

Figure 27 Schematic representation of disc unit showing how TRACTION moves disc material centrally due to straightening action of peripheral ligaments.

Currently promoted back pain management practices almost uniformly exclude traction as a modality largely because a few studies comparing traction to simple bed rest purported to demonstrate no benefit. The most recent[10] is no different. A cynical suspicion would conclude that these studies were avariciously funded and accepted by the hospital bill payers because they saw a large amount of money being spent on patients simply sitting in a hospital bed with a costly, complicated, device that may or may not have helped. Nevertheless, these studies were, in fact, valid representations of reality because they accurately elaborated the failure of the then state-of-the-art of traction as applied with ropes pulleys and weights, **proving in the offing, that, if one does something wrongly or badly, one can expect to achieve no better results than doing nothing, regardless of the motivation.** It could also be that any coincidental benefits that were being observed were offset by the actual increase in pain created by traction applied in the absence of a competent, rational, understanding of Lumbar mechanics.

Traction in these studies was also applied while the person was flat on their backs. No effort to insure that the ideal Lumbar curvature was maintained; so, as the spine was stretched with a good old-fashioned traction device, it only managed to flatten the Lumbar curve into the equivalent of flexion. For an injury that was initially a flexion injury, **conventional traction**, combined with the weight of the body in the absence of Lumbar support or insuring the MAINTENANCE OF EXTENSION, **opened the**

posterior intervertebral space, thereby, allowing the disc material to migrate posteriorly (if it moved at all). Additionally, traction was applied to the entire spine without regard to the discomfort inflicted by its effect on normal discs. In this scenario, just as many people were probably made worse by traction as were made better.

Traction's abandonment as a successful modality was also due, in part, to the perceived excessive amount of traction believed necessary to successfully separate vertebral bodies. It was argued that one third of the weight of the body was usually necessary to effect sufficient force to separate vertebrae. The classical application of traction was deemed too difficult to administer realistically with weights, pulleys, and ropes; so, again, the "baby was thrown out with the bath water." For years, traction (especially administered in the hospital for days at a time) was, therefore, viewed as unnecessary. Probably this decision was partly influenced

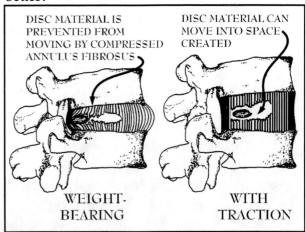

Figure 28 Diagram demonstrating effect of TRACTION on disc unit

by third party payers who jumped at any opportunity to kick patients out of the hospital and supported by the desire to decrease spending as much as possible--a mentality that persists to this day. This, in retrospect, may have been coincidentally better for patients; however, the motivation, nonetheless, can still be looked upon as suspect.

This problem was magnified by an absence of good diagnostic methods to accurately determine which persons would benefit by traction when properly applied. For instance, traction can be seen to aggravate back pain originating from facet joint inflammation to which some (but not I) attribute as much as 20% of low back pain. Any sore joint in the body would not improve if it were constantly stretched by a weight attached to it. People with arthritis of the elbow would rightfully complain bitterly if caused to hang a weight from their arm rather than rest the joint when it is acutely painful.

Suffice it to say that *The O'Connor Technique (tm)* does not apply traction in the manner described in classical orthopedic usage. **The O'Connor Technique (tm) is novel in that, through a logical approach to the physical mechanics of identified discogenic pain, it applies an expedient, gentle, self-administered, focused, weight-of-body-parts traction to effect the re-centralization of displaced disc material.** While the traction is applied, it is used intentionally to give the displaced disc material a volume of space into which it can re-centralize.

TRACTION as utilized and applied in *The O'Connor Technique (tm)* takes advantage of two effects that occur when traction is placed upon a disc unit. Foremost, **there is a centrally-pushing effect on disc material generated when the peripheral ligamentous structures of the disc are pulled tight and straight**. The effect is similar to when a basket or Chinese finger trap is stretched. The edges of any basket-like structure will deform centrally when stretched, going from a concave to a straight or even a convex configuration. The similarly designed disc unit's annulus fibrosus and capsule are pulled taut during traction. When the outer bands of the capsule

153

(and especially the posterior longitudinal ligaments) are straightened, peripheralized disc material is pushed centrally (See Figure 27).

TRACTION allows disc material to move centrally largely because a space was created when the nucleus pulposus herniated through the annulus fibrosus at the time of injury. This space is composed of the (previously described) fissures and tears through which the displaced disc material moves. When TRACTION is applied the "roof and floor" of these tunnel-like channels separate giving a larger space as the vertebral bones move away from each other. This increased space created in the center of the disc gives the displaced disc material a place to go (See Figure 28) that it otherwise would not have. **Without TRACTION the weight of the body above the disc serves to compress the potential space making it, for the most part, impossible for disc material to relocate so long as weight-bearing is occurring.**

This is the main reason why exercises that allow for flexion and extension during weight-bearing can be ineffective, futile and unnecessarily painful. Without a place in the central part of the disc for the displaced disc material to migrate into, the material stays in the painful configuration or is pushed more peripherally during exercise.

Secondarily, **a suction-like mechanism (Figure 29) is acting when TRACTION is applied that serves to draw peripheralized disc matter centrally due to the negative pressure generated as the vertebral bodies separate.** Just as a balloon glued to two spools will deform with the peripheral contents moving centrally to fill the void created when the spools are pulled apart, nature's abhorrence of a vacuum causes the more fluid-like components of the nucleus pulposus to be drawn centrally.

It would probably be more "scientifically appropriate" for me to say "possibly" and "it appears", etc. because I have not actually had the opportunity to stick needles into damaged discs and measure the pressures. However, I can feel this happening in my own discs when just TRACTION is applied, the rest is simply a logical series of assumptions based upon an observation combined with a knowledge of physics and anatomy. In the final analysis, it works! *O'Connor Technique* **TRACTION is actually very simple to implement. It is only a matter of hanging a part of the body from another part of the body until such time as the muscle, tendons, and ligaments acting on a particular disc unit are stretched to their comfortable maximum.** It is the application of specific stretching techniques combined with proper timing in relationship to other movements that causes the capsule to act on the disc material to move it centrally. During the MANEUVERS sections of the book, the reader will be given the directions on how to apply the TRACTION by positioning the body, when to apply it, and when to release it. It is only necessary to apply and maintain TRACTION until the vertebrae can be positioned so that when

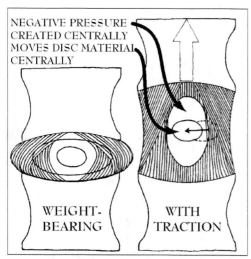

Figure 29 Schematic representation of disc unit showing how TRACTION creates a negative pressure capable of moving peripheralized disc material centrally

the TRACTION is released, the re-weighting forces will further serve to position disc material away from the point where it is generating pain. After the TRACTION has achieved its maximum effect (usually on the order of seconds to minutes rather than hours or days), it need not be sustained any longer.

The force necessary to bring about sustained, comfortable *O'Connor Technique (tm)* TRACTION is supplied by the individual's body without the need for complicated devices, pulleys or weights. To successfully open and separate the disc unit, usually the weight of that part of the body superior or inferior to the level of the affected disc is usually sufficient to satisfy this requirement. If not, the strength of the arms, legs, or an assistant can be used to increase the tractive force for short periods of time. An extended period is not usually necessary to maximally separate the vertebral bodies and coax the disc material to migrate back to the disc's center. So, the practitioner of *The O'Connor Technique (tm)* is not required to remain restrained in a complicated apparatus.

O'Connor technique TRACTION is also applied slowly and gently with a pain-mediated damage-prevention control built in. If it hurts, you don't do it, and you are able to stop before any potential damage can be done. This unique application of TRACTION allows the elastic portion of the disc to come to full length in a relatively short period of time; and, in most instances, when it has reached its maximum benefit length, it need not be prolonged.

There is little or no benefit to be gained by persisting with the maximum TRACTION after it has arrived at its maximum therapeutic effect. To do otherwise can be unnecessarily uncomfortable such as in the case of being strapped into orthopedic bed weights and pulleys for days at a time. It's easy to see why the old, conventional, traction methods actually increased the discomfort of enough patients to result in the study showing that just as many people did better with bed rest alone. It is reasonable to assume that a statistically significant number of patients got worse and ruined whatever benefit traction gave to those who were lucky enough to be positioned in such a manner that traction helped them

Perhaps thankfully, the effect of classical traction was nearly impossible to maintain because, in actual practice, the weights pulled the patient to the end of the bed whenever they attempted to adjust their posture. Frequent changes in posture were nearly impossible to prevent since the pain induced by prolonged traction, especially at unaffected joints, forced constant adjustment. After only a short time, the actual traction was non-existent, and it was no great feat of intellect that studies concluded the only benefit probably came as a result of the enforced bed rest that being attached to the apparatus engendered.

With *The O'Connor Technique (tm)* maximum TRACTION is applied largely only at the site of the problem and not necessarily along the entire spine. Sometimes it is unavoidable; however, there is no requirement to apply TRACTION to unaffected discs. It is any wonder why traction studies showed no increased benefit. Weights were strapped to a person's waist and every vertebrae below the center of gravity was stretched to straighten the spine beyond the neutral (mildly extended) configuration. Thereby, the discs were allowed to move further posteriorly-- negating any benefit gained by the stretching that would have moved them centrally by the negative pressure created.

The TRACTION employed in *The O'Connor Technique (tm)* eliminates the counter-productivity of conventional traction yet maximizes the beneficial and therapeutic effects of the simple act of traction when intelligently and appropriately applied. **Throughout this book, TRACTION will be referred to and employed by various positionings that place the specific problem areas of the spine in true traction causing them to be stretched for therapeutic benefit.** As these positions are mastered, the pain relieving result will convince even the skeptic that traction, still, (despite "scientific evidence" to the contrary) exists as an age-old, long-ignored, therapeutic modality if properly employed.

Although, for the most part, it is with precise positioning of only the weight of body parts that TRACTION is employed to affect specific disc units; **sometimes, PASSIVE TRACTION supplied solely by the weight of the body (albeit necessary) is not sufficient.** In those difficult cases requiring TRACTION to be maximized, the **other muscular areas of the body (such as the hands, arms, or legs) can be used to push or pull the body away from the putative disc.** This would best be considered as ACTIVE TRACTION. By experience, I have found that **sometimes the weight of the body has to be assisted into generating the tractive force capable of moving particularly difficult-to-centralize, herniated, disc material.** During the MANEUVERS Chapter, attention will be directed towards the ways the arms, legs, or other parts of the body can be brought to bear, producing ACTIVE TRACTION at the point in the MANEUVER's directions where it becomes pertinent. However, in general, it is worthwhile to understand that, **if a particular disc problem is not being solved, it could be that you are not generating sufficient TRACTION or you are not allowing yourself to relax properly** to let the body's weight succeed in the TRACTION effect. I would recommend that the reader be cognizant of this reality, and consider the need for increasing ACTIVE TRACTION to its bearable maximum whenever doing the MANEUVERS that rely upon TRACTION for success.

FLEXION IN TRACTION is the positioning that accounts for the most influential movement of disc material; so it will be covered first. However, in order to maximize the stretching, a short course in RELAXATIONAL BREATHING is necessary to insure that, in every MANEUVER in which you apply TRACTION, it is done efficiently with the highest probability of benefit.

RELAXATIONAL BREATHING

It may, at first, sound like something more befitting a yoga book, but **the controlled and intentional practice of effective breathing contributes greatly to the success of TRACTION** during nearly all of the MANEUVERS in *The O'Connor Technique (tm)*. For brevity's sake, I have elected to make a separate heading to talk about its importance so that it can be applied during all the times when maximum relaxation wishes to be achieved to effect a maximal TRACTION whether ACTIVE or PASSIVE.

While attempting the MANEUVERS, **if the muscles acting on a disc unit are not totally relaxed during the TRACTION phase, the paraspinous musculatures' contraction will prevent the disc spaces from opening to allow for movement of the discs.** For a lot of patients and for a variety of reasons, relaxing the muscles of the spine during the MANEUVERS is easier said than done. It is unrealistic to expect a simple telling-of-yourself to relax to be effective, especially when in painful spasm or fearful that any movement will result in increased pain. Therefore, learning <u>how</u> to relax the spinal muscles becomes imperative.

I have found that the act of exhaling, for some, undoubtedly necessary, physiological, reason, is naturally, automatically, and fortuitously coupled with a generalized relaxation of the spinal musculature. Perhaps it is necessary to have this involuntary mechanism operative to insure that the body is capable of exhaling without active muscular contraction commands from the brain. As the process of exhaling proceeds, it appears necessary for the body to relax muscles in order to effectively achieve the automatic exhaustion of gases from the lungs. One doesn't have to consciously tell one's muscles to exhale, nor does it require the contraction of any muscles. It proceeds automatically, once the action of exhaling is initiated, through a generalized relaxation of the breathing muscles as well as the numerous other muscle groups of the body attached to the spine.

This effect on the spinal muscles can be capitalized upon to achieve a prolonged moment of near total spinal musculature relaxation which, when applied in combination with some form of sustained TRACTION, allows for the necessary separation of vertebral bodies. I have termed this concept RELAXATIONAL BREATHING.

The synchrony of this RELAXATIONAL BREATHING, combined with TRACTION, is probably one of the easiest, yet most important, techniques to master. First, one must assume the TRACTION position best suited for whatever level of the spine is being worked upon (these are provided during the MANEUVER directions). The tractor weights of the body on either side of the disc in question for PASSIVE TRACTION or a preparation of the arms, legs, etc. for the application of ACTIVE TRACTION through the use of other muscle groups must be pre-positioned before initiating the process. Once the body is positioned to allow for TRACTION by gravity or by the active use of the extremities to separate the spinal vertebrae, a deep breath is taken by inhaling air until the chest is fully raised and as much air fills the lungs as comfortably possible. This volume of air is held for a second while a conscious effort to relax the muscles surrounding the affected segment is initiated. After the mental command is given to relax the segment, then exhale deeply, slowly, and automatically. By that, I mean to say, do not forcefully blow the air out (that would require an active contraction command to the chest muscles); rather, just close your mouth and let the breath escape through your nose by letting the chest wall relax. The natural recoil of the chest walls will (without effort) allow the air to be expelled.

It is during the time that exhaling is occurring that the spinal muscles automatically relax because, while the chest wall muscles are totally relaxing to let the air out, the remainder of the muscles of the spine also coincidentally relax. It is almost as if the instant that the command from the brain goes out to let the chest wall relax, a wave of relaxation continues on to other muscle groups of the spine. This wave of relaxation can actually be felt and encouraged to increase its duration by intentionally and consciously prolonging the duration that the chest wall stays in relaxation. The longer it takes for the air to get out, the longer the "command" of relaxation is in force and, consequently, the longer the duration of spinal relaxation. Letting the air out very slowly by limiting the flow as it passes through the back of the mouth can prolong the time the muscles are caused to stay in relaxation. The practical maximum amount of TRACTION can only be achieved by performing this sequential breathing/relaxation method while coordinating it with the TRACTION effort.

Now, it is important, once the relaxation is achieved, to not destroy the effect by

immediately tensing up again. Once the relaxation has occurred at a particular segment, the goal is to maintain that relaxation by consciously avoiding any contraction of muscles acting at that segment. If you are going to gently perform any therapeutic MANEUVER such as THERAPEUTIC CIRCUMDUCTION, NARROW-ARC ROCKING, etc. (as described later), try to move only the body parts distant to the actual disc in question so as to **move the putative disc unit without actually using the muscles** attached to it. This is not as confusing as it sounds. In the case of a Lumbar disc, you can simply move only the muscles of hip girdle and legs or use the arms when the Cervical vertebrae are in TRACTION. When you move the upper trunk or legs, by default, the spinal segment in question can be made to circumduct without contracting muscles attached to it. **As soon as the CIRCUMDUCTION is finished go right back to consciously relaxing.** If the relaxation or subsequent TRACTION is not complete, **repeat the breathing sequence again and again until the disc unit is fully relaxed before proceeding with the movement.**

The significance of this manifests itself later, but when one is using an ACTIVE TRACTION such as in the case of pulling one's head and neck off of the shoulders for a Cervical disc traction or pushing the hips away in a hip hang to effect a maximum amount of inter-spinous separation, **the lifting or pushing should be done at and during the time that the air is being expelled from the lungs.** Immediately, as the initial volume of air is exiting the lungs, begin the active TRACTION and continue to apply force until the air is completely expelled. Then, for the few seconds following the complete expulsion of air, the spinal segment in question should be at its maximum amount of relaxation and, therefore, separation. Every effort should be made to keep this maximum amount of traction applied while relaxation is in effect. This is the best time to expect the peripheral ligaments of the annulus fibrosus to come to their maximum longitudinal or axial length, the central suction of the nucleus pulposus to occur, and any THERAPEUTIC CIRCUMDUCTION to begin. The consequent centralized movement of the disc material can be aided by gentle THERAPEUTIC CIRCUMDUCTIONAL and rotatory twisting movements, wriggles, gyration-like, or "hula" dance-like motions while TRACTION is sustained.

Actually coordinating the THERAPEUTIC CIRCUMDUCTION IN TRACTION with a long-exhalation makes it more effective. You take a big breath, start to exhale, then do the THERAPEUTIC CIRCUMDUCTION while you apply TRACTION. You continue to slowly exhale while you apply more traction and continue the THERAPEUTIC CIRCUMDUCTION. Then, as the last of the air is leaving, you stop the CIRCUMDUCTION and let the last bit of relaxation take advantage of a sustained TRACTION. Then, go on with whatever other motions are required by the particular MANEUVER while keeping the segment relaxed as long as needed.

This maximum effect cannot last forever. After all, you have to take another breath eventually. After the TRACTION is completed is an ideal time to initiate small, non-forceful and gentle contractions of the extensor muscles described later under the general heading of THERAPEUTIC EXTENSIONS but also includes the SEQUENTIAL ARCHING EXTENSIONS. This helps to "milk" or squeeze the disc material centrally if you imagine that you are trying to "trap" the disc material with the peripheral edges of the adjoining vertebral bodies of the disc in question as described in the "INCH-WORM" technique. By practicing and repeating this RELAXATIONAL BREATHING method in conjunction with the TRACTION and EXTENSION techniques, the efficiency of these MANEUVERS can be increased. With repetition, you will learn to coordinate the RELAXATIONAL BREATHING with the TRACTION so that you can instantly relax any particular segment, put it in maximum traction; and, then, perform an EXTENSION MANEUVER rapidly, effectively, and with little effort, whenever and wherever you need. If your disc material has not migrated "out" very far, this is often all the effort it takes to put it back "in."

Anytime you recognize disc discomfort, this combination of moves can be done while sitting in a chair with your arms holding your upper body off the surface, against a table while standing, or against a horizontal railing you are leaning your back against. You can use the fender of a car, a playground raised pull-up bar, or the back of a car seat. Whenever and wherever it is necessary and appropriate to reposition disc material. For instance, with a Lumbar disc herniation problem, just before getting up from an, unintentional, seated slouch posture and is causing discomfort, you can do a light un-weighting TRACTION with your arms. Then, a RELAXATIONAL BREATHING coordinated with a CIRCUMDUCTION MANEUVER (while hanging your spine as shown in the top photo of Figure 22 in this Chapter) would best be followed by an ACTIVE EXTENSION then a RE-WEIGHT BEARING before you get up as in the middle photo in Figure 22. It's hard to imagine, but something as simple as this can stop and prevent the onset of Lumbar back pain. The RELAXATIONAL BREATHING combined with TRACTION gives you that instant of maximum disc opening you need to allow displaced disc material to be manipulated centrally when followed immediately by EXTENSION.

FLEXION IN TRACTION

Even though WEIGHT-BEARING FLEXION is decidedly contraindicated, **FLEXION IN TRACTION is the most effective means by which extremely peripherally displaced disc material is moved sufficiently to allow for its ultimate re-centralization.** I regard it as one of the techniques that make *The O'Connor Technique (tm)* unique since I know of no patient-performed physical therapy currently in practice intentionally employing this method.

It is not simply a stretching of the spinal ligaments to increase mobility. It is a specifically directed NON-WEIGHT-BEARING FLEXION designed to stretch select ligaments that will intentionally move disc material centrally. What ligaments need to be stretched depend upon where the disc material is situated. The location and orientation of the displaced disc material determines precisely what direction is ideal to physically push the displaced disc material deeper into the central disc space from whence it came.

Most people can perform FLEXION IN TRACTION as an initiating action in any MANEUVER, and everyone who wants to be certain that they have done everything to maximize success should be able to do it without fear of damaging their backs further (pain will be your guide in that decision). However, it probably isn't necessary for those with just slightly off-center discs that don't prolapse or extrude so much as to put direct pressure on the capsule. **I have found that, for most people with significant disc disease that does not respond to simple EXTENSION MANEUVERS, this FLEXION IN TRACTION is necessary for consistently achieving relief.** I have even gone so far, in my clinic, as to initiate every manipulation I do with a FLEXION IN TRACTION because I have found that it is largely painless, does no observable harm, and I have had to resort to it so often that I just find it more efficient to prepare the disc for the compulsory EXTENSION MANEUVER that should follow. In that way, I less often have to repeat an EXTENSION MANEUVER because the first one failed due to not being properly prepared by a preliminary FLEXION IN TRACTION.

Later, when these MANEUVERS are described in detail, I start with a FLEXION IN TRACTION movement for each area of the spine so as to educate the reader in the technique, provide the highest probability that the MANEUVER will be successful, and insure that the reader knows how to perform the whole sequence in one series of movements. **Then, if the problem is found to respond sufficiently to only the EXTENSION IN TRACTION components, the FLEXION IN TRACTION can be dropped from the regimen.**

Due to the importance of this concept and the fact that it may only apply to the more difficult back pain problems, I elected to dedicate a separate section describing the process; yet it can be used to initiate every MANEUVER with little harm to be expected except for the need not to stretch the posterior peripheral ligaments unless it is necessary because, by so doing, you reduce the capsule's capacity to maintain a closed position with scarring contractures. The amount of flexion to which any damaged posterior peripheral ligaments are exposed after they have been torn may theoretically inhibit them from forming a tight scar if they are repeatedly stretched. Unfortunately, a person given the choice between staying in pain or fear the theoretical consequence of stretching a scar too much, uniformly selects the immediate pain relieving option. I have seen too many people who cannot get out of pain without using FLEXION IN TRACTION to not recommend it as an initiating movement in any MANEUVER strategy.

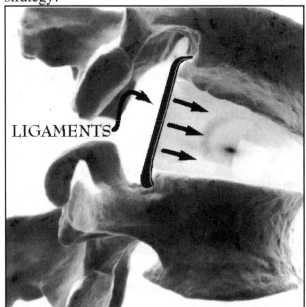

Figure 30 Anterior FLEXION IN TRACTION selectively tightens posterior ligaments pushing adjacent material centrally.

Another reason I treat it separately is because flexion can sometimes seem to be an ubiquitous enemy. Say, for instance, a person has several disc protrusions in the same general area of the spine but at different levels from separate injuries. In one instance, **the flexion (even unweighted) necessary to put "in" one disc may push an adjacent disc "out," especially if its decentralization or herniation propensity is towards the opposite side.** This should be anticipated, especially if there is a history of several significant traumatic events causing pain in the same general area yet on opposite sides. Often when this is the case, pain at a different level is induced when flexion is forced. **If this is the case, proceed with caution and stop if any excessive pain is induced by FLEXION IN TRACTION.** In that case, it may be better for that person to rely just on the TRACTION/EXTENSION components of the MANEUVERS; however, I think this is an uncommon enough situation to only mention it in passing.

Theoretically, **in order for a piece of fragmented central disc material to cause persistent pain (enough to seek medical attention), the herniation has to have put sustained, non-spontaneously-remediable, pressure on the peripheral ligamentous structures** because that is the only portion of the disc that is innervated and capable of experiencing direct pressure pain. If it is putting that much pressure on the peripheral ligaments and hasn't improved with bed rest, chiropractic manipulation, or "conservative management," then it probably must be lodged between the rim portions of the vertebral bodies. When that is the case, a patient usually needs that extra FLEXION IN TRACTION "push" to get the disc material ideally positioned for the EXTENSION MANEUVERS to be effective.

The mechanism by which FLEXION IN TRACTION functions is purely mechanical and equivalent to the way in which an Eskimo blanket toss game works. An object (the Eskimo=disc material) comes in contact with a piece of fabric (the blanket=the peripheral ligamentous capsule) causing it to bow away from the object. The bowed piece of fabric is pulled straight and an object in contact with that fabric is moved in the same direction that the fabric pushes it when the fabric is pulled to its full length.

As seen in Figure 30, when a disc unit is anteriorly flexed, the posterior ligamentous elements are caused to tighten. This tightening brings the ligaments to full length causing whatever adjacent material to feel pressure to move anteriorly. In the weight-bearing state, FLEXION is to be considered the enemy of a herniation damaged disc; however, this is not ordinary FLEXION. This FLEXION is combined with TRACTION and is very specific in the ligaments that are stretched. **The traction component of FLEXION IN TRACTION separates the vertebral bodies and gives the peripheralized disc material a space into which it can be moved more centrally.** The space is created when the tunnel of the fissure through which the disc material originally traveled to get to the periphery is opened as traction separates the vertebral bodies. Otherwise, the weight of the body would keep this space closed. TRACTION opens it; and FLEXION maximally stretches the posterior ligaments more so than just TRACTION alone.

The specificity of the direction in which the FLEXION IN TRACTION is aimed determines which ligaments are tightened the most and, consequently, the direction in which the disc material is moved. If one flexes to the right anterior, the left posterior ligaments would be tightened the most. So, to get disc material that has herniated or protruded to the left posterior (as in Chapter 2 Figure 17) periphery

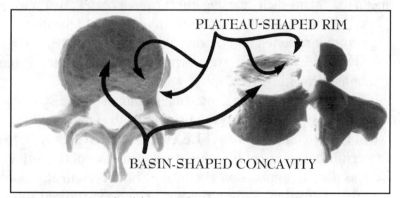

Figure 31 Vertebral bone's disc surface anatomy

to move more centrally, one would want to FLEX IN TRACTION to the right anterior.

Physically, the disc material isn't moved more than a few millimeters, but it doesn't have to be moved much at all. It only needs a little nudge to get it into position for other MANEUVER actions to complete the re-centralization. The reasoning is as follows.

When the central disc material becomes herniated so severely through the annulus fibrosus that it is protruding onto or outside of the cylindrical plane of the plateau-like peripheral rims of the vertebral bodies, causing the ligamentous component of the peripheral annulus fibrosus (the capsule) to bulge outwardly or to abut against the posterior longitudinal ligament, simple UNWEIGHTING or TRACTION is often insufficient to accomplish a re-positioning of the disc towards the center enough to allow an EXTENSION MANEUVER to be successful.

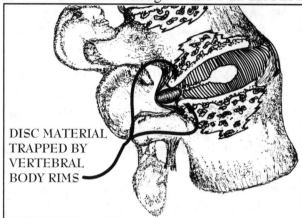

Figure 32 Disc material trapped in WEIGHT-BEARING EXTENSION due to its position beyond rims of vertebral bodies

You see, the vertebral bodies have rims of somewhat flattened surfaces forming plateau shaped surfaces before becoming the basin-like concavity towards the center (See Figure 31). The displaced disc material can become lodged in this narrow but important region, and unaided EXTENSIONS will not be sufficient to mobilize it. EXTENSIONS rely, in large part, upon the effect the basin-like, bi-concave, vertebral surfaces have on relatively solid materials. When the edges of two basins are brought closer together like clam-shells closing, as in a WEIGHT-BEARING EXTENSION, material just inside the edge of the concavity will move centrally towards the region of the greatest concavity.

Just as if a clam were biting down on a piece of rubber, if it captures the bulk of it inside the rims, the rubber will continue to move centrally due to the curvature of the two shells' surfaces physically directing its movement by virtue of their shape. If the solid disc material is lodged too peripherally in the areas where this concavity is not present, this EXTENSION-mediated "clam-shell" closing effect cannot occur. In a sense, the clamshell's rims unfortunately "bite" down on it and prevent it from moving. In the disc, when rubbery disc material is in this region or more peripherally, using only a WEIGHT-BEARING EXTENSION can sometimes even pinch or squeeze the material causing it to bulge further against whatever capsular ligaments are retaining it (See Figure 32).

In these situations, a maximum amount of FLEXION while the disc unit is in TRACTION needs to be applied first to re-position the disc material more central to this rim region. That's why I refer to this action as "FLEXION IN TRACTION." **In order to move decentralized disc material enough to get it within the concavities of the adjacent vertebral bodies, tension must be specifically applied on the lateral intervertebral, posterior peripheral ligaments of the annulus, capsular, and/or the posterior longitudinal ligaments so they will push (by their straightening) the disc material inward to a more non-painful, central, position.**

Only extreme FLEXION IN TRACTION will tighten the posterior longitudinal ligaments and the peripheral ligamentous bands of the annulus fibrosus enough to push the disc material closer to the center so that a, later, EXTENSION will be successful in moving the disc material the rest of the way to a re-centralized position.

When all else seems to have failed with simple TRACTION followed by EXTENSION

MANEUVERS, this exaggerated FLEXION IN TRACTION may be the only means to mobilize the displaced disc material. Agreed, it is, in essence, a FLEXION which stretches scarred posterior peripheral ligamentous structures thereby potentially increasing their laxity: however, there seems to be no other way of reconciling this dilemma when the disc material has moved to that "no-man's land" area of the disc. By far and away, though, to do so is not nearly as detrimental as WEIGHT-BEARING FLEXION.

It is important, therefore, to use FLEXION IN TRACTION judiciously and limit its use to only when pain makes it necessary. Remember, these movements are not exercises. They are only required when the disc material has been displaced sufficiently to cause pain. **To determine if your particular disc material has migrated into that narrow, yet exceptionally important region that requires FLEXION IN TRACTION, there are a few findings that can lead you to conclude it has**. First of all, simple TRACTION/EXTENSION MANEUVERS (like the one described above referencing Figure 22 in this Chapter) don't work to immediately and remarkably alleviate the pain. Second, if the disc material is in this position, **an EXTENSION to the same side as (or directly over) the protrusion/herniation will result in a pinching or wedge-like pain upon RE-WEIGHT-BEARING IN EXTENSION at the end of a MANEUVER**.

Recall, **when CIRCUMDUCTING after a simple TRACTION/EXTENSION MANEUVER to test the MANEUVER's successfulness, you run into the same ARREST OF CIRCUMDUCTION motion in EXTENSION, it is because you have not sufficiently centralized the disc material.** The most plausible reason for these failures is because the decentralized disc material is situated too far peripherally and is being compressed by the flat surfaces of the peripheral rims of the vertebral bodies. In these instances, the best recommendation I can give is that **FLEXION IN TRACTION must be used whenever simple TRACTION going into EXTENSION MANEUVERS give no relief**. In actual practice, for the first-time MANEUVER user and the patients I see in my practice, I have learned that the FLEXION IN TRACTION is so often necessary that I nearly always recommend its initial use.

Whenever FLEXION IN TRACTION is used, **the anterior spinal flexion at the putative disc level should be aimed 180 degrees away (that is, directly opposite) from the center of the area of arrested DIAGNOSTIC CIRCUMDUCTION**. This may sound technical, but it only means that the maximum amount of FLEXION should be focused such that the posterior ligamentous structures are maximally stretched directly over the site of the herniation/protrusion and, by definition, that would be the site of the most pain and arrest in DIAGNOSTIC CIRCUMDUCTION.

For example, if the disc material is protruded to the left posterior, DIAGNOSTIC CIRCUMDUCTION should be arrested in this area (as depicted in Chapter 3 Figure 6) and pain should be felt more on the left than the midline or right. When the disc is protruding to the left, the left posterior ligaments should be the ones purposely caused to stretch when FLEXION IN TRACTION is employed by flexing to the right anterior because when you flex to the right anterior, the left posterior ligaments are maximally stretched. The more to the left the pain is felt, the more you would want to stretch the posterior left-sided ligaments by flexing more to the right.

The ideal to be sought here is to preferentially stretch those ligaments directly abutting against the protruded disc material so that the stretching achieves its maximum, directed, efficiency at moving the disc material more towards the center of the disc. Stretching other ligaments serves little purpose, so **a person should try to become sensitive and cognizant of the exact position of the displaced disc material so that a FLEXION IN TRACTION can be accomplished directly "over" the prolapsed or herniated material.** This is the reason why it is important to understand the concepts of DIAGNOSTIC CIRCUMDUCTION in Chapter 3. Unless you can picture in your mind where the displaced disc material is resting relative to the vertebral bodies, you can't logically approach the correction. Of course, you can still do the appropriate MANEUVER without really understanding what is going on at a logical, anatomical, level; however, if you do understand it to that extent, the task is made much more easy and you can usually think your way around any difficulties, seeming inconsistencies, or times when improvising becomes necessary.

ROPE-ASSISTED TRACTION

Achieving the sufficient TRACTION force for either FLEXION, EXTENSION, or CIRCUMDUCTION and sustaining it long enough to be effective is not always a simple task. **When a segment of anatomy has not been moved in a particular manner for a long time or if it is painful, it takes gentle, controlled, and judicious forces applied patiently over a time period long enough to effect change.** Most often, this requires assistance since, oddly enough, humans were not born with all the devices necessary for a comfortable life nor were they all born with enough money to make life as comfortable as they would like. That's why I've chosen to write the following, simple and cheap method to effect self-induced TRACTION rather than engage in the development of expensive devices which most people couldn't afford.

Don't be instantly put off by the complexity of the directions. You may not even require the use of such a degree of TRACTION. Too, after awhile, you may not need to use the rope at all because you will get so good at doing it by yourself. Whatever, don't assume that it is too complicated and turn yourself off to learning it. If you look at the diagrams, the whole thing is quite simple. My only vice in writing this is that I have tried to cover every contingency. You may not even need to get this complex to solve your problem if it is simple and not requiring of a lot of TRACTION. **The problem without using the loop-knotted rope method that I describe here, though, is that when you try to hold on to the bed sheets or a simple length of rope, you may end up inadvertently contracting the muscles of the back. This can defeat the TRACTION effect on the separation of the disc space; yet some people (including myself) are often able to sufficiently relax the back muscles while simply grasping a length of rope secured to the bed frame.** You could try to have someone hold onto your legs or arms; however, even the most devoted helper gets tired and bored long before you have hung long enough to achieve the effect. So, all things considered, the reader is best served using the loop-knotted rope method described below. I have tried to make it as simple as possible.

The **most effective and cheapest traction assistance device** I could conceive of is a bed and a rope or, more comfortably, a mover's-type strap. The bed needs to be a standard box-spring and mattress type with at least one free side over which you can hang your body (preferably a side with enough adjacent room to allow you to exit that side or end of the bed in the mornings when getting out of bed). The bed should be high enough off the floor so that you can hang half of your body over the edge yet not hit the floor with your knees. This is the standard height of a bed and mattress such that the mattress surface is about 6-10 inches above the knees.

The strap or rope should be strong enough to support the entire weight of the body if necessary. A woven nylon strap is ideal, but as this might incur greater expense than necessary, any rope, the thicker the better, will suffice. It should be somewhat longer than twice the length of the bed but not nearly three times its length (too much rope gets in the way). The blanket can be used to wrap around the rope to prevent it from digging into your flesh if you can't find a mover's strap. Heavy clothing will also do, and if you use a strap it is less likely to apply a sharp pressure to the skin.

One end of the rope needs to be secured to the opposite side of the bed from which you intend to hang over. This can be done easiest by tying one end to the frame underneath the head of the bed and draping the rest of the rope over the bed so you can hang over the foot. **At about the top third of the bed, make a loop out of about two feet of the rope and tie a knot with the loop** (See Figure 33). **The free end is then passed through the knotted loop making a large lasso/sling.**

Lumbar and Lower Thoracic

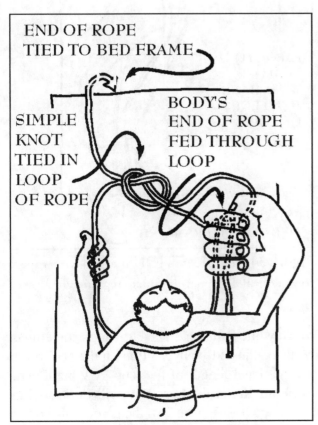

Figure 33 Rope with loop-knot in bed for Lumbar and lower Thoracic TRACTION.

Text inside figure:
END OF ROPE TIED TO BED FRAME
SIMPLE KNOT TIED IN LOOP OF ROPE
BODY'S END OF ROPE FED THROUGH LOOP

To achieve traction of the Lumbar and Lower Thoracic spine, the large lasso/sling is **slung over the back and under the arms**. The length of the sling component of the rope can then be adjusted by pulling on the free end after it passes through the small loop. **Grasping the rope at the point where it passes through the small loop lets you hold yourself at any particular position on the bed while only having to contract the muscles of your strongest hand.** By simply relaxing your grip, you can let out more rope as you start to hang to adjust the point where your body is hanging over the edge of the bed. The point where the body bends over the edge of the bed is the site where the FLEXION IN TRACTION of the spine will occur. **By adjusting your position on the bed (superiorly or inferiorly), you can change the spinal level at which the maximum amount of FLEXION IN TRACTION is applied. To observe this rope apparatus in proper use, turn to the first few Figures in the MANEUVERS Chapter's "HIP-HANG"** Section.

Disc pain in the **Cervical and Upper Thoracic regions** require you to **hang your upper body over the edge of the bed with the legs fixed so you don't slide off the edge of the bed**. The simplest way to accomplish this is by tying a knot in a loop of rope and fastening one end of the rope to the bed frame. The loop, created with a single over-hand knot, need be only just wide enough to slip your foot through. The rope should be tied to the bed frame so that the loop is positioned at about the site your foot would rest when you are hanging your head over the edge of the bed.

In another, more complicated method (that allows you to more accurately adjust the length of the rope) the rope is knotted in basically the same way as described in the Lumbar and Lower Thoracic method above, only, instead of looping the large lasso/sling around your body, you **pass your foot through the large loop and hook the heel** or the knee with it. The foot is better to hang from than the knee because you can then use flexion of your knee to generate more traction and you can roll easier if hanging by your heel. However, hanging with your heel takes dexterity and calf strength. If you find using just your heel to hang by too uncomfortable or too much of an energy expenditure, the lasso loop can be made so small that the foot is trapped from leaving the loop. This may require some adjustment of the length of the end tied to the bed frame, but it lets you hang more freely.

Now, getting to the point where you can hang by your heel may take some adjusting to accommodate for the length of your body. You can adjust the size of the larger loop to the point where it can easily be kicked off of the foot yet be small enough to

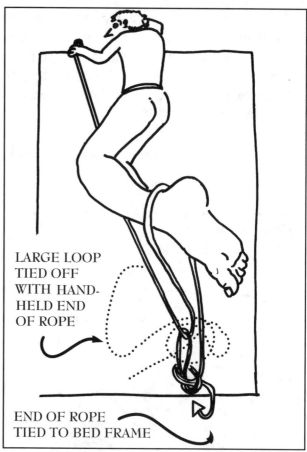

LARGE LOOP TIED OFF WITH HAND-HELD END OF ROPE

END OF ROPE TIED TO BED FRAME

Figure 34 Bed TRACTION method with rope for Cervical or upper Thoracic regions.

be able to stop the foot and heel from slipping through while hanging. The large loop sometimes needs to be tied off at the proper length once you have adjusted your position on the bed to the ideal configuration. You can test the set-up to find the ideal length of the loop by lying down, **hanging your head over the end of the bed to about the site where you will be inducing TRACTION while holding onto the free end of the rope** (See Figure 34), then, you **tighten the free end of the rope to the point where it is comfortably able to hold your body at the right position relative to the edge of the bed. After you have arrived at the ideal loop size and** length, you can get up, tie off the large loop so it won't act like a lasso to freely increase its size when your weight is on it and **adjust the entire apparatus if necessary to be certain that you can hang your head and shoulders over the edge at the right site**. The loop of rope's size usually needs to be fixed with another knot made with the free end of rope (as indicated by dotted lines in the Figure 34 diagram) so that it can hold you without the use of your hands, since both hands will be needed for generating TRACTION at the neck. This heel-loop knot apparatus in use is portrayed in the Thoracic (Chest) Pain Maneuvers Section's Figure 5 and the Cervical (Neck) Pain Maneuvers Section's Figure 8.

BE VERY CERTAIN THAT YOU ARE CAREFUL USING THE ROPE. UNTIL YOU ARE COMPETENT AND ABSOLUTELY COMFORTABLE WITH USING A ROPE FOR TRACTION, IT SHOULD BE ONLY DONE IN THE COMPANY OF SOMEONE WHO CAN COME TO YOUR AID IF YOU GET TANGLED OR DISTRESSED IN ANY WAY. IF HANGING OVER THE EDGE OF THE BED WITH YOUR HEAD DOWN CAUSES DIZZINESS OR VERTIGO, STOP AT ONCE. YOU MAY HAVE SOME BLOOD VESSEL PROBLEM IN YOUR NECK OR BRAIN. SEE A DOCTOR BEFORE ATTEMPTING IT AGAIN.

The intensity of the traction is controlled by how much weight the hanging part of the body is allowed to apply to the rope-fixed part. The weight of the body that hangs over the edge of the bed supplies the tractor force, but the legs' or arms' bearing some of that weight can control how much force is exerted on any specific segment.

NARROW-ARC ROCKING

NARROW-ARC ROCKING is a rather simple but effective technique that relies upon applying progressive areas of tension on the peripheral ligamentous capsule to partially centralize disc material. When a disc is placed in FLEXION IN TRACTION, the up-side ligaments are stretched to their full length and, in so doing, peripheralized disc material is moved centrally a small amount, enough to get it out of the plateau like rim area and into the concavity so that an EXTENSION, performed later, will work.

Unfortunately, one cannot be certain that the ligamentous structures are directly over the particular piece of disc material that needs to be centralized. Due to the inaccuracy of sensory input, one could be ineffectively stretching ligamentous material adjacent to the ideal ligaments that would be able to put direct pressure on the protruding disc material. Therefore, it is necessary to "hedge" your anatomical "bets." By that, I mean that you must make every effort to insure that the precise ligamentous fibers directly over the displaced disc material are brought to full length so that their centrally directed pressure can move the disc material centrally.

This is insured by rolling <u>the entire torso</u> on both sides of the problem disc slightly in one direction through a short arc, stopping, and then rolling in the opposite direction in a sort of rocking motion while FLEXION IN TRACTION is maintained (See Figure 35). On a micro-anatomical level, when a disc unit is placed in FLEXION IN TRACTION only the uppermost ligamentous structures are stretched maximally. As the roll is executed, fibers of the ligamentous capsule adjacent to those being stretched in simple FLEXION IN TRACTION are

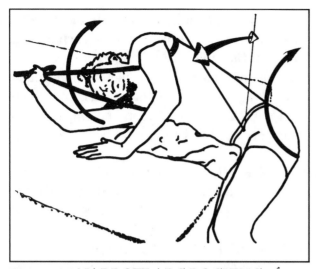

Figure 35 NARROW-ARC ROCKING of Lumbar disc

stretched more than previously. Even though only millimeters apart, each degree of the arc through which the disc unit is rolled causes progressively adjacent capsular fibers to be stretched in succession (See Figure 36). Instead of just a few fibers being stretched, ultimately, when the rolling completes an arc in one direction and then the other, the whole of the segment of the peripheral capsule that constitutes the "up" side of the disc's periphery is brought to full length. This insures that the whole of the area capable of having sustained a herniation is afforded the benefit of a stretching of the peripheral capsule directly contiguous with the herniation or protrusion.

Stretching the peripheral ligaments, as one may recall, pushes the adjacent peripheralized disc material more centrally. It doesn't have to push it much, but when the disc material is that far "out" it needs that little push to get it closer to the center enough for other strategies to work.

In other words, NARROW-ARC ROCKING can be envisioned as if a preferential area of maximum tension is being placed upon the "up" side of the disc and passed back and forth over its surface in a circumferential pattern to push peripheralized disc material centrally.

This NARROW-ARC ROCKING while the disc is in FLEXION IN TRACTION with the painful side up is very closely related to, and could be defined as a subtype of PASSIVE THERAPEUTIC CIRCUMDUCTION because, in essence, this is a circumduction effected without the use of muscles contracting at or near the problem disc site. More explicitly and technically it should be termed SHORT ARC PASSIVE THERAPEUTIC CIRCUMDUCTION IN TRACTION; however, it is so much easier to describe it as simply "ROCKING." It is just as adequately described as a "rocking" and "rolling" of the disc rather than a "hula" dance because with the "hula" the circumduction is more of an active motion because the muscles of circumduction contiguous with the disc unit are being activated. In contradistinction, when NARROW-ARC ROCKING is accomplished, the muscles that would otherwise perform ACTIVE THERAPEUTIC CIRCUMDUCTION are relaxed. With the muscles relaxed during NARROW-ARC ROCKING, the disc is afforded the highest possible amount of TRACTION to be co-existing with movements that do not require the contraction of muscles. This increases the probability that disc material will be centralized because the maintained traction insures that the mobilized disc material has a volume of space to move into.

When performing a NARROW-ARC ROCKING motion, it is only necessary to roll through a short or narrow arc of movement. The arc is, in this case, defined as if the disc were a circle and the range of motion through which one rocks or rolls is like a pie section of this circle with the center of the disc at the pointed part of the pie shape and the arc of movement is described as the distance traveled along the circumference. The associated angle (See Figure 35)

168

of this arc is the angle through which the entire torso travels. Since the spine is in a lateral bend (FLEXION IN TRACTION), the disc is not just rolling, but CIRCUMDUCTING back and forth through a described arc usually no greater than 60 degrees.

Allowing the roll to proceed into a prone or supine position (90 degrees of arc) or into full EXTENSION (180 degrees of arc) is not desired nor achieved during this movement. The full roll serves a different purpose. The purpose of NARROW-ARC ROCKING is to preferentially tighten a specific area of the uppermost component of the disc's peripheral ligaments to insure that prolapsing disc material is replaced into the concavity region of the adjacent vertebrae. This small but significant component of the total movement of the decentralized disc material is often essential for successful pain relief.

THERAPEUTIC CIRCUMDUCTION

As mentioned earlier, in SELF-DIAGNOSING YOUR DISC a circumduction is utilized to determine the site and orientation of displaced disc material. In that context, circumduction can be considered "DIAGNOSTIC CIRCUMDUCTION;" however, circumduction will be put to an additional use during *The O'Connor Technique (tm)* MANEUVERS described later. These are referred to more specifically as "THERAPEUTIC CIRCUMDUCTIONS" because they are capable of relieving pain. **THERAPEUTIC CIRCUMDUCTIONS are more often used concurrently with TRACTION but can be used as well in concert with WEIGHT-BEARING situations, all with the same purpose intended--to intentionally and specifically move disc material.** Just as in DIAGNOSTIC CIRCUMDUCTION, there are ACTIVE and PASSIVE forms. The ACTIVE form would be when you are using your paraspinous muscles associated with the problem disc to effect the movement, and the PASSIVE form would be when the muscles are relaxed such as when you are lying down and rolling over while keeping those muscles relaxed.

Perhaps the most beneficial THERAPEUTIC CIRCUMDUCTION, as you will learn later, is done when the spine is relaxed in TRACTION (hanging over the edge of a bed) and you roll from a prone to a supine position. This is most accurately referred to as a PASSIVE THERAPEUTIC CIRCUMDUCTION because the muscles contiguous with the disc being circumducted are not actually activated during the rolling in TRACTION; rather, they are relaxed and that particular disc going through the circumduction does so passively.

Understanding the function and usefulness of THERAPEUTIC CIRCUMDUCTION to centralize disc material is sometimes essential because, as you will learn later, it is not always possible to move a disc centrally with a straightforward, isolated, TRACTION, FLEXION, or EXTENSION MANEUVER. The displaced disc material did not always migrate "**out**" simply by a straight path as it "tunneled" through the broken layers of the annulus fibrosus. Many times, (as in Figure 7, Chapter Three) the disc material is trapped by laminations of annulus fibrosus and prevented from moving along a straight path to the center again. THERAPEUTIC CIRCUMDUCTION overcomes this difficulty and is one of the only ways to move disc material circumferentially.

However, one relative certainty is that the quasi-Newtonian/Monty Python axiom applies here: **What goes "out" must come "in."** One must solve or master the "puzzle" or find the "combination" to this natural "lock mechanism." There are a few assumptions that, if you make within reason, you can be sure that you will have given yourself the best probability of figuring out the right combination of movements. First, when central disc material migrates, **one must assume that it has moved from the center to a position more towards the posterior periphery**. It can be somewhat laterally positioned as is probably more often the case; but, by and large, it is most often situated posterior to the central region it once occupied. **Whenever the displaced material has a lateral component to its position (that is, any herniation other than directly to the midline posterior), one may assume that the laterally directed damaging forces have more than likely moved the discs posterio-laterally by a straight path through a radial tear (fissure). However, additional damaging forces could have caused the disc to dissect laterally along a circumferential tear to become lodged within layers of the annulus fibrosus.** In the latter case, when an attempt is made to use a simple EXTENSION to replace it, its movement can be blocked by contact with more centrally placed laminations of the annulus fibrosus. So, to move it ultimately centrally, one must first move the errant disc material along the circumferential tear in the opposite direction that it originally traveled when it became lodged out of place in the first place. Once it returns to the area of the radial tear, it then can be moved centrally with a straight EXTENSION along the axis of the radial tear (See Figure 40). The reader can refresh the memory of this phenomenon by reviewing the mechanism of damage elaborated in Chapter II's section on Disc Herniation Pathology.

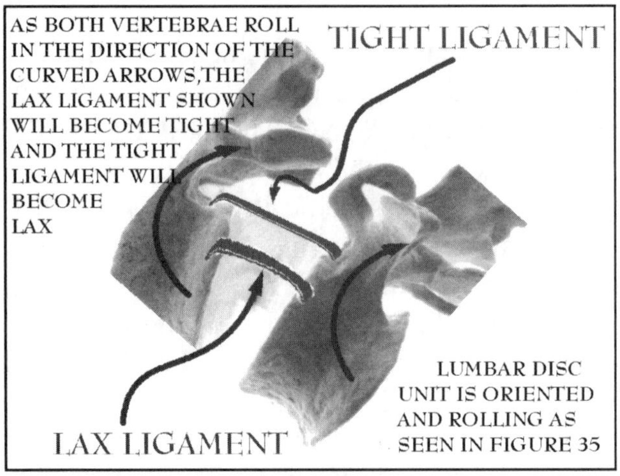

AS BOTH VERTEBRAE ROLL IN THE DIRECTION OF THE CURVED ARROWS,THE LAX LIGAMENT SHOWN WILL BECOME TIGHT AND THE TIGHT LIGAMENT WILL BECOME LAX

TIGHT LIGAMENT

LAX LIGAMENT

LUMBAR DISC UNIT IS ORIENTED AND ROLLING AS SEEN IN FIGURE 35

Figure 36 Close up view of disc unit's posterior ligaments as NARROW-ARC ROCKING puts maximum TRACTION IN FLEXION on upper most ligament.

This may seem exhaustingly complicated to attempt to figure out exactly which direction it moved and, in essence, the design of the "maze." **Yet, you don't really have to figure it out exactly to get the disc material to return to the centrum. Basically, as you perform a THERAPEUTIC CIRCUMDUCTION while the disc is in TRACTION, unweighted, or sometimes while weight-bearing, the progressive pressures created in an ever-advancing posterior direction usually squeeze the disc material centrally because in most instances you are dealing with a simple, straight radially aligned fissure.**

CIRCUMDUCTING clockwise if the displaced material is on the right or counter clockwise if on the left, will serve to force the material back along the axis of the most common simple radial tear through which it previously traveled, by insuring that the forces on the disc material always have a centrally directed vector as a component. The best initial direction of CIRCUMDUCTION is determined by the side to which the pain radiates. **A good rule of thumb is to first CIRCUMDUCT in the direction towards the pain.** By that, I mean that **if the pain is referred to one side (rather than the posterior midline) your first circumduction should be in the direction of that side.** You would, of course, initiate any THERAPEUTIC CIRCUMDUCTION by flexing slightly anteriorly and then "gyrate" towards the side of pain. **If the pain is felt on the right side of the body, you would circumduct the part of the body above the lesion clockwise (that is, if you were looking inferiorly on a clock face superimposed on the disc as delineated in Chapter Three Figure 3), the direction your upper body would be circling would be clockwise. Conversely, if the pain is more on the left side, the upper part of the body should be circumducted counterclockwise.**

I have found this to be correlated with the highest probability of success in actual practice. The rationale for specifically choosing these directions is based upon their having the greatest probability of moving the disc centrally because regardless of any other type of tear of fissure, the herniated disc has to have a radial tear and most likely it is located in the posterior lateral quadrant of the disc.

For instance, if the pain radiates to the left (due to a herniation as pictured in the Figures 17 & 18 in Chapter II) and the site of arrested motion is on the left, the herniation is most probably to the posterior and left of the disc's midpoint. To get it to re-centralize requires that some vector of the force you place on it to move it must come from the far peripheral left and be directed towards the center (which, in this case, is a right-ward moving force). Only forces from the left or posterior moving to the right (midline) and anterior will work to centralize the peripheralized disc material in this instance. The more laterally the disc material has dissected, the more from the left side towards the center the forces must progressively move. In Figure 37, as a counterclockwise circumduction is accomplished, the peripheral parallel surfaces of the vertebral bodies squeeze together in continuous succession from point (A) to point (B), to point (C). Due to the circular shape of the vertebral body's edges, this results in forces that would always tend to move an object at points A, B, or C, in some fashion, centrally along any radially oriented line or tear (fissure).

However, in the same situation, counterclockwise circumduction forces as they proceed around the disc would tend to cause a piece of disc material at points D, E, or F to be moved to the right. This would tend to not cause the displaced disc material at sites D, E, & F to centralize; rather, they would be moved towards the periphery. This is why it is best to start with a counterclockwise circumduction if the pain is on the left and a clockwise CIRCUMDUCTION if on the right.

Similarly, for disc material dissected predominately to the right, a clockwise CIRCUMDUCTION would be best to move

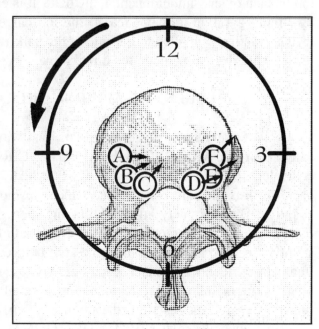

Figure 37 Diagram showing effects of counterclockwise circumduction on disc material at lettered points to move in direction of arrows.

171

disc material centrally. Alternatively, if a clockwise circumduction were tried, for disc material dissected to the left, the successive forces applied would be directed from right to left. As before, this would counter-productively serve to push a left-sided disc protrusion further to the left periphery along a simple radial tear. Theoretically, in the majority of cases involving simple radial tear type fissures, this probably would be counterproductive.

In a slightly different manner in which disc material can be moved circumferentially, this same effect can be accomplished during the MANEUVERS by what is best called ACTIVE THERAPEUTIC CIRCUMDUCTION in which one **progressively changes the point where maximum EXTENSION force is applied in a circumferential pattern by contracting the muscles of extension. In this manner, the FULCRUM EFFECT (described and depicted in Chapter Three, Figure 2) is put to beneficial use by the surfaces of the vertebral bodies putting pressure on disc material to move it. The major difference, here, that doesn't result in pain as the product of this endeavor, is because usually TRACTION is being employed to give the disc material a space to occupy and there is a directionally appropriate force applied. This is accomplished by CIRCUMDUCTING while simultaneously extending, first in one direction (from the most lateral aspect of the painful side to the midline) then, if unsuccessful, trying in the opposite direction.**

To elaborate on this action, if your pain is more on the left, you should start the leaning EXTENSION as far to the left of the midline as possible, you would then circumduct the upper torso counterclockwise towards the midline (as if looking down at a clock face superimposed on the disc) while maintaining the arch so that each point where the maximum EXTENSION force is applied on the vertebral bodies moves progressively closer to the midline as the circumduction proceeds. It is as if one had the task of moving a baseball trapped between two drums stacked on top of each other without touching the ball. It is easy to see that the ball could be moved around by simply gyrating (circumducting) the top barrel. As the pressure increased when the most weight was being applied to the side of the ball, the ball would move circumferentially one way or the other depending upon the direction you gyrated the barrel.

SEQUENTIAL ARCHING THERAPEUTIC CIRCUMDUCTION

Alternatively, to achieve the same end with increased force, you can use an action I call SEQUENTIAL ARCHING THERAPEUTIC CIRCUMDUCTION. "Arching" in this context is equivalent to an ACTIVE EXTENSION , which means contracting the posterior muscles of the back towards the side of reference which, in most instances, is to the posterior, even if only slightly. By alternately arching, relaxing then circumducting a little, arching, relaxing, and circumducting a little more along an arc-like path from one side towards the posterior, each time slightly closer to the midline than the arch before, you can move disc material very selectively. In an almost identical manner, each time you use your back or neck muscles to contract into an arch, you can follow by circumducting a small increment while in full EXTENSION, then relaxing the arch and restarting the arching, again, only the next time moving closer to the midline by an incrementally small CIRCUMDUCTIONAL movement. After each time you arch, you then move the point where the vertebral bodies pinch together an increment more along the periphery of the disc, and then arch again. With each arching movement, you squeeze disc material from

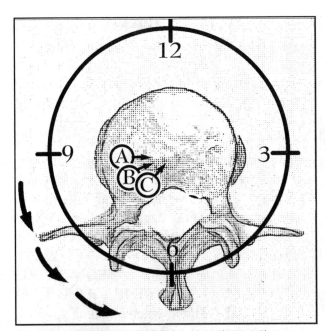

Figure 38 SEQUENTIAL ARCHING
THERAPEUTIC CIRCUMDUCTION
diagram

the periphery towards the center.

As an example of how this would be accomplished, Figure 38 shows a diagram of a disc looking down on it from above. Presuming that the pain is to the left (due to a herniation as pictured in the Figures 17 & 18 in Chapter Two), by arching directly towards the left side of your body (the 9 o'clock position), you would be compressing the vertebral bodies' peripheral rims immediately adjacent and peripheral to point A, serving to push an object at point A centrally. Then, relaxing so as to reduce the degree of lateral bending and EXTENSION you then circumduct slightly towards the posterior to bring you similarly over point B (approximately the 8:00 position). Arching in EXTENSION and leaning directly over point B would compress this point with forces that would move it anteriorly and centrally. Circumducting on to point C (at approximately 7:00) an EXTENSION would serve to move an object at point C more anteriorly towards the center.

If point A had a piece of disc material, the arching would squeeze it, and it would be moved more towards the midline of the body. Then, doing the same thing over point B, would tend to move it towards the midline also. By so doing repeatedly in a counterclockwise sequential pattern, one could move a piece of unseen material within the confines of the disc capsule from left to right (towards the center) and from posterior to anterior (also towards the center) depending upon the path of least resistance. If there were a channel that limited and defined the path the piece of material had to follow as it moved centrally, the squeezing would have to move the material along that path centrally. If the path led directly to the center of the disc because it was a radial tear type of fissure, within which the disc material moved peripherally in the first place, the disc material can expect to be centralized by the sequential squeezing that occurs with the SEQUENTIAL ARCHING THERAPEUTIC CIRCUMDUCTION technique.

In order to completely understand the manner in which this technique functions to move disc material, look above at Figure 38, paying attention especially to point B. This point B is re-represented in Figure 39 where it is superimposed upon a disc in which a herniated piece of disc material is shown. This type of herniation should give pain on the left side. When one arches (extends) towards the 8:00 position during a SEQUENTIAL ARCHING THERAPEUTIC CIRCUMDUCTION the vertebral bodies would preferentially compress directly over point B. When this arching and compressing is directly over point B, the consequence is that disc material should move centrally back along the path it traveled when it displaced. In fact, it would also have been helped on its way by arching at points A and C as well; yet as the SEQUENTIAL

173

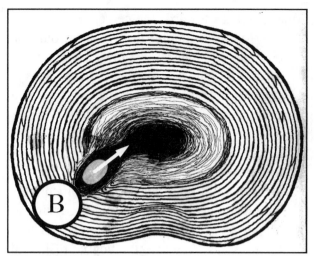

Figure 39 Diagram of disc with simple herniation of disc material that would be moved centrally by compression over point B

ARCHING THERAPEUTIC CIRCUMDUCTION progresses to point B (by virtue of this particular herniation pathway) the disc material is given an in-line straight shot to the center of the disc by the existing radial fissure.

For a clearer picture, Figure 40 shows a three dimensional disc unit arching (extending) towards the left posterior (8:00) position. It demonstrates how arching in that configuration would cause a piece of disc material to move centrally from point B as the schematic diagrams in Figures 38 & 39 describe. During the act of SEQUENTIAL ARCHING THERAPEUTIC CIRCUMDUCTION, when reaching the 8:00 position, the most pressure would be applied immediately peripheral to point B in the diagrams. If the fissure happens to be in line with point B, then the disc material will have little or no resistance and should move centrally when that particular spot is compressed.

Since it is difficult to determine exactly the orientation of the fissure without a painful, costly and invasive diagnostic test (the discogram), using SEQUENTIAL ARCHING THERAPEUTIC CIRCUMDUCTION moves the points where pressure is applied through an arc-like pattern that, in all probability, will eventually apply the necessary pressure at the ideal location to cause disc material re-centralization especially if it wouldn't move with a more simple rolling-in-TRACTION type of PASSIVE CIRCUMDUCTION as described at the beginning of this section.

This works because if all the possible points on the periphery are compressed, it is difficult to miss the ideal one, in spite of not being able to actually see the fissure. By the pain pattern and the results of a DIAGNOSTIC CIRCUMDUCTION one should be able to roughly determine the site of the disc material's displacement and (in the uncomplicated case) it is only a matter of directing your EXTENSION directly over it to squeeze it centrally.

Also, this same sequential arching that moves along points of the periphery of the disc can gently force and move the disc material around between layers of ligamentous tissue in

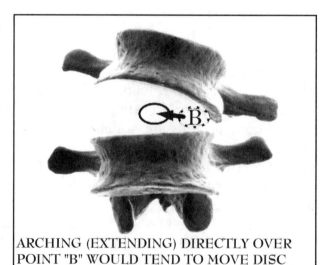

ARCHING (EXTENDING) DIRECTLY OVER POINT "B" WOULD TEND TO MOVE DISC MATERIAL CENTRALLY

Figure 40 Anterior to Posterior view of disc unit shown in EXTENSION towards left posterior

174

a concentric fashion as well. If doing this in one direction isn't helpful, try arching first laterally on the other side and progressively direct the force towards the midline or start at the midline and progressively direct the arch to one side or the other. Feel free to experiment so long as nothing induces pain that shoots down the legs or increases its severity. Make an effort to remember whichever seems to result in favorable disc movement or relief of pain so you can reproduce the same movement again in the future, should the same pain pattern recur and this technique found to be necessary and successful.

This technique is very similar to the PASSIVE THERAPEUTIC CIRCUMDUCTION method. This ACTIVE THERAPEUTIC CIRCUMDUCTION is combined with arching that allows a certain measure of force to be applied, but it is not really much weight-bearing force. It is only the force that your back muscles can generate. If any pain were to intervene, you can instantaneously stop the contraction of muscles to unload the vertebrae a lot easier than UNWEIGHTING after weight-bearing.

Unfortunately, in nature, statistical probabilities are not always applicable to the individual. A person could have a piece of disc material positioned, in a complicated fissure, mostly to the left that dissects into a wing of a "L" shaped circumferential tear which tracts towards the midline (as in Figure 41). In that event, (a counterclockwise THERAPEUTIC CIRCUMDUCTION may only force it to the end of the "L" and not centrally along the radial tear. Therefore, initiating with a clockwise THERAPEUTIC CIRCUMDUCTION (as in Figure 42) would be better to move the disc back to the radial tear. Then, it would take an EXTENSION towards the 8:00 position (directly over point B in Figure 42) to squeeze the disc material centrally along the radial fissure.

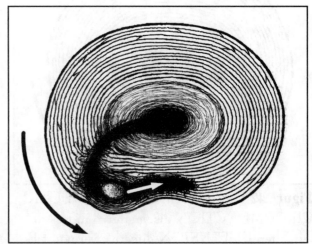

Figure 41 Disc herniation with disc material trapped in a circumferential tear where counterclockwise THERAPEUTIC CIRCUMDUCTION would cause it to move to right.

However, one must assume that complicated tears are in the minority and the result of multiple injuries. In this case, it would have required a forceful traumatic flexion injury with the Lumbar spine having been flexed to the right anterior to create the radial component of the tear and while the disc material was displaced peripherally a flexion injury to the left anterior creating the circumferential tear.

Most readers need not concern themselves with this level of complexity; therefore, only after failing at the THERAPEUTIC CIRCUMDUCTION (which has the highest probability of success) should you feel the need to adopt a more complex strategy.

Nevertheless, the inner sanctum of the degenerating disc could be a quirky, maze-like gamish of broken annular fibers and fragmented disc material that defies description. In that case, clockwise and counterclockwise movements can be alternately tried with various wiggles and EXTENSIONS to try to jiggle the pieces centrally.

175

This descriptive level of complexity may be seen as far too complex to have pertinence to the average reader's disc problem and reading frustration level; so, a simple take home message can make it much simpler: **First try the THERAPEUTIC CIRCUMDUCTION direction that has the highest probability of success (that being if the pain is to the left a counterclockwise CIRCUMDUCTION and if to the right, clockwise) followed by the rest of the EXTENSION/WEIGHT-BEARING MANEUVERS (to be described later), if that doesn't work, then try in the opposite direction and alternate between the two.** Too, one should pay attention to the pain sensations you evoke when doing a PASSIVE THERAPEUTIC CIRCUMDUCTION in any given direction. If the pain appears to move more laterally or medially, then there is a good possibility that you have a piece of disc material moving within a circumferential tear. Then, you will have to play the "BB"-in-the-maze game to re-centralize the disc material, but try to remember (take notes if necessary) the way you did it so that you don't lose the advantage of reproducible results. If still no success, just keep wiggling and jiggling in hopes that random activity will prevail.

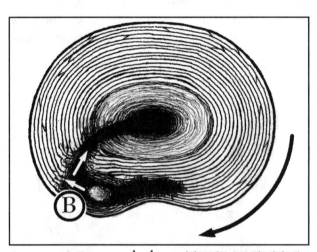

Figure 42 During clockwise THERAPEUTIC CIRCUMDUCTION disc material moves to left, then EXTENSION directly over point B moves material centrally

You may not be able to recall exactly what works because you only "know" it works when you have completed the entire MANEUVER several steps down the way. But, a good policy is that if you feel the "knuckle crunch" of cartilage moving on cartilage at the site you are working, you can assume that you have moved the disc material. If it suddenly makes you feel better, you have done the right thing so be sure to jot down on paper what movements you were doing immediately before achieving success. If a particular series of movements doesn't result in pain relief, keep trying. It should not require forceful action, gentle rolling (PASSIVE THERAPEUTIC CIRCUMDUCTION) in TRACTION, successive contractions and relaxations of the muscles necessary to execute a MANEUVER, or a standing WEIGHT-BEARING THERAPEUTIC CIRCUMDUCTION will usually squeeze the disc material in the direction you wish it to travel.

If one were to observe a person doing these CIRCUMDUCTIONS for a Lumbar disc, the best way of describing the way the hips and back move is to call it a "Hula Dance." When TRACTION is applied it could be called a "Hanging Hula." So, when performing the CIRCUMDUCTION at the Lumbar vertebral levels during the MANEUVERS, one should get into a position that puts TRACTION on the disc unit in question and move your hips as though you were doing a "hula" dance. These ACTIVE THERAPEUTIC CIRCUMDUCTIONS can be tried when you are in FLEXION IN TRACTION, EXTENSION IN TRACTION, or at the very end when you are terminating the whole MANEUVER process in a partially weight-bearing upright EXTENSION "bump and grind" to finally "seat" the disc in its central location.

As will be described later in the MANEUVERS sections, a THERAPEUTIC CIRCUMDUCTION can be used as a final "*coup de grace*" when you are upright. For the Lumbar and Thoracic spine, it is prevented from being a full-weight-bearing event by the placement of the hands on the hips (akimbo) and pushing downwards with the arms. This action lifts the upper torso off of the hips which results in a partial weight-bearing. For the Cervical region the hands can be used to lift the head off of the shoulders. Understand that an injudicious use of full weight-bearing THERAPEUTIC CIRCUMDUCTIONS can potentially move the disc material forcefully into a place that you don't want it to go. By unloading the spine, you have a better chance of getting disc material to move anyhow, because it has some place to migrate into if the disc unit is unweighted. Finally, for the Lumbar spine, a CIRCUMDUCTION IN EXTENSION is performed that looks a lot like a saucy, strip-tease dancer who is showing the audience her anterior pubic region. The hips are thrust forward for the "bump" and the circumduction is the "grind" in the "bump and grind" portion of the dance. Sorry, gentle reader, if this description is not deemed politically correct, but I just can't think of any better way to describe it that is more universally envisionable.

For the Cervical and Thoracic region THERAPEUTIC CIRCUMDUCTIONS, the "hula" analogy doesn't fit. So, the best way I can describe it is to act as though there were a long, imaginary, pencil extending perpendicularly from your forehead with the point on the ceiling. Then, you move as if attempting to draw large ovals on the ceiling. To achieve the UNWEIGHTING when called for, one can hold onto the head and lift it off of the neck with your hands and arms. For UNWEIGHTING the Thoracic region, leaning back on a bed, on the arms of a chair, or some other means so that your elbows are supporting your weight and your upper torso in EXTENSION . In this instance, the movement of circumduction is performed by figuratively drawing the ovals on the ceiling with the entire segment of the torso above the site of pain doing the drawing.

In all instances, the UNWEIGHTING component is gradually and finally withdrawn allowing the disc segment to become progressively more weighted and you determine first, if a fully weighted circumduction can be accomplished in EXTENSION without arrested motion or pain (for all intents and purposes identical to the DIAGNOSTIC CIRCUMDUCTIONS done when determining the site and direction of a protrusion as described in Chapter Three's section on SELF-DIAGNOSING YOUR DISC). If weighted DIAGNOSTIC CIRCUMDUCTION ending in full posterior EXTENSION can be done free of pain and arrest, the disc is probably back "in." If not, keep trying with combinations or MANEUVERS which will be described later.

Do not be concerned if some of this seems too abstract and difficult to understand, as you read the MANEUVERS sections, the conceptual nature of THERAPEUTIC CIRCUMDUCTIONS becomes more concrete. After you have performed the MANEUVER most fitting for your particular disc problem, you can later return to this section for review to better understand the theory of their functioning.

EXTENSIONS

Spinal "EXTENSION" is the opposite of "FLEXION" and constitutes an increase in the angle between two vertebral bones such as when one bends backwards from the anatomical position towards the posterior. If a person bends backwards or posteriorly, the spine is said to perform "EXTENSION;" but here we are largely concerned only with the particular disc unit having a herniation to the posterior. **An EXTENSION movement is one of the more integral components of *The O'Connor Technique (tm)* because it can be employed to move decentralized disc material centrally**. It is covered here as a general principle because it usually follows the FLEXION IN TRACTION MANEUVER, although in reality, **it is probably the most important movement in its ability to efficiently re-centralize disc material**. The manner in which this is accomplished is divided herein into three basic categories: EXTENSION IN TRACTION, WEIGHT-BEARING EXTENSION, and WEIGHT-BEARING HYPER-EXTENSION.

EXTENSION IN TRACTION

EXTENSION IN TRACTION is the position of being in an extended posture while at the same time in TRACTION. In the context of this section it concerns itself only with the disc unit containing decentralized disc material; however, when speaking of EXTENSION in the usual

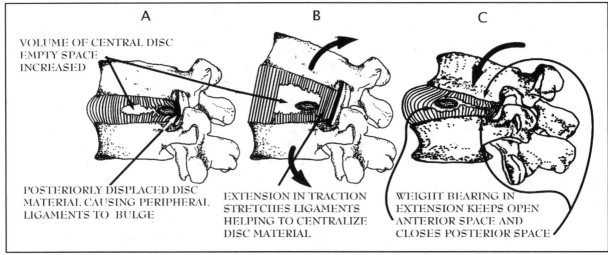

Figure 43 Lateral view of disc unit going from neutral with displaced disc material (A) to EXTENSION IN TRACTION (B) and then to WEIGHT-BEARING IN EXTENSION (C)

sense, the whole spine is usually described as being "extended."

For the purpose of explanation, I would ask the reader to first contemplate the damaged disc unit when it is in the neutral position while weight-bearing. The vertebral bodies are bearing weight and closing the central space or cavity which the solidified nucleus pulposus once occupied before it was displaced to the posterior. The surfaces of the vertebral bodies which are contiguous with the disc are, so to speak, parallel (Refer to Figure 43A).

The action of TRACTION has already previously been discussed in its ability to cause a negative pressure to be generated in the center of the disc as well as with the stretching of the sides straightening the ligaments which push material inwardly. These two actions serve to centralize disc material. Now, while TRACTION is maintained and the disc unit goes into EXTENSION (See Figure 43B), you will note that the central space is increased in volume; however, the posterior space which constitutes the fissure is relatively more closed as the surfaces of the vertebral bodies are relatively closer at the posterior periphery. Any displaced (peripheralized) disc material that has migrated through a tunnel in the annulus fibrosus now is faced with the posterior aspect of that tunnel being closed as EXTENSION occurs, reducing its ability to move both posteriorly and, especially, peripherally. This is the principle action of EXTENSION IN TRACTION. It closes the fissure in the annulus fibrosus at its posterior aspect and gives the displaced disc material no other place to go except anteriorly and centrally because the rims of the vertebral bodies have closed peripherally and posteriorly.

Also, the posterior ligaments are stretched, assisting the anterior movement of the disc material by pushing on them as they straighten. Because TRACTION is maintained, the displaced disc material is insured that it has a place to go further posteriorly. This is why simply extending while weight-bearing as advocated in other programs is not as successful and can even increase the damage. In a large percentage of disc herniations, the disc material is so far peripherally that when an unreasoned WEIGHT-BEARING EXTENSION is accomplished, it can result in the disc material being squeezed further peripherally, causing greater pain or increasing the extent of the protrusion. EXTENSION IN TRACTION prevents that to a large degree.

Additionally, **the simple act of maintaining EXTENSION while IN TRACTION removes hydraulic pressure and FULCRUM EFFECT forces from the disc. Putting a painful disc unit into this configuration has the effect of decreasing pain and serves as one of the best positions of comfort. Not only does the pain become reduced due to the lack of pressure, but the simple positioning, with the disc's posterior periphery being closed and the anterior open, predisposes the displaced disc material for spontaneous centralization.** As the body makes postural adjustments, the disc material has the highest probability of moving centrally due to the random motions of an unweighted disc.

This effect can be achieved at any disc level by supporting the part of the body superior to the disc in question with properly positioned pillows (preferably the large, firm couch cushion type) and allowing the inferior aspect's weight to provide TRACTION. More on this later in the section titled DYNAMIC POSITIONING.

WEIGHT-BEARING EXTENSION

Now comes the more powerful, intentional, moving force. The **EXTENSION IN TRACTION is replaced by WEIGHT-BEARING while EXTENSION is maintained**. This is the **WEIGHT-BEARING EXTENSION** component of *The O'Connor Technique (tm)* and differentiates this books methods from simple extension exercises (like McKenzie's) because, there, the weight-bearing component is generally preceded by an ill-conceived WEIGHT-BEARING FLEXION or no preparatory action at all. In other programs, the extension exercise is likewise usually initiated in an isolated and unprepared manner which predisposes the disc to not only failure at decentralization but potential harm if the disc material has nowhere to go when

179

it is exposed to force.

The EXTENSION IN TRACTION components of *The O'Connor Technique (tm)* MANEUVERS insure that during the transition from EXTENSION IN TRACTION to WEIGHT-BEARING IN EXTENSION the disc always has a place into which the displaced material can migrate because TRACTION is judiciously maintained. With just an unprepared extension, the disc material can move posteriorly to be crimped (See Crimping Pain in Chapter Two) into a more significant protrusion or not move at all, making the exercises a waste of time.

By observing Figure 43C, one can see that, as the disc material feels the weight of the compressing vertebral bodies during WEIGHT-BEARING EXTENSION, the disc material is squeezed centrally with the force of the weight of the body parts above the affected disc coming down on the other vertebral body with its layer of annulus fibrosus beneath and above the displaced disc material. As these forces progress, the anterior and central region of the disc stays open because both EXTENSION and TRACTION are maintained until the disc space closes with weight-bearing. Since the fissure/tunnel is the path whereby the disc material moved peripherally in the first place, in most cases, the disc material must travel in a reverse direction along that same tunnel to get back to the center. Maintaining EXTENSION while the WEIGHT-BEARING is ongoing insures that the tunnel's anterior is kept open; and the disc material has no where else to go except anteriorly and centrally.

Understand that **if you have figured out (through a DIAGNOSTIC CIRCUMDUCTION) where the displaced disc material is located, you can specifically direct your EXTENSION to the medial posterior or laterally to target the precise end of the fissure. It is not necessary or advised to simply extend directly to the posterior in every case unless your pain and arrested circumduction is** actually **centered directly in the posterior midline. It is better to aim your EXTENSION in the direction of the pain and towards the site of arrested DIAGNOSTIC CIRCUMDUCTION so that the herniated disc material is specifically targeted for central movement.** Only after you have positioned yourself in EXTENSION, while maintaining TRACTION directly over the disc material, should you accomplish the WEIGHT-BEARING component. This insures that the WEIGHT-BEARING IN EXTENSION compression forces are purposefully directed to move the disc material within the radial fissure back to the center of the disc.

Quite frequently, one sees "unenlightened souls" who suffer from chronic neck pain sitting upright, gyrating, crooking, or rapidly twisting their heads from side to side with the chin up. They usually refer to it as "cracking their neck." It is apparent to me that they are unwittingly performing WEIGHT-BEARING THERAPEUTIC CIRCUMDUCTIONS IN EXTENSION. Undoubtedly, this behavior must provide some measure of relief or so many people would not be practicing it. In most cases, they probably have only slightly off-center discs that are amenable to such a self-designed maneuver. However, the relief is obviously short-lived; and they must repeatedly persist in it because, although limitedly helpful in alleviating minor disc displacements, it fails to address the larger problem of a significant herniation, prolapse, or peripherally displaced disc material. Unfortunately, due to their lack of knowledge, they injudiciously employ weight-bearing forces that act to their mechanical disadvantage.

When one witnesses someone doing this over and over again it evidences that it doesn't provide sustained relief. Most probably in these cases, what they are doing is slightly moving the displaced disc material only enough to relieve the FULCRUM EFFECT pain or pressure on the peripheral ligamentous structures yet never truly centering the displaced disc material. If this doesn't convince the reader as to the failed efficacy of this measure, then considering the physiology, mechanics, and anatomy of the activity should.

First of all, without UNWEIGHTING the head, even if they do manage to successfully move disc material, the disc material has little or no central space to enter. The weight of the head and neck compress the disc spaces making any attempt at centralization of disc material, solely in this manner, exceedingly difficult. In this event, the weight-bearing works against centralization.

Also, **without making the effort to first position the disc material so that it is inside the rim of adjacent vertebral bodies' peripheries, weighted MANEUVERS (EXTENSION or flexion) can cause the disc material to become forced away from the fissure canal (that allowed it to move off center in the first place) making it more difficult or unlikely to re-centralize.** If a weighted MANEUVER is attempted in this instance and significant force is applied, the displaced disc material can advance a circumferential or radial tear, becoming lodged in such a manner as to be much more difficult to re-centralize.

Too, with badly applied weight-bearing forces, a piece of disc material that was partially protruding could be crimped by the rims of the weighted vertebral bodies into a position outside the plane of the outer circumference of the vertebral bodies causing a herniated fragment to become protruded and trapped outside of the plane of the vertebral bodies' peripheral margins. This is probably one of the worst events that could happen to a neck pain sufferer. This is a reason why chiropractors can be harmful without traction. The disc material has no where to go except to put pressure on an already weakened capsule.

Despite all these scenarios, it may seem inconsistent or paradoxical; however, **there is a justification and legitimate role for WEIGHT-BEARING EXTENSIONS in the alleviation of disc pain under certain specific circumstances, at the ideal time, in the correct sequence, and only after certain criteria are satisfied.** The satisfaction of these criteria comes only after you have become capable of identifying your displaced disc's position as within the capability of the concavities of the vertebral bones to move it centrally when they come together during weight-bearing. This can be done very easily with little extra effort.

The O'Connor Technique (tm) MANEUVERS, later to be described, were designed to align the disc material in such a way so that the disc can beneficially sustain the forces generated by correctly applied WEIGHT-BEARING EXTENSION. If the MANEUVERS are done correctly, the disc material's environment should be idealized for a centralization of mobile disc material when the bi-concave surfaces of the vertebral bones experience EXTENSION forces and the force of gravity.

Whether or not the earlier components of a total MANEUVER have been successful in accomplishing this end is usually determined at the end of any given MANEUVER accomplished to re-centralize the disc; yet, it is prudent and necessary to **test the success of the MANEUVER by circumducting the affected segment of the spine at the disc level in question in a similar fashion as though you were trying to locate the position of a displaced disc fragment.** The manner in which this is done is, in principle, identical to that method described in the chapter on SELF-DIAGNOSING YOUR DISC. Review that section, if necessary.

In short, **a circumductional effort (particularly WEIGHT-BEARING THERAPEUTIC CIRCUMDUCTION IN EXTENSION) should be done immediately preceding the final gesture of every MANEUVER because, at the same time, you are gently testing whether the disc is in and you are assisting its movement centrally by the partial WEIGHT-BEARING EXTENSION aspect of the final movements.**

Circumducting through the 180 degrees of EXTENSION after a MANEUVER, if you pivot at the disc level and gyrate the body around the affected segment, you are, in essence, determining if the same arrested motion that was present before the MANEUVER is still present afterwards. In the process of so doing, a partially WEIGHTED EXTENSION fortuitously can function to completely centralize a disc fragment that is just slightly off-center and prepared to go "in" by the previous MANEUVER so long as you limit the CIRCUMDUCTION to EXTENSION. **This type of CIRCUMDUCTION should always be limited to the 3:00-6:00-9:00 range of motion. WEIGHT-BEARING FLEXION (circumduction through the 3:00-12:00-9:00 positions) has no place here.** Ideally and theoretically, this THERAPEUTIC CIRCUMDUCTION should, also, first proceed in the direction of the painful area. For example, for a right-sided pain, one should circumduct from the 3:00 towards and to the 6:00 position.

In the case of a Upper-to-Mid Cervical disc, circumducting the head and neck above the problem disc level without UNWEIGHTING it is not particularly problematic or dangerous since the weight of the head is not that great; however, it is probably better to reach up and lift the head off of the shoulders to insure that initially no weight-bearing is felt. It may not always be necessary to unweight the head for this; but it is better to be safe than sorry if you are unsure of the status of the disc material. After you have circumducted enough to convince yourself that the disc is safe to bear weight, you can release your lifting effort and let the full WEIGHT BEARING IN EXTENSION occur.

However, a disc problem in the Low Cervical or Upper Thoracic region is a different animal because the shoulder muscles attach to these vertebrae. Attempting to lift the head off of the shoulders with the arms causes weight to be felt at disc levels where the anchoring shoulder muscles originate and defeats the UNWEIGHTING process. This can be overcome by, instead, planting the elbows on some surface (such as a large cushion, desk, or back of a couch) and carrying the weight of the head and neck with the hands so that the Low Cervical or Upper Thoracic discs are unweighted for the CIRCUMDUCTION IN EXTENSION attempts. Usually, this is functionally accomplished during the pertinent MANEUVER itself while reclining, but we are, in this case, talking about the upright posture when the head would have otherwise been in a weight-bearing condition.

Incidentally, this type of technique, in and of itself, can be used to independently centralize disc material quickly and efficiently at a moment's notice without any preparation. With UNWEIGHTING, the same activity that was described above in the "unenlightened soul" becomes a safer and more efficient means to effectively centralize disc material while seated so long as it is accompanied by UNWEIGHTING and the assurance that the disc material is not peripherally protruded.

A Mid-to-Low Thoracic disc and the Lumbar discs definitely should be unweighted by pushing down with the arms and hands on the hips while pivoting at the appropriate level of the problem disc if standing. When you place the hands on the hips, by pushing downwards, you lift the upper portion of your body off of the problem disc and pivot at the region of the problem disc level. If seated, lifting oneself off of the chair with elbow-locked arms will do. UNWEIGHTING before allowing weight-bearing circumduction makes the testing aspect (DIAGNOSTIC CIRCUMDUCTION) of the action only partially weighted so that in the event pain ensues, you have not risked any additional harm by prematurely putting too much weight-bearing force on the damaged disc.

Now, this may have the appearance of getting highly technical and sophisticated; however, it is really conceptually very simple. When I am able to completely circumduct the vertebral bodies at the affected disc through their full range of motion without arresting pain, I, then, am certain that the disc material is not impeding that range of motion and, therefore, is sufficiently centralized to not fear the potential consequences of full weight-bearing on a displaced fragment. By slowly relaxing the arms, the weight-bearing is gradually experienced in such a way that all the previous effort at moving the disc centrally is not wasted by too soon an attempt to "seat" the disc with a WEIGHT-BEARING EXTENSION.

Oftentimes, even when the criteria referencing the absence of pain or arrested motion are satisfied, something still feels slightly "out." In that event, the final performing of the WEIGHT-BEARING EXTENSION focused in the direction of the previous source of herniation pain often serendipituously results in a complete "seating" of the residually off-center disc fragment.

To achieve this added benefit when I have someone in my office, who I take through an entire MANEUVER to re-centralize an acutely painful displaced disc, I usually always have them stand up carefully afterwards and perform a PARTIAL WEIGHT-BEARING or UNWEIGHTED CIRCUMDUCTION IN EXTENSION advancing to a FULL-WEIGHT-BEARING CIRCUMDUCTION IN EXTENSION both of which are simultaneously THERAPEUTIC AND DIAGNOSTIC to document for my satisfaction (and theirs) that the disc no longer arrests movement. Quite often during the process, an audible "crunch" can be heard indicating that the final re-centralizing event has taken place. In that case, the DIAGNOSTIC CIRCUMDUCTION serendipitously becomes an ACTIVE THERAPEUTIC CIRCUMDUCTION. This has been followed, so often, by a look of surprised disbelief, as they recognize that they are indeed able to move their back again and the wedge-like pain has subsided, that I am forced to conclude that **a controlled and carefully administered WEIGHT-BEARING CIRCUMDUCTION IN EXTENSION is a necessary terminal component of every MANEUVER.** The reader will note later in the book, when reading about MANEUVERS, that such an action finalizes every MANEUVER. For each MANEUVER, photographs are provided which demonstrate the proper performance for every respective spinal area so they need not be included here.

It is essential to recognize, however, **if a WEIGHT-BEARING EXTENSION or HYPEREXTENSION (HYPEREXTENSION** being an exaggerated EXTENSION beyond the normal range of motion of the joint) **results in a pinching pain or an arrest of motion, then discontinue the effort immediately and return to the neutral position as painlessly as possible and either repeat the MANEUVER series until the pinching is relieved, or give yourself a break and try again later**. In the interim, it is best to avoid any WEIGHT-BEARING EXTENSION so long as this pinching pain is present when EXTENSION is attempted. To persist might make the problem worse.

WEIGHT-BEARING HYPEREXTENSION

Another category of EXTENSIONS is best considered as a **WEIGHT-BEARING HYPEREXTENSION, because it actually takes the disc unit beyond its usual range of motion in EXTENSION while bearing weight so as to more forcefully maximize anterior movement of the displaced disc material**.

This technique can be looked upon as an improvement upon the original Yoga posture and McKenzie extension exercise (Chapter One, Figures 3 & 4) which, in my estimation, serve only a limited purpose because I find them, without the preliminary FLEXION IN TRACTION and EXTENSION IN TRACTION, to be inefficient and too frequently unsuccessful a means of re-locating displaced disc material to make an isolated recommendation of them.

McKenzie pioneered the extension exercise as a means of reducing back pain by discovering that a patient got relief when inadvertently left in a prone position with the head of the exam table elevated so that the Lumbar spine was maintained in WEIGHT-BEARING HYPEREXTENSION without the use of the back muscles hence the appellation, "PASSIVE EXTENSIONS." These exercises, however are not consistently or uniformly successful because of two basic reasons.

One, many people's decentralized disc material has migrated so far off center that simply extending only traps the disc material by pinching it between the outer aspect of the annulus fibrosus and the posterior longitudinal ligament. In this case, not only is no relief experienced; but more pain and further herniation can result if the MANEUVER is forced before being certain that the disc material has previously been moved to within the confines of the vertebral bodies' bi-concavities. It is to satisfy this variable of the pain equation that I have added the concepts and permutations of FLEXION IN TRACTION prior to EXTENSION to push the disc material sufficiently centrally so an EXTENSION will be successful.

Two, McKenzie's extension exercise is routinely portrayed as properly done when the body is flatly in the prone position and the arms are used like a push-up to bring the torso above the hips up like a seal. This posture is fine for a disc that has not protruded out very far from the center and remains close to the midline of the body, but neglects the reality that if the disc is protruding more laterally and rests near the periphery, a straight upwards extension serves to push pieces of disc material more directly anteriorly. For a lateralized piece of disc material located within a circumferential tear, this can cause it to dissect further into the laminations of the annulus fibrosus where it can become increasingly difficult to re-centralize. That is why I recommend that an *O'Connor Technique* EXTENSION MANEUVER should always be intentionally directed so that it aims the compression forces such that the disc material is moved in the most likely direction to effect its re-centralization.

The O'Connor Technique's (tm) major improvement on the aforementioned methods consists of directing the HYPEREXTENSION in the direction of the disc herniation or site of pain. For a lateralized disc herniation that radiates pain to the lateral aspect and arrests weighted circumduction more laterally than at the midline, the WEIGHT-BEARING HYPEREXTENSION, or for that matter any EXTENSION MANEUVER should be aimed laterally. This requires that one bend towards the side and site of pain when extending regardless of the spinal level involved.

The more laterally the pain, the more laterally the EXTENSION should be aimed. During the descriptions of the MANEUVERS, I often refer to this action as extending directly over the painful site or the herniation. This can often require the EXTENSION component of a MANEUVER to look more like an actual bending to the side than what most people would consider a simple EXTENSION. However, discs rarely herniate in any way anteriorly; so there is usually always a posterior vector to the bending which technically makes it an EXTENSION.

One can also combine the WEIGHT-BEARING HYPEREXTENSION with a directional CIRCUMDUCTIONAL component (see above THERAPEUTIC CIRCUMDUCTION) to meet the challenge of those discs in which the solidified nucleus pulposus becomes trapped within the circumferential laminations of the annulus fibrosus. It may become necessary to exert force to cause the material to move circumferentially before it can re-trace its path back to the center of the disc, because it may not move centrally without being pushed and an EXTENSION will just produce more pain due to the FULCRUM EFFECT if it is trapped between a laminations of the annulus fibrosus. When resorting to a WEIGHT-BEARING CIRCUMDUCTION IN HYPEREXTENSION, it should be preceded by a few CIRCUMDUCTIONAL as well as a TRACTION efforts. The CIRCUMDUCTION will give the disc material an opportunity to move circumferentially before WEIGHT-BEARING is applied. The TRACTION component attempts to insure, first, that the center of the disc is cleared of any interference caused by the force the weight of the body above the disc will apply on the central structures of the disc. Also, the TRACTION actually can have sucked any of the liquid nucleus pulposus material centrally and have assisted to insure the migration of the solidified component back to the center.

Years ago, I utilized and advocated the simple McKenzie extension approach because it was all that I knew and found its success very limited. With the additions described above and its elevation to a <u>DIRECTED</u> WEIGHT-BEARING HYPEREXTENSION, the effectiveness of this technique can be vastly increased by selecting the ideal sequence and the most opportune time to engage that type of MANEUVER. When the MANEUVERS are described, later in the book, this technique is incorporated where it is most appropriate; and its use is not limited to just the Lumbar spine. It also finds a relevant application within the modality termed DYNAMIC POSITIONING, especially when the disc material is difficult to centralize yet it is not in a position to be crimped.

I have even resorted, in frustration, to lifting a heavy weight while in strenuous lateralized HYPEREXTENSION to force a piece of my own disc material centrally on several occasions. I even once got "mad" at my back after concluding that some lamination or piece of torn disc material was preventing the full centralization of the mobile disc fragment, and I put my neck in EXTENSION over the site of persistent discomfort and jumped up and down while in HYPEREXTENSION to "ram" the material totally into the fully centralized position because the disc material kept popping out too readily. It worked, and the disc seated centrally enough to not go "out" for an extremely long time. My belief is that from then on, the disc components that were preventing its centralization thereafter assisted similarly in retaining it in its centrality. It is important to understand that before I did it, I convinced myself that the disc was within the rim of the vertebral bone's "lips" by careful application of the DIAGNOSTIC CIRCUMDUCTION principle. I wouldn't recommend doing the same to anyone who is not fully cognizant of the entire theory, principle, and practice of *The O'Connor Technique (tm)* and willing to take the risk and live with the consequences. I can do that to myself; but I cannot recommend it to anyone else. Instead, I present the following less vigorous means of centrally seating disc material.

SEQUENTIAL SEGMENTAL EXTENSIONS

SEQUENTIAL SEGMENTAL EXTENSIONS are movements that sequentially extend the disc units of a painful region of the spine. There are two basic types, CASCADING, a passive technique and INCH-WORMING, an active technique.

The "CASCADE" Technique

Throughout the MANEUVERS sections of the book, the reader will find references made to the CASCADE technique. **This technique employs the edge of the bed (or platform) to serve as a point over which the spine hangs to effect a HYPEREXTENSION without the use of muscular contraction. It can also be described as a SEQUENTIAL SEGMENTAL PASSIVE EXTENSION because it entails the gradual hanging EXTENSION of each disc of the spine, one after the other, moving in a sequence from one vertebral body to the next.** Usually the point of support applied to the spine by the platform, as it flows over the edge like a waterfall, is from inferior to superior; however, it can be equally effective when practiced by sliding the spine from a superior to inferior fashion. In essence, it amounts to nothing more than letting the spine spill over the edge of whatever platform you are using until a relevant body part lands on the floor. By its passivity, a HYPEREXTENSION can be affected which does not cause a reduction in the size of the space into which the displaced disc material needs to return until the posterior aspect of the disc space is closed by the EXTENSION.

Since the technique involves sliding over the edge of a platform like a couch or bed and CASCADING, it is a kinetic process that allows for the application of innumerable angle and pressure changes to act upon the not only one disc in particular but numbers of discs with one common factor--EXTENSION. By causing a lengthy segment of the spine to CASCADE, there is a greater chance of effecting the ideal EXTENSION at the precise disc and put the ideal EXTENSION pressures on it as well, should it prove difficult to exactly determine at what level the actual problem disc exists. By CASCADING into a WEIGHT-BEARING EXTENSION, **this technique makes sure that the segments that have just sustained the maximum HYPEREXTENSION are kept in TRACTION and EXTENSION until they actually experience the WEIGHT-BEARING which puts anteriorly and centrally directed compression forces on them.** This prevents the disc material from moving posteriorly until there is a physical certainty that it cannot escape the effect of anteriorly directed forces.

CASCADING is routinely practiced immediately before any RE-WEIGHT-BEARING of the affected disc occurs, terminates when the WEIGHT-BEARING is maximized, and generally follows the THERAPEUTIC CIRCUMDUCTION component of a MANEUVER. Such is the ideal time for it to function. Necessarily, one must eventually return to weight-bearing after an attempt to re-centralize disc material. The CASCADE makes certain that the disc material is given every opportunity to re-centralize, even to the extent of insuring that every move made, especially the dismount from bed or couch, serves that purpose.

Each MANEUVER that employs the CASCADE has an accurate description of how such a technique is practiced when the MANEUVER is described. Since the MANEUVERS are so specific and well-described, it would be repetitious to engage, now, in such an articulate description of every one of its uses; so, the reader is directed to the individually pertinent MANEUVER for explicit directions in how and when to proceed with the CASCADE. However, it need only be looked upon as something as simple as sliding off the edge of what ever platform you are on, to the ground, relaxed in the EXTENSION posture.

The "INCH-WORM" Technique

To avoid repetition and because this technique can be used in conjunction with just about every MANEUVER, THE "INCH-WORM" TECHNIQUE warrants a separate heading. Technically speaking, it could be better termed, SEQUENTIAL SEGMENTAL ACTIVE EXTENSIONS; however, it is best described by the former because most people can relate to and mimic how an "inch-worm" moves. It can be applied to all levels of the spine and should be used during most of the MANEUVERS while relaxed in TRACTION; however, **whenever one is in EXTENSION and needs to move superiorly or inferiorly or when simply adjusting position, the spine should be made to move like an "inch-worm" so as to maximize the probability of moving disc material centrally.**

For the non-entomologists, the "inch-worm" is actually a caterpillar and because it only has legs at the distal aspects of its long segmented worm-like body it is mistakenly referred to as a "worm." To move, it first raises up the end of its body in the direction it plans to move, stretches the body away from the fixed point, then plants the moved terminal section of its body, gripping the surface with its feet and contracting its muscles to arch the mid-section which brings the other, more distant, part of the segmented body closer to the newly fixed end. This formerly distant part, which is now closer, is then planted and fixed. Then, the grip of the recently-fixed section end is released. This previously planted end is again moved a distance away from the whole by elongation away from the newly fixed end, and planted again. This process repeats so that the worm moves in one direction along the axis of the animal.

The spine is segmented like an inch-worm and can be made to move like one. People move like an inch-worm quite often while lying on their backs in bed, reading, when they want to move superiorly in the bed without letting go of their book. They usually elongate the neck, plant the back of the head on the pillow, push their elbows into the mattress away from the head, contract the erector spinae (which causes the spine to arch into an EXTENSION configuration), push with their legs, and they move towards the head of the bed. And thus, as this is repeated, the spine acts like an inch-worm, moving them superiorly (See Figure 44). This also can be done while lying on the side or in a supine position.

187

To accomplish this action for the Lumbar spine, a site above the painful disc is fixed and the aspect of the spine inferior to that point is allowed to hang in a mild EXTENSION IN TRACTION. This, as will be described later in the "Hip Hang" MANEUVERS, can be done by hanging over the edge of a bed's mattress or large pillows on the floor . Once TRACTION IN EXTENSION is achieved, the erector spinae muscles are contracted which puts the affected disc in an ACTIVE

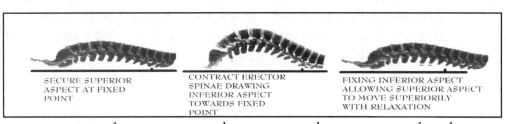

SECURE SUPERIOR ASPECT AT FIXED POINT

CONTRACT ERECTOR SPINAE DRAWING INFERIOR ASPECT TOWARDS FIXED POINT

FIXING INFERIOR ASPECT ALLOWING SUPERIOR ASPECT TO MOVE SUPERIORILY WITH RELAXATION

Figure 44 Spine functioning as inchworm (note relative position of marker on line as spine moves from Left to Right)

EXTENSION. The spine is then relaxed and allowed to go back into a TRACTION IN EXTENSION and the process is repeated. It can be done in the recline or while lying more to one side or the other depending upon the presence of a lateral component to the pain. Most often, the painful site is aimed towards the floor. An important consideration is that when the spine is hanging in TRACTION the arching contraction of the erector spinae muscles should be aimed towards the painful site, directly over the herniation site. This allows the maximum amount of squeezing or milking action to be applied along the axis of the radial fissure. A diagram demonstrating the spinal configurations for a directly posterior midline Lumbar disc herniation is seen in Figure 45 with a mattress diagramed as the means to fix the Lumbar spine's superior aspect.

To accomplish this action for pain in the neck and upper thorax, start by lying face up. Bringing the chin closer to the neck, elongate the neck by lifting up the shoulders and moving the head to a position as far superiorly as possible on the mattress, then, by planting the posterior aspect of the head against the mattress to grip it, you contract the erector spinae muscles (the muscles of the posterior neck). This causes the neck and upper thorax to arch into EXTENSION, pulling the rest of the body below the neck superiorly. With the head planted, the rest of the body below the area you are contracting wants to move superiorly. This can be assisted by pushing gently with the lower extremities, or if you want to induce a TRACTION effect, the legs can be left to drag and this forces the neck muscles to pull the body superiorly, creating TRACTION at those disc units inferior to those disc units that are contracting.

The same type of action can be performed with any part of the spine simply by planting the body part most superior to the disc in question and contracting the extensors of the back above the disc in question

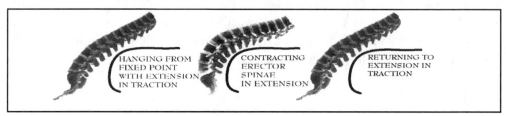

HANGING FROM FIXED POINT WITH EXTENSION IN TRACTION

CONTRACTING ERECTOR SPINAE IN EXTENSION

RETURNING TO EXTENSION IN TRACTION

Figure 45 "INCH-WORM" technique for Lumbar spine while hip-hanging over the edge of a mattress

to pull the most inferior body part superiorly. If you are careful to only use the muscles superior or inferior to a given disc unit, while keeping the actual disc unit's muscles relaxed, a very effective type of SEQUENTIAL TRACTION can be generated.

By analyzing this movement as you do it, you will find that if you do contract the muscles that surround the disc's posterior aspect, you can also induce very effective EXTENSIONS at successive levels of the spine in a rhythmic and sequential manner. As these EXTENSIONS are activated at a given segment, adjacent and distal segments are caused to experience TRACTION due to the weight of the body that is literally being dragged towards the fixed end, as the muscles of extension superior to it contract. Now, any particular segment is usually not strong enough to move the entire body while in the recline especially when in pain. So, it is usually necessary to help the movement along with the legs if your intent is to actually move; however, you do not necessarily have to change your actual position on the surface you are on to achieve the beneficial effect.

In fact, to maximize this method's effectiveness, make a point to sequentially perform ACTIVE EXTENSIONS and alternate them with a relaxation of the segments of the spine that are painful. By positioning your spine just right while hanging, you can relax back into PASSIVE EXTENSION while keeping the part of the body being dragged unmoved; yet, at the same time, maintain a positioning that sustains a TRACTION so that, when you relax, the disc unit experiences TRACTION when you relax. This may sound complicated, but I have actually incorporated this into the design of the MANEUVERS you will be practicing later by my choice of when I recommend using an "inch-worm" technique.

In this manner, the individual disc units with posteriorly displaced disc material can be caused to "milk" that disc material centrally. When you are said to "milk" something you are alternately squeezing and relaxing a liquid filled space such that liquid would move through the channel because it is stopped from moving at one end and squeezed in a direction away from the stopped area during the contracting action; then the chamber is allowed to re-fill during the relaxation phase. Well, that is exactly what you are accomplishing during this movement at the central disc space level. As you are in a PASSIVE EXTENSION IN TRACTION and relaxed, the "channel" that constitutes the radial tear (fissure) through which the disc material had migrated is filled with disc material. Then, as you gently and not too forcefully contract the back's extensor muscles, you close a posterior part of the space between the vertebral bodies. Because the muscles are at the posterior aspect of the spine, the compression starts from the posterior aspect and moves anteriorly. As the surfaces come together, the material between them (the pieces of fractured desiccated disc material as well as the residual liquid components of the nucleus pulposus) is squeezed anteriorly and centrally.

Again, this action can also be compared with a sort of "nibbling" at the pieces of disc material on the periphery so that they are "ingested" centrally. Thinking of the two adjacent vertebral bodies' concave surfaces as a pair of clam shell-like "mouth parts" aimed posteriorly, the posterior peripheral rims of the vertebral bodies as its "teeth", and the space between the bi-concave surfaces of the vertebral bodies that interface with the annulus fibrosus as the "mouth" cavity, this movement can be likened to a clam taking small bites at the posteriorly peripheralized disc material. As the posterior rims of the vertebral bodies "teeth" close upon pieces of disc material during ACTIVE EXTENSION, the inside curvature of the "clam-shells" force it deeper

189

into the center. Each time TRACTION/relaxation opens the "mouth," peripheralized material is drawn into the cavity by the negative pressure created, then again with muscular contraction of the erector spinae, the "teeth" close on the material, allowing it to only move anteriorly and centrally.

Either looking upon it as "nibbling" or "milking," the de-centralized material is little by little moved centrally through a process that is not forceful nor violent. **You don't need to actually move upwards on the bed if you are in the ideal position for EXTENSION IN TRACTION; however, any time that it is your intention to move into that ideal position from a less ideal position, you can do it in an "inch-worm" manner; and, as you are doing it, you will be accomplishing countless numbers of EXTENSION IN TRACTION combined with ACTIVE EXTENSION MANEUVERS similar to repeating the actions depicted in Figure 44, over and over.** These EXTENSIONS are very similar to WEIGHT-BEARING EXTENSIONS, only in this instance, the "weight-bearing" is not supplied by gravity but only by the force of contraction of the erector spinae musculature.

When you become experienced and comfortable with this technique you can expect to utilize it whenever you feel that displaced disc material is causing discomfort. When seated, upon sensing that the disc material has slightly moved posteriorly because you have inadvertently been in WEIGHT-BEARING FLEXION, you can unweight with your arms and employ the same "inch-worm"-type movement a couple of times before getting up. You should be able to feel the disc material move centrally. Finishing the MANEUVER with a WEIGHT-BEARING EXTENSION should leave you immediately pain-free. Or, upon waking in the morning and feeling the same sensation of discomfort due to a night of unconscious flexion, you can roll to one side (the painful side up), place your up-side hand on your hip, pushing away to induce TRACTION, you can sequentially extend towards the same side as the herniation pain and often feel the disc material of each successive disc move centrally as you "INCH-WORM" your way to a spine prepared for weight-bearing the rest of the day. You may only need this as a morning EXTENSION technique, but if it is insufficient, a CASCADE technique can follow as previously described.

DYNAMIC POSITIONING

As previously discussed in the section on WEIGHT-BEARING FLEXION, the reader should accept that certain positions, predominately WEIGHT-BEARING FLEXION (forward flexion while weight-bearing), whether instantaneous or maintained for long periods, predispose a damaged disc for posterior migration of disc material and frequently results in pain. The important consideration is that, a given flexion position, with even a small amount of weight, when maintained for a lengthy period, can be as pain-inducing as a great weight for a short period of time. In other words, **a small force applied over a prolonged period can be seen to effect as great a movement of the disc material in a previously damaged disc as a great force applied over a short period of time**. As elaborated above, the small force over a long period of time can be something as simple as leaning over a counter to do dishes for a half an hour; yet, it can be equally as pain-inducing as a garbage can lifting accident.

Everyone with a "bad back" would agree that bending very far forward and trying to lift a heavy weight rapidly can result in pain. Most would also agree, in the same sense, that bending over with a small weight for a prolonged time can accomplish the same amount of discomfort. So much as being caused to lean forward carrying only the weight of the upper body for a prolonged period can be sufficient to bring on pain in the presence of a disc herniation. Quite often, the pain is experienced when one tries to straighten up after bending over for a long time.

The consideration reconciling this reality is that **the migration of the discs is a function of time duration and degree of flexion as well as a magnitude-of-force (weight-bearing) dependent phenomenon.** By that, it is usually possible for the average occasional back pain sufferer to slightly bend forward at the waist quickly and return to the erect position without pain. Now, take the same person (or yourself if you feel the need to prove this to yourself) and have them bend over to the same degree whilst holding a twenty pound bag of potatoes. If that isn't sufficient, try thirty. It is a guarantee that if you continue to increase the weight, even while holding the degree of flexion constant, you will increase the likelihood and severity of pain.

So too, the longer you hold the weight while the back is in flexion, the more likely you are to induce pain. You may be able to hold the weight for a few seconds in 45 degrees of flexion; but after a while, pain intervenes and you will be forced to give up. Not just because of muscle strain, that will certainly be acting; but, here, I am talking about reproducing the pain of a disc migration event.

Now, consider that the quantity, quality, time, and degree of forces capable of creating a great deal of spinal discomfort can be produced while simply sleeping in the wrong position. **Just as increasing the weight or degree of flexion, holding even an inconspicuously small weight in a small degree of flexion for a period of hours can result in sufficient disc material migration to cause pain due to slow and steady disc displacement.** In keeping with this reality, sleeping eight hours with only the weight of the body acting upon a damaged disc qualifies as a likely situation capable of producing pain despite its seemingly innocuous character. Anyone who went to bed without pain and woke up inexplicably in it can testify to this reality.

Numerous patients of mine, as well as myself, have awakened with a "stiff" neck or back and can't recall any event that could have precipitated the pain. Although frequently attributed to "over doing it" the day before because no other explanation seems tenable, this phenomenon can be understood by considering that it was most likely caused by extensively prolonged mild flexion at the level of a previous injury that allowed the disc to migrate to the periphery during the prolonged flexion occasioned by sleep in the "wrong" position.

Sleeping for hours in relaxed WEIGHT-BEARING FLEXION at any spinal level, such as when you sink into a soft mattress or support your head too high with a pillow, supplies sufficient total force to put a previously damaged disc "out". Since you are asleep, you do not have the benefit of being able to recognize a painful position nor are you able to guard your back with muscle control. This force applied over such a prolonged time, combined with the gentle twitching and contorting of sleep, constitutes a cumulative force and set of circumstances equivalent to most any other recognizable situation readily seen as capable of displacing disc material.

The principle of DYNAMIC POSITIONING relies upon the logical converse of this reality such that maintaining a position most likely to reproduce the equivalent mechanical forces in reverse should have the opposite effect--and it does! In other words, **if even a small amount of force can <u>unintentionally</u> cause pain due to prolonged WEIGHT-BEARING**

FLEXION, then, by the same mechanism applied in reverse, <u>intentionally</u> directed **EXTENSION IN TRACTION or UNWEIGHTED EXTENSION can create an environment of forces over time that lend themselves towards spontaneously moving disc material centrally and anteriorly, resulting in an alleviation of the painful condition**. The process of so doing I have termed **"DYNAMIC POSITIONING."**

The basic tenet of **DYNAMIC POSITIONING** is that for each level of the spine involved with disc disease, there are distinct body positions and postural techniques that provide the most optimal **UNWEIGHTING** and maintenance of properly directed forces that can lead to spontaneous centralization of the disc material and consequently pain relief. These positions, when prolonged sufficiently, can be capitalized upon to gently and almost effortlessly coax the back into a pain-free state as well as give the back pain sufferer practicing the technique the best chance of maintaining it that way.

DYNAMIC POSITIONING serves at least two functions depending upon when and how it is applied. One function places the particular spinal segments in the most mechanically advantageous position for prolonged periods of time so as to allow for the disc material to gradually migrate back to the ideal central position after acute episodes of pain or in chronic situations in which the disc material has been persistently de-centralized and is otherwise difficult to re-centralize. A second function serves to keep the spine in the most advantageous position so that it can heal, reshape, and contour, affording the least probability of allowing a future protrusion event to occur. These functions are both suited to relieving sporadic events of pain as well as effective in stopping prolonged painful episodes, but the first function is better suited for relieving the acutely painful episode.

The first function served by **DYNAMIC POSITIONING** is best looked upon as a **short-term, immediately gratifying, solution, utilizing either FLEXION or EXTENSION while MAINTAINING TRACTION.** It is best employed to get out of immediately occurring pain.

The second function, later more intricately described as **MAINTENANCE OF EXTENSION,** is more appropriately seen as a **long-term one employing EXTENSION principally to keep out of pain once you are pain-free.** The persistent EXTENSION assumes that if this position is maintained consistently over a prolonged period, the spinal anatomy will eventually acclimatize to this position and preferentially re-model the bones, ligaments, and muscles to accommodate to this posture rather than an alternative flexion position which is more likely to result in pain. The long term effect is designed to promote a more permanent stability of the back and maintain a prolonged pain-free existence; therefore, it is best used to stay out of pain. This component has basically two subheadings which are more precisely categorized as an AVOIDANCE OF FLEXION and MAINTENANCE OF EXTENSION.

Actually, justification for the ability of the long term component of the concept to prevent disease is quite simple. Look at a lot of elderly people. More often than not, you will see that they are markedly hunched over at the base of the neck and bent forward at the Thoracic and Lumbar spine. This is termed **kyphosis** and is accepted as **a consequence of gravity acting upon the spine for years. Due to human anatomical design, flexion is the default posture in which humans inadvertently spend most of the time**. In order for kyphosis to occur, at least one disc unit has to occupy most of its time in flexion. Most probably, the initiating process is due to the disc's central material migrating posteriorly followed by levels of successive discs having to occupy most of their time in flexion due to the carriage of the superior aspects of the body more anteriorly. This relentless cycle persists eventually resulting in major segments of the spine being molded and fixed in flexion.

This probably is the most influential precipitating factor dictating the chronically flexed demeanor because, with each movement of the central disc material posteriorly at any level, the ability to painlessly extend is slightly reduced and thereby increases the time spent in relative flexion. This state of affairs lasts for so long that the spine re-models into a posture of constant flexion; and, terminally, the spine becomes physically and mechanically unable to extend even to a neutral position.

Regardless of what initiates this process, it is obvious that the spine becomes permanently fixed in flexion because it is in flexion most of the time. However, there is no reason to regard this process as immutable or inevitable. There are many equally-aged counterparts who do not suffer from this malady, and their lack of kyphosis predominately **can be attributed to the relatively increased amount of time they spend in extension or neutrally as opposed to flexion.** Years of mechanically disadvantageous "poor posture," extension causing pain while upright, lying in bed 12-16 hours a day propped up by pillows, and flexion being the only comfortable position for ambulation cumulatively conspire to create the permanent spinal flexion of old age.

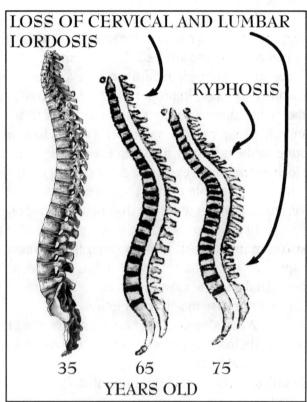

Figure 46 Spinal kyphosis

Conversely, if constant unconscious flexion can be expected to bend a back forward over a period of years, then consciously positioning one's self in the opposite configuration can certainly be expected to prevent it. By continuously **maintaining EXTENSION and preventing the flexion** one can expect to **prevent** the likelihood that the discs will fall victim to the **posteriorly directed migration of disc material** to which gravity, in combination with the general structure and function of the aging body would otherwise predispose them.

The point to be made here is not so much that a person can prevent kyphosis by maintaining an EXTENSION posture (they most probably can); but that **the extent of time a person spends in a particular posture is exceedingly influential in the shape the spine adopts** over time. It is based upon this obvious conclusion that DYNAMIC POSITIONING theoretically functions.

DYNAMIC POSITIONING'S successful re-modeling of the spine depends mostly upon the individual arriving at the understanding necessary to adopt various methods and

comfortably constant positions capable of effecting a prolonged and properly directed UNWEIGHTED EXTENSION (or UNWEIGHTED FLEXION in certain cases) at the level of the putative disc and sustaining them without the expenditure of muscular energy. It is not enough to be simply able to attain any given posture, it must be comfortably maintained for prolonged periods and at every reasonable opportunity. The most comfortable period in a person's life should be sleep; so, it seems most appropriate that one should take advantage of this time period wherein the body is committed to 6-8 hours/day (a third of your life) of relative inactivity. For that reason, the next treatment of this subject begins by discussing how sleep time can be used to your advantage.

If properly-executed MANEUVERS are not immediately successful, often it is because the ideal position has not been achieved, it is not maintained long enough, or not enough TRACTION is placed upon the affected disc system largely due to pain preventing any additional immediate force to be applied, regardless of eventual benefit. Ineffective results can also be due to an inability to relax, improper MANEUVERING, disc material that cannot easily migrate towards the center due to portions of the annulus fibrosis that interfere with its travel, or spasm of the muscle group preventing proper TRACTION to be successful. These situations often persist in spite of the necessity for sleep even though the mechanical pain is still present. Often, pain and sleep are mutually exclusive events. You can't sleep because you are in pain and unless you sleep you won't be able to relax spasmed muscles enough to allow for TRACTION to separate the vertebrae enough to let the disc material migrate to a non-painful position.

In order to give the disc material the best probability of migrating, **the back or neck pain sufferer must learn how to sleep in the most mechanically advantageous position** that will capitalize upon the relative paralysis of sleep. This is where DYNAMIC POSITIONING is beneficial because most people can learn to sleep in the postures that afford the highest probability for anterior disc material migration.

When sleeping, the skeletal muscles achieve a degree of relaxation unmatched by even the best medicinal muscle-relaxants. Once sleep's relaxation is achieved with TRACTION applied, the vertebral bodies can be expected to separate further than when awake. The goal then becomes to utilize a comfortable position that relies upon gravity to provide TRACTION to separate the vertebral bodies. The position chosen need only satisfy a few criteria. It must be easy to achieve and maintain as well as comfortable enough in which to sleep. Without this relaxation afforded by sleep the vertebral bodies sometimes cannot achieve the degree of separation necessary to allow disc material to centralize.

If one can be DYNAMICALLY POSITIONED advantageously for 6-8 hours a day, the cumulative effect can be expected to be beneficial especially in light of the alternative--allowing the opposite, improper, mechanically disadvantageous, position to be maintained so that the time spent is counter-productive from a spinal structural perspective. **Practicing this doesn't mean that you must necessarily dedicate only sleep-time specifically for this endeavor; rather, the time you ordinarily spend in a position for routine reclining purposes can be simply modified to incorporate the ideal position for your problem disc instead of just randomly assuming an alternative position that can be predictably and ultimately painful.** The important consideration above all others is that, **after the most mechanically advantageous position is achieved, you relax, and remain in that position for a reasonably prolonged period.**

194

Discs don't always just easily slip back in. It often takes time for all the paraspinous muscles to relax sufficiently to allow for the intervertebral space to enlarge or stretch to the fully open configuration. Also, the basket weaved fibrous component of the disc itself, the annulus fibrosus, cannot be brought to its full longitudinal length too rapidly without constant steady tension. This tension is difficult to achieve in the presence of pain and spasm so it must be accomplished slowly and carefully without rapid movements or sudden jerking. There is no reason to fear this endeavor, because **DYNAMIC POSITIONING amounts to nothing more than resting in a particular position for a prolonged period so as to position the body in the most advantageous alignment for a re-centralization of the displaced disc material**.

If the spasm is too intense and it is impossible to relax, this may be overcome with prescription muscular antispasmodic medications like Valium (tm) (=diazepam) or Soma (tm) (=roboxaine); but if the desire to avoid pharmaceuticals is elected, most health food stores carry herbal preparations containing herbs such as Camomile, Kava-Kava, Valerian root, Mugwort, Skull Cap, Wild Lettuce, etc. which, rumor has it, accomplish a similar function albeit without the FDA's approval, the quantification exactitude, or scientific reassurances engendered in alternative products. I cannot make recommendations for their use or imply any benefit; however, some people claim them to be effective, benign, relaxants. Regardless of the substance used or not used, a minimum requirement is that constant TRACTION forces must be applied to bring all the involved muscles, ligaments, and tendons to full length in order for the central area of the disc unit to be maximally opened and made ready to accept the displaced, de-centralized disc material.

The simplest way of describing the most advantageous position for sleep, or for that matter any DYNAMIC POSITIONING, is to **make it the most comfortable position such that the affected segment of the spine is placed in slight TRACTION as well as mild EXTENSION (or FLEXION depending upon the location of the displaced disc material)**.

DYNAMIC POSITIONING, in a figurative way, can be seen as a slow motion MANEUVER; however, it is unrealistic for a person to sleep in some of the positions described in the MANEUVERS' instructions to achieve the maximum amount of EXTENSION or FLEXION simultaneously with TRACTION. So, some realistically optimal compromise must be reached between comfort and the degree of sustainable TRACTION because **too much TRACTION, EXTENSION, or FLEXION for too long can, in and of itself, be uncomfortable and, thereby, self-defeating**.

Finding the optimal position in which to sleep is best approached by identifying which spinal segment is affected and specifically directing your efforts towards putting that particular segment in the ideal amount of **FLEXION or EXTENSION while simultaneously maintaining TRACTION** during a sufficiently prolonged period that will allow for sleep to occur.

Now comes the most technical component of the whole chapter. **You must decide whether you should DYNAMICALLY POSITION yourself in EXTENSION or FLEXION while in TRACTION.** The TRACTION (or UNWEIGHTED) component is indispensable for the beneficial effect. **Sleep and prolonged motionless positioning in TRACTION is what painlessly allows the disc space to widen so as to allow for re-centralization to occur.** The disc material has to have a space to go into before it can move. It takes time for these ligaments to come to full length and for the muscles around them to relax enough under the pull of sustained TRACTION to stop spasming in contraction and simply to come to their full length also. So,

some degree of TRACTION, however slight, should be maintained no matter what else you do because the disc unit cannot be weight-bearing if an anterior migration of disc material is to be expected.

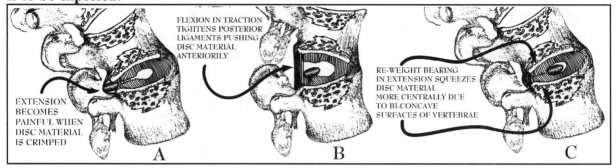

Figure 47 Cut-away view of disc unit depicting disc material trapped at periphery (A) requiring FLEXION IN TRACTION DYNAMIC POSITIONING (B) to position it so that a RE-WEIGHT-BEARING IN EXTENSION (C) has the opportunity to move disc material

Unfortunately, there is a heightened level of complexity involved. **The individual has to determine whether to DYNAMICALLY POSITION in EXTENSION or FLEXION and (if appropriate) towards the proper side.** To understand the distinction, we have to refresh ourselves as to the anatomy of the decentralization process. Recall in the FLEXION IN TRACTION chapter that it is necessary to move the disc material centrally by stretching the posterior peripheral ligamentous structures to get the fragments of disc material beyond the "rims" of that narrow peripheral plateau region immediately peripheral to the concavities of the vertebral bones. It is when the disc fragments are in this region, or more peripherally, that EXTENSION can be expected to cause pain. This pain is the same type of pain that a standing DIAGNOSTIC CIRCUMDUCTION (weight-bearing) causes when motion is arrested in EXTENSION and is either caused by a crimping, pinching, or FULCRUM EFFECT. If disc material is being pinched or crimped (See Figure 47A), pain and the resultant wedge-like motion arresting pain probably won't go away with simple EXTENSION IN TRACTION MANEUVERS or DYNAMIC POSITIONING and a preliminary FLEXION IN TRACTION may be required before relying upon EXTENSION IN TRACTION.

DYNAMIC EXTENSIONS

Although there is a distinction to be drawn between the optimal choices, **the singular most often successful method of DYNAMIC POSITIONING is EXTENSION IN TRACTION**. So much so, it could be referred to as the "default" position because it is the best position if you have any doubt as to the relative position of the displaced disc material or if you want to adopt the best position for the long-term benefits of DYNAMIC POSITIONING.

If you do not get a pinching pain while extending towards the site of pain, you can be reasonably certain that the displaced disc material is positioned somewhat within the peripheral rim; but not so centrally that EXTENSIONS won't be effective. So, now, a prolonged EXTENSION posture that positions your disc for only centralized movement can be effective.

196

Even if the most appropriate MANEUVER or FLEXION IN TRACTION-type DYNAMIC POSITIONING is unsuccessful in relieving pain, the EXTENSION IN TRACTION DYNAMIC POSITIONING can be employed; and, at the very least, it is the best pain-stopping device in *The O'Connor Technique (tm)* armamentarium. The reason this is so is because the **EXTENSION component always functions to direct the displaced disc material centrally** at the same time **the TRACTION component serves to prevent possible trapping of the disc material that would otherwise occur in a WEIGHT-BEARING EXTENSION.** This also allows for even extremely peripheralized disc material to be predisposed to central movement, albeit not as effectively as a FLEXION IN TRACTION effort. For de-centralized yet not totally peripheralized disc material, EXTENSION IN TRACTION is ideally suited; but even if there is a pinching discomfort in full EXTENSION, the pain is usually relieved when the disc unit is placed in mild EXTENSION combined with TRACTION. **So, it can be viewed as a caveat that a mild EXTENSION simultaneously with TRACTION can almost always be employed without too much discomfort and with a reasonable probability of relieving pain and centralizing disc material.**

Your level of comfort can dictate the predictable degree of success. If the EXTENSION IN TRACTION position is too exaggerated, you probably won't be able to relax comfortably let alone sleep because of the positional discomfort. If it is comfortable, you can probably be certain that the optimal position has been achieved. Keep in mind that simply putting yourself in any comfortable position is not sufficient, since lying on one's side during back pain episodes with pillows between the legs is often described as the most comfortable position. However, this position doesn't lend itself mechanically to allow for the migration of the disc material into the ideally centralized configuration. It may be comfortable, but you have little hope of finding pain relief when you wake up, whereas DYNAMIC POSITIONING often results in waking without pain because the disc material centralizes during the sleeping event.

EXTENSION IN TRACTION is also one of the easiest positions to adopt because it may only require something as simple as a pillow positioned near the site of pain while lying on your back. The pillow puts the involved spinal segment in PASSIVE EXTENSION and simply relaxing puts the disc unit into a mild TRACTION supplied by the weight of the body on either side of the disc unit that is draped over the pillow. Alternatively, a large pillow (and/or couch cushion) can be used to support an entire large section of the spine allowing the segment of the spine on the other side of the damaged disc to hang over the edge of the pillow. This increases the degree of EXTENSION and TRACTION, both of which can be modified by changing the size of the pillows.

For instance, in the presence of **Lumbar pain**, large couch cushions stacked on a couch so that the hips can hang in EXTENSION constitutes the most comfortable and effective means of dealing with the pain of acute injury. Putting a pillow under the upper (superior) thorax with its edge at the level of the problem disc unit so that the neck and head hang over the edge is one of the most effective means of dealing with **low neck and shoulder pain of spinal origin**. For the **mid-to upper neck** region, the placement of a soft towel rolled to a size that fills the curvature of the neck seems to fit the problem best. More on this later will be presented in sections dedicated to specific areas of the spine.

DYNAMIC FLEXION IN TRACTION

When discogenic pain is present and simple TRACTION/EXTENSION MANEUVERS are unsuccessful, DYNAMIC POSITIONING should be directed to FLEX WHILE IN TRACTION to cause the peripheral ligamentous structures to move the disc material slightly more towards the center (Figure 47B) so that eventually an EXTENSION can be successful. This sometimes requires patience and a relatively prolonged time period to move trapped disc material. DYNAMIC POSITIONING fulfills that requirement so that afterwards an EXTENSION IN TRACTION MANEUVER followed by WEIGHT-BEARING (Figure 47C) will allow the "clam-biting" action of the bi-concave surfaces coming together to squeeze the disc material back into the exact center from which it originated.

This FLEXION IN TRACTION DYNAMIC POSITIONING, like simple FLEXION IN TRACTION, should be aimed in a direction directly away from the area of pain. For example, if DIAGNOSTIC CIRCUMDUCTION reveals that the pain and, therefore, the herniated disc material is in the 7 o'clock position (to the left and posterior), you must FLEX IN TRACTION for a prolonged period towards the one o'clock position (anterior and to the right). In the same sense, if the pain is in the 5 o'clock position, you would have to direct your FLEXION towards the 11 o'clock position.

The ideal DYNAMIC POSITIONING type of FLEXION IN TRACTION can be accomplished by following the vertebral level specific FLEXION IN TRACTION directions given in the specific spinal region's MANEUVERS section. It would be unnecessarily redundant to repeat each one here. At this point it is only necessary to understand the basic principle. When the MANEUVERS are later described, **one can pause for a prolonged period at any point in the MANEUVER to take advantage of the DYNAMIC POSITIONING effect**. Depending upon what vertebral level your pain is located, to find the ideal DYNAMIC POSITION you can turn to that specific area of the MANEUVERS section and **find a means to recreate, as closely as possible, the same positions that are described.**

The "MANEUVERS" section of the book instructs you in the adoption of specific positions and postures to effect disc material movement. It is simple enough to stay in any given described position for a longer period than the MANEUVER would require. For instance, **when doing a MANEUVER that asks of you to adopt a FLEXION IN TRACTION, all you need to do is prolong that component of the MANEUVER to accomplish the appropriate DYNAMIC POSITIONING. These should be positions comfortable enough that they can be maintained for a long period of time, even to the extent of sleeping in them.** This is important because the MANEUVERS usually describe positions which are intended for use for only the duration of the MANEUVER. The same positions of the MANEUVERS can and should be modified to adapt to whatever environment you have chosen and be **maintained less vigorously (with less TRACTION or flexion) or more comfortably for as prolonged a period as necessary until you have successfully caused enough migration for a later-coming EXTENSION-type MANEUVER or EXTENSION-type DYNAMIC POSITIONING to be tried**.

The reader should understand that one may not have to incorporate a FLEXION IN TRACTION type of DYNAMIC POSITIONING into MANEUVERS if you have a simple, non-complicated disc problem. However, for protrusions or very old injuries, one may have to practice FLEXION IN TRACTION-type DYNAMIC POSITIONING for night after night or repeatedly until the disc material moves centrally enough for the other EXTENSION-type DYNAMIC POSITIONS to be tried. However, **do not assume that if you haven't succeeded in this preliminary component that you can't go on and try the EXTENSION type actions and other MANEUVERING.** You can rely upon discomfort to tell you if you are premature in the use of EXTENSIONS because the positioning in EXTENSION will be especially uncomfortable if the disc material's peripheral positioning makes WEIGHT-BEARING EXTENSION not yet ready to be applied.

The FLEXION IN TRACTION-type of DYNAMIC POSITIONING may be also uncomfortable as the inflamed ligamentous structures are stretched and caused to increase their pressure against the protruding disc material; however, this is not usually as painful as the constant pinching pain of a trapped piece of disc material being crimped off by EXTENSION. Since the TRACTION component usually makes it less painful than the untreated condition, whatever discomfort you may experience usually pales in significance compared with the original weight-bearing pain. In the FLEXION IN TRACTION scenario, the TRACTION component usually allows a space to be created so that when the tightening ligaments abut against the disc material, it moves centrally without an obstruction to induce pain as flexion would otherwise cause when weight-bearing.

In EXTENSION, the pain can come from a trapped piece of disc fragment. There is nowhere else for the pieces to go, and they have to further bulge, stretching the pain receptors. The presence of this pinching pain while in EXTENSION can be your most accurate guide to help you determine whether FLEXION IN TRACTION should be initially employed or whether to use EXTENSION IN TRACTION as your choice of DYNAMIC POSITIONING. Also, the presence of referred pain (pain felt in another part of the body despite originating in the disc) indicates that pressure is being felt on the capsule. Any time a disc material fragment is touching the capsule, there is a reasonable indication for at least a trial at FLEXION IN TRACTION.

As an example of how DYNAMIC POSITIONING can be accomplished when the disc material is peripheralized far posteriorly, you can perform this simple procedure. You start by lying face down (supine) on a mattress which places you in a mildly weighted EXTENSION as you sink in to the mattress. To be certain you find the displaced disc material, you can roll such that the painful site is up, aimed at the ceiling. If this is uncomfortable and results in a crimping type of pain, it most likely means that displaced disc material is being trapped as the source of pain. To determine the precise location of the decentralized disc material, refer to the section on DIAGNOSTIC CIRCUMDUCTION and then position yourself over the edge of the mattress, with pillows or some other positioning techniques as if you were going to perform a FLEXION IN TRACTION (see FLEXION IN TRACTION section of Chapter Four). Then, you simply put the painful disc unit into a flexed non-weight-bearing configuration and relax into a mild, non-painful, comfortable position that closely approximates a FLEXION IN TRACTION MANEUVER but to a much lesser degree of both FLEXION and TRACTION. It is only necessary to insure that enough FLEXION and TRACTION is applied sufficient to place only mild pressure on the peripheralized disc material. You may adjust your position with pillows as necessary to insure that it is comfortable because, if it is uncomfortable, you would not want to go to sleep in that position lest you may awake in greater discomfort. Once comfortably positioned, you may lie for a long time or even sleep in that position. As you sleep, even if only for an instant, the position of FLEXION IN TRACTION predisposes the migration of the peripheralized disc material centrally as you breathe, make postural alterations, or adjust yourself for more comfort as time goes on.

Nothing says you have to spend the entire night in that position, nor do you have to actually sleep, you may simply lie there until you have been successful or you feel you have been successful enough to change your position with an EXTENSION MANEUVER or to DYNAMICALLY POSITION yourself in EXTENSION IN TRACTION. You can even arrange yourself in this position to read or watch TV, just so long as the problem disc is in FLEXION IN TRACTION long enough to effect movement of the disc material.

Once you have used FLEXION IN TRACTION-type DYNAMIC POSITIONING (as depicted by Figure 47B), immediately upon ending the DYNAMIC POSITIONING component of the effort, you should follow with an EXTENSION IN TRACTION component then go on to a WEIGHT-BEARING EXTENSION (as depicted by Figure 47C) to capture the disc material before it can again migrate peripherally. This usually can be done simply by rolling towards the painful side and using the same pillows that were used to keep you in FLEXION to assist you, now, in EXTENSION.

To elaborate exactly how to accomplish this for every section of the spine would be redundant; so, for details, the reader is referred to the section that describes the area-specific MANEUVERS and encouraged to **apply the DYNAMIC POSITIONING methodology to these specific regions of the spine as though it were just a prolonged component of that action of the MANEUVER.** This activity requires careful re-positioning and constant vigilance to insure that you **do not flex while weight-bearing in the same direction you were flexing during the DYNAMIC POSITIONING because that may just push the disc material right back into the rim area or beyond.** If that happens you will have defeated your purpose and previous effort. Therefore, after a FLEXION IN TRACTION, without delay, you should re-position yourself (while maintaining TRACTION at the site) until a "clam-biting" type capture of the disc with the concave surfaces of the vertebrae through an EXTENSION MANEUVER with a WEIGHT-BEARING follow-through can be completed. Read this section again if you don't completely understand the concept or if you were confused (or bored) by all the movement terminology. Rest assured, when a person follows the MANEUVER directions and adheres to the proper sequence, they can't go wrong. These MANEUVERS will be described in the so-named chapter, later.

So as to clear up any confusion and not make this seem too complicated, **DYNAMIC POSITIONING can be looked upon simply as any other back pain alleviating technique** (especially, but not exclusively, FLEXION IN TRACTION or EXTENSION IN TRACTION) described in this book, **only maintained over a prolonged period so that the gentlest of motions will suffice and time can be used to your advantage**. If, by virtue of your symptoms and the principles described in this book, you feel a FLEXION IN TRACTION MANEUVER would be most appropriate to alleviate pain, then DYNAMIC POSITIONING in that configuration would be the most appropriate choice. The same goes for EXTENSION IN TRACTION or other positions and postures described in the MANEUVERS. It's basically that simple and need not be looked upon as too complicated or intricate to practice.

SELECTING THE IDEAL DYNAMIC POSITION

If some thought is given to the selection of the ideal DYNAMIC POSITION to accomplish a slow steady movement of the disc material back to its centralized location, one might readily discern that such a goal can be accomplished in any number of ways. As previously indicated, the two main choices are EXTENSION IN TRACTION or FLEXION IN TRACTION; however there are, within these categories, alternative means to reach the same mechanical goals.

For instance, when a Lumbar pain radiates directly to the posterior, DYNAMIC EXTENSION can be accomplished by reclining with a large pillow(s) in a configuration placed so that the posterior body surface is bowed over the pillow as in Figure 48A. In this configuration, the painful site is aimed towards the ground such as in a standard EXTENSION IN TRACTION position. TRACTION, in this case, is supplied by the weight of the body pulling away from the site of pain due to the force of gravity on body segments superior and inferior to the problem disc unit. This TRACTION opens the disc unit by separating the parallel dish shaped surfaces of the vertebral bodies that enclose the disc, allowing the disc material to travel, with less impediments, centrally. Additionally, the angulation of the EXTENSION makes it nearly impossible for the disc material to move in any other direction than centrally. It is also easy to see how if the hips were allowed to slide off of the pillows to the floor, the weight of the body superior to the disc in question would then be brought to bear on the disc unit. Thereby, a simple shift of the body inferiorly from this position can convert an EXTENSION IN TRACTION-type DYNAMIC POSITIONING to a WEIGHT-BEARING EXTENSION in a near effortless sliding movement. The choice of this position rather than an alternative makes such a movement exceptionally easy, and depending upon the ideal individualized movement that might be necessary to move a particular disc, this version of EXTENSION IN TRACTION might be found to be more advantageous for any given person. However, another option exists to effect a DYNAMIC POSITIONING in EXTENSION IN TRACTION at the same disc level by positioning the posterior side facing **upwards** with postural support applied along the spinal axis both superior (the pillows) and inferior (the floor) to the painful disc at enough distance from the painful site such that the segment is still being extended (bent) towards the posterior (See Figure 48B) even though one is facing towards the floor. The weight of the superior aspect of the body above the disc unit can be fully supported by high pillows to allow the inferior aspect of the body to hang from it thus creating an EXTENSION IN TRACTION. From this position, the upper body can be slid off of the pillows, when necessary, so that its weight is felt by the disc unit thereby generating another means of WEIGHT-BEARING EXTENSION. In this way, gravity serves to compress the posterior portion of the disc unit together in such a manner as to squeeze the de-centralized material centrally much as the final weight-bearing components of the therapeutic MANEUVERS are accomplishing when they are used.

The point to be made here is that an EXTENSION IN TRACTION that is easily converted into a WEIGHT-BEARING EXTENSION can be accomplished in at least two separate and distinct means. One is in the supine and the other is in the recline; yet the principle and mechanical effect is equivalent. The only difference is in how the pillows are used as supports.

In all cases of EXTENSION, the vertebral components of the disc unit posterior to the herniation are brought closer together so as to trap the errant disc material and give it no other

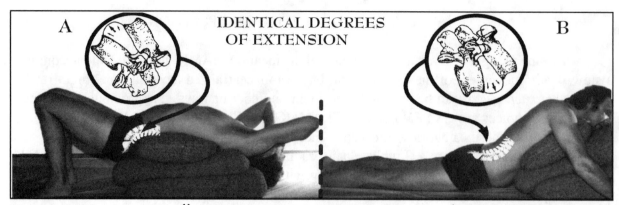

Figure 48 Two means to effect DYNAMIC POSITIONING in Lumbar EXTENSION

avenue of travel other than towards the central region of the disc. In the first case (Figure 48A), TRACTION is causing the entire vertebral surface to separate, but the anterior (aimed upwards) aspect is separated more than the side aimed towards the ground. In the second case (Figure 48B), the posterior aspect of the vertebral bones' surfaces are compressed together by gravity acting on adjacent portions of the body inferior and superior to the disc while the lower aspect is spread apart as the disc unit "hangs."

In either case, by sliding inferiorly and weight-bearing, the upper body's weight can be used to develop more force to squeeze the disc material centrally and is putting into practice the beneficial aspect of the WEIGHT-BEARING HYPEREXTENSION previously mentioned.

As an aside, it should be re-emphasized that WEIGHT-BEARING EXTENSIONS should be reserved only for those situations in which the disc is definitely capable of moving only centrally and cannot be trapped between the rims of the vertebral bodies and the peripheral ligamentous "capsule" where it can be pinched or crimped. If this position causes a pinching discomfort, this should indicate that the disc material is too far peripheralized for this method and that an alternative positioning be utilized until such time as it can be done. However, once that the disc material has been successfully moved centrally beyond the plateau/rim, WEIGHT-BEARING EXTENSION-type DYNAMIC POSITIONING IN EXTENSION is an excellent means of re-seating the disc material deep into the central area from whence it originally came.

Of course, if the pain radiates to one side more than the posterior, the same choices present themselves except that when employing EXTENSION IN TRACTION one would necessarily lay on one's side. The easiest to accomplish DYNAMIC POSITION, when pain radiates to one side, is with the spine draped over a pile of large pillows positioned directly under the painful segment while the painful side is aimed downwards.

When pain radiates to one side, to effect WEIGHT-BEARING EXTENSION DYNAMIC POSITION, one could, instead, lie on the opposite side with the entire region of the spine containing the painful segment bowed downwards between a pair of pillows placed on either end of the spinal region distant from the painful disc unit. Alternatively, you can achieve the same goal by choosing to use a large stack of pillows upon which the aspect of the body superior to the problem disc unit rests letting the inferior aspect hang from near the site of the herniated disc. So long as the painful side is kept largely aimed upwards, hanging in this position provides an

EXTENSION IN TRACTION; then, when sliding the upper body off of the pillow stack, you can go into WEIGHT-BEARING EXTENSION simply by letting the disc unit bear the weight of the body above it.

Additionally, by controlling the spinal contour relative to its position on the pillows, the amount of WEIGHT-BEARING on the disc can be changed. With minor dexterity and a little practice, a person can go from TRACTION into WEIGHT-BEARING in a smooth motion without giving the disc material an opportunity to escape your control over its centralized movement. The spinal region-specific directions for that sort of effort will come in the sections dedicated to MANEUVERS, and to individually elaborate upon them here would be premature and repetitive.

Nevertheless, what is being accomplished is not all that difficult, if you can picture it in your mind what is happening within the disc, the **choice you make usually amounts to the environmental appurtenances you have at your disposal and whether you find it easier, more comfortable, or more successful to aim the herniated fissure/canal upwards toward the ceiling or down towards the ground**. In each case, you **take advantage of gravity to leisurely coax a movement of the disc material along the axis of the fissure**. Either way will suffice, but it is good to know you have a choice, depending upon the setting in which you find yourself.

Oftentimes, convenience dictates the form DYNAMIC POSITIONING takes. The position shown in Figure 48A can be adopted while reading a book, while that of Figure 48B can be adapted to watching TV on the floor, or at an outdoor camp out, you can be "making your bad back better" atop a sleeping bag while enjoying the starlit sky and no one would know it unless you told them.

The selection of the precise positions you choose at any given time depends also upon the desired practical outcome. **If the disc is far enough herniated that extending towards the same side of the protrusion while WEIGHT-BEARING causes pain but you are uncertain as to whether the nature of the pain is indicative of a piece of disc material contacting the capsule, the choice of either FLEXION IN TRACTION or EXTENSION IN TRACTION might be equally as appropriate, since either would engage the effects of TRACTION to stop the pain, yet allow nonetheless for migration centrally.** In this event, starting with FLEXION IN TRACTION and changing to EXTENSION IN TRACTION can be the most effective strategy. One may find that, at first, DYNAMICALLY POSITIONING draped over a pillow with the pain site aimed upwards in FLEXION IN TRACTION gets the disc material to move centrally just enough to allow for a roll over so that the pain site gets aimed downwards in TRACTION IN EXTENSION to squeeze it into the fully centralized position. Once the disc material is fully centralized, the choice of position would then be changed to the one most comfortably apt to keep it there by using WEIGHT-BEARING EXTENSION. If this sequence is employed, what you will be accomplishing, in essence, is a long, drawn-out, MANEUVER, nearly identical in practice and principle to what will be discussed in a spinal region-specific fashion, later, in the next upcoming chapter of the book. The beauty of DYNAMIC POSITIONING, however, is that you use time to your full advantage, because, as stated at the outset of this section, the movement of disc material is a time-dependent phenomenon. Sometimes, it simply takes extra time to achieve the sought-after results.

The choices should be experimented with, and the future decision as to which one, or combination, is best should be outcome-mediated. **The way that gives the most relief should**

be applied most frequently because there are numerous other factors which can account for why one method works better for one area of pain in a particular individual rather than another. I explain this varied success by considering that the pre-, intra-, and post-positioning muscular actions can make subtle differences in the alignment of the vertebral bodies and consequently result in slightly different disc fragment movements.

Take for instance the process of getting into a particular position. This activates one set of muscles and relaxes the opposing muscle groups. The very opposite is true when positioning so that the other side of the body faces towards the force of gravity. Different and opposing muscle groups selectively contract and relax in sequences largely the opposite of what the other positioning event evoked. This alternative fighting-against-gravity and using gravity to your advantage places different stresses on the disc unit so that when positioning is complete, a different set of circumstances are presented to the disc unit--some of which assist and others hinder the centralizing movement, depending upon the exact circumstance of the intra-disc environment.

The take home message, however, is that **by experimenting with the basic variations on the same principle you will eventually find the ideal means to position yourself such that the maintenance of that position will eventually lead to relief and, with continued use of that positioning, will prevent future escape of the disc material to the periphery**. This process need not be particularly complex or energy intensive. As alluded to above, it can simply be a matter of how you position yourself on a couch to watch TV, on the floor while reading or resting, or in bed before falling asleep. If pillows are not available, for lateral lesions, the shoulders and the hips themselves can be incorporated into the positioning to serve the same function as pillows due to their lateral surfaces being so distant from many areas of the spine.

I have found that DYNAMICALLY POSITIONING myself while reading in bed can be an excellent means of killing two birds with one stone. For Cervical pain, as I read, I hang my neck and arms over the edge of the mattress in FLEXION IN TRACTION and lie there for a while until all the muscles come to full length; then I change position as if I'm going through a THERAPEUTIC CIRCUMDUCTION MANEUVER, only in slow motion, to end up in EXTENSION IN TRACTION. Once I'm certain the disc material is "in," I go into the ideal DYNAMIC POSITION to keep it centralized. This is usually an EXTENSION IN mild TRACTION; however, if I want to use some applied force, a WEIGHT-BEARING EXTENSION is not out of the question.

Understand that the practice of DYNAMIC POSITIONING can be incorporated into the, later to be described, THERAPEUTIC MANEUVERS such that at the end of the MANEUVER a properly planned DYNAMIC POSITION leaves you in the ideal position for central migration of disc material. Towards this end, I tell almost all of my patients to **practice their most beneficial MANEUVER before going to sleep at night then leave themselves in a supine position with the problem disc unit supported by and slightly draped over a pillow in a near-universally helpful EXTENSION IN TRACTION posture. The pillow need only be high enough to put the disc unit in slight TRACTION and EXTENSION. In the Cervical region this amounts to sleeping with a pillow supporting the natural Cervical curvature and for the Lumbar region, the pillow supports the Lumbar curvature. For Low Cervical/High Thoracic discs, a firm pillow placed under the painful side's shoulder blade is ideal. In all** cases, the problem disc unit is kept in slight **TRACTION and EXTENSION by the pillow.** I personally find this method the most successful and for this reason, notwithstanding all the intricacies elaborated immediately above, **I usually advocate EXTENSION IN TRACTION as the most frequently successful method of practicing DYNAMIC POSITIONING** because I am more sure of its success rate and unsure whether patients truly understand the deciding factors that would dictate a different option.

Too, at any time during a MANEUVER you find a position that is extremely comfortable, that results in immediate or routine pain relief, or that results in what appears to be an advantageous movement of disc material (wherein a painless crunching sound like a knuckle cracking is heard and relief of pressure or discomfort occurs) stay in that position for a while, and rely upon the gentle, tiny postural adjustments to increase the probability of complete central disc migration. Take notes of this exact position and how you got into it so you can use the same DYNAMIC POSITIONING again in concert with the MANEUVERS that preceded or followed it when the identical pain presents itself in the future.

MAINTENANCE OF EXTENSION

MAINTENANCE OF EXTENSION, can be looked upon as the more long-term, dimension of DYNAMIC POSITIONING; however, due to its importance, it deserves special attention. It is another one of the principles advanced in this book that differentiates it from most other back pain programs in that *The O'Connor Technique (tm)* recognizes the functional role of **maintaining all levels of the spine (damaged or otherwise) in relative EXTENSION as much of the time as possible.** The major reason for advocating this posture is because the majority of back pain results from flexion damage. **Keeping the back from flexing by MAINTAINING EXTENSION not only prevents flexion damage but insures that the conditions predisposing to it are constantly minimized.** One thing for sure, if you're in EXTENSION you can't be exposing the disc unit to WEIGHT-BEARING FLEXION stresses. A **MAINTENANCE OF EXTENSION positions and maintains the posterior aspects of the vertebral bodies closer together, thereby mechanically preventing or physically dissuading the disc material from migrating to the posterior periphery for both the short and long term.** The longer EXTENSION can be maintained, the lower the probability disc material has to migrate posteriorly.

Now, it may seem obvious, but **if people have pain in EXTENSION, they shouldn't maintain this posture because that can mean the disc material is being crimped, there is facet arthritis, or spondylopathy.** I am as much a realist as anyone; and I, too, advocate, if it hurts, don't do it. The reader may at this point conclude that I'm guilty of an inconsistency. After all, pain in EXTENSION is one of the principle means one has of identifying whether a disc is at fault. If a disc is protruding, it should hurt when extending, so how can I also say don't extend if it hurts. It sounds like I'm telling you what to do when I, by my own definition, know you can't do it. Hold on, I'm not advocating the opposite of what I was advocating.

One of the hallmarks in identifying whether a disc is the problem (as I explained in Chapter Three, DIAGNOSING YOUR DISC) is pain in EXTENSION during DIAGNOSTIC

CIRCUMDUCTION. When the disc is "out" far enough, WEIGHT-BEARING EXTENSION will hurt as the herniated disc material is compressed sufficiently. But, when the disc is back "in" it won't hurt or pinch in EXTENSION posturing. Therefore, if it does hurt and arrests motion, then the disc is most probably still "out," and EXTENSIONS involving too much weight-bearing pressure or a high degrees of EXTENSION can reasonably be expected to be painful. **However, once it is "in," maintaining EXTENSION keeps the de-centralized disc material "in" by at least preventing flexion (after all, if you are in EXTENSION, you can't be in flexion).**

This MAINTENANCE OF EXTENSION policy pertains to those instances and patients who can do it comfortably and non-painfully. For the most part, those who have self-manipulated their discs "in" by using the principles of this book should have little or no discomfort even in high degrees of EXTENSION. **The MANEUVERS are designed to get the disc "in" so that EXTENSION can be comfortably maintained to keep it in.** For that time period until it goes "out" again, they should not have pain or arrested CIRCUMDUCTION IN EXTENSION any longer. When the disc is "out" one cannot be expected to place oneself in a position of pain and remain there for prolonged periods. **The degree of the EXTENSION can be tempered and modified with the addition of TRACTION to accommodate or avoid any pain.** Again, **if it hurts, don't do it**. You don't need to experience pain to practice *The O'Connor Technique (tm)*.

Over the long term, **by staying in some degree of EXTENSION for most of the time you are alive, the body can be expected to re-model itself into that position rather than the kyphosis of aging.** As mentioned in the beginning of the DYNAMIC POSITIONING sections, Kyphosis is the outcome of constant flexion as one ages. If EXTENSION is MAINTAINED, it is reasonable to assume that less kyphosis will occur.

EXTENSION MAINTENANCE is especially pertinent with injuries to the spine. Think about what happens during every flexion injury. The posterior soft tissue elements of the vertebral disc system (not only the posterior ligamentous capsule, but the facet joints' capsules and the interspinous ligaments) are stretched to the breaking point in many places. All of the ligaments have a capacity to be torn and probably are damaged to one degree or another.

When the disc herniates through the peripheral layers of the annulus fibrosus and capsule, the capsule repairs itself with "gummy bear" consistency granulation tissue that eventually turns to scar, like any other damaged tissue with a good blood supply (as opposed to the more central components of the annulus that do not have an adequate blood supply and do not heal). The scars forming while the back is maintained in EXTENSION, and flexion is avoided, will be a different scar from one that is constantly stretched in flexion. **The scar formed while the disc is MAINTAINED IN EXTENSION will tend to keep the posterior elements of the vertebral column closer together and thereby reduce the probability of future openings that will allow additional herniations protrusions.**

On the other hand, if the scar is constantly stretched by flexion, it will become a more flaccid, elongated, scar that is more apt to predispose to an opening of the posterior periphery of the annulus fibrosus and thereby allow for a higher probability of additional herniation. This is one of the reasons why ligament tears in other parts of the body are splinted by physicians, so as to allow the scar to form without motion that would otherwise stretch it, making it less tight.

The take home message here for an herniated disc is to **get the disc material "in" as fast as possible and keep it "in" during the healing stage. In order to do that, the herniation or** protrusion must be localized, identified (diagnosed), as soon as tolerable after an injury; and attempts to re-centralize it must be made intelligently and effectively so that painless EXTENSION can be MAINTAINED as soon as reasonably possible and for as long as necessary.

Being realistic, it may never go back "in" or may require surgery to remove the disc material that has escaped the capsule, compresses a nerve, or generates debilitating pain. In either case, you have to accept the probability that your disc may not be able to be put "in" by yourself or through a manipulation along the theoretical principles designed in this book; however, those are the odds you are stuck with. It doesn't mean that forcing your way through with a painful EXTENSION is the solution. I would never advocate that. **If attempting to MAINTAIN EXTENSION hurts, it probably means that the disc has been extruded to the point that an EXTENSION actually increases the bulge pressure (by a crimping action) causing the disc to have a good chance of totally becoming a full extrusion or sequestration.** So, if that appears to be happening, more manipulative MANEUVERS are necessary to recruit what ligaments remain to aid in centralizing the disc material. Recall in the chapter on FLEXION IN TRACTION that the success depended upon the disc material still being retained by the remaining elements of the ligamentous annulus fibrosus and peripheral disc capsule to be able to push the disc material centrally as tension is applied to them. **So, if no matter what MANEUVER you do doesn't end in successfully allowing you to extend without pain, you really shouldn't persist in WEIGHT-BEARING EXTENSION attempts and consider the options of seeking medical consultation, imaging studies, or surgery, whatever is most appropriate.** Only after imaging studies have shown that there is no actual protrusion, should you then persist in MANEUVERS to mobilize the disc material.

You can, however, and should by all means, **attempt to maintain the greatest degree of pain-free EXTENSION as possible at all times,** especially if it can be done in the non-weight-bearing condition or in some mild degree of TRACTION. This **MAINTENANCE OF EXTENSION insures that if you do move just right or the conditions that were preventing the disc from centralizing change to allow a re-centralization, the probability of the disc material being spontaneously re-centralized will be increased because you are in the ideal position for it to happen**.

Too, a **MAINTENANCE OF EXTENSION policy will keep the injured segment of the disc unit's posterior elements in a closed position for a majority of time thus predisposing them to heal and remain in that configuration**. I explain the manner in which maintaining EXTENSION can re-configure the damaged disc unit most convincingly by asking the reader to consider why a person having been placed in a cast experiences an arrest of muscle mobility and can only move an extremity a short distance before it is stopped by contractures after the cast is taken off. If one understands what physiological principles are acting in these instances, one can be given hope that, by using *The O'Connor Technique (tm),* eventually, the future events of back pain will be fewer and far between than otherwise.

This is reasonable to assume because, in the case of the casting, the patient is prevented from moving an extremity for a prolonged period of time. The muscles and ligaments acting on the immobilized joint undergo transformations known as contractures. **That is, if a muscle, tendon, or ligament is not allowed to function at its full length nor caused to be stretched to**

full length because of the muscles on the opposing side of the arm or leg never fully contract to let that movement happen, they are replaced by non-contractile, poorly elastic scar-like material in an evolutionarily successful mechanism designed to perpetually "take up the slack" in order to adjust to varying mechanical conditions. In persons with cerebral palsy, due to a neurological inability to move one muscle group, these detrimental connective tissue tightenings in the opposing muscle group are known as flexion contractures; but in the presence of Lumbar or Cervical EXTENSION with the intentional avoidance of flexion, the same mechanism can function advantageously to a degree. Call them, if you will--EXTENSION contractures.

The back's connective tissues can be expected to perform similarly over the long term if they too are prevented from flexion and maintained in an extended position. Just as in the case when the muscles are unable (due to damage) to be stretched to their originally designed length, if a person intentionally never lets the erector spinae muscles be stretched to their full length during full flexion, they will contract to a shorter length and ultimately inhibit a full length response when flexion is performed. Instead, they will restrict the movement of the spine so as to keep it predisposed to a constant state of relative extension due to the intentional infrequency of flexion that would otherwise allow them to be stretched to their greatest length. In a figurative sense, by MAINTENANCE OF EXTENSION, you are putting your damaged disc unit in an "intellectual" cast while it heals and a "cognitive" splint whenever it is painful.

PREFERENTIAL STRENGTHENING/SELECTIVE HYPERTROPHY OF EXTENSOR MUSCULATURE

This discussion now evolves into another closely-related phenomenon that eventually can automatically assist you to MAINTAIN EXTENSION and act to keep disc material centrally located. This equivalently-important physiological mechanism is revealed when a "muscle-bound" body builder relaxes his arms. They do not usually rest as flat against his sides like a "normal" individual. Rather, their arms stay bent at the elbow several inches from the body. Consider that in the body builder's situation, continually strengthening the biceps (a larger muscle than the triceps) causes it to HYPERTROPHY or get relatively stronger and larger than the opposing muscle group--the triceps. This results in the arm's configuration being predominately flexed at the elbow towards the biceps (anterior) side of the arm when at rest. Similarly, when the extensor muscles of the back are likewise caused to HYPERTROPHY through repeated, PREFERENTIAL STRENGTHENING, they, too, can be expected to inhibit a spinal flexion at rest. The inhibition of spinal flexion reduces the probability of the disc material moving posteriorly.

This evolutionarily programmed physiological response to exercise in concert with an AVOIDANCE OF FLEXION can theoretically be exploited to your advantage in the presence of a weak or damaged disc system. If the erector spinae muscles are never allowed to come to full flexion length by meticulous avoidance of FLEXION (especially hyperflexion and WEIGHT-BEARING FLEXION, unless necessary, such as in the case of recruitment of these ligaments as elaborated in FLEXION IN TRACTION to mobilize disc material) and never allowed to perform

208

continuous repetitive flexion as in exercises, the muscles of extension can be expected to remain shorter than they otherwise would. **The avoidance of the use of the spine's flexors combined with a preferential strengthening of the muscles of extension then can serve to re-model the spinal architecture (especially the Cervical and Lumbar spine) into an extended configuration to help prevent the posterior disc spaces from opening more than they otherwise would in the unaltered condition.** If the torn ligamentous structures on the periphery of the posterior disc area can be allowed to scar down in extension, the paraspinous ligaments and tendons allowed to undergo a minor degree contracture, and this is constantly maintained by the relative increased strength of the extensors, the back can be expected to respond by not decentralizing its disc material nearly as often. Over the "long haul" that is life, adhering to this policy reasonably stands to result in less pain.

Due to my previously stated contention that *The O'Connor Technique (tm)* is not an exercise program, I can't philosophically make too large a demand on an exercise component for relief. Exercise requires an application of force and an expenditure of energy. People in pain fear the former's risk and most working people have little of the latter commodity to spare. Exercise, all too often, is unnecessarily painful and exhausting for people who are caused by their economic condition to exercise (labor) for a living. These are usually the people who routinely suffer from back pain because they realistically have to use their backs to keep food on their tables and roofs over their heads. That is why I felt the need to advance a non-exercise method of restoring backs to functional status. However, I would be remiss in not at least offering the reader an opportunity to better their condition by **intentionally strengthening muscle groups that both prevent flexion and maintain EXTENSION. I term this concept PREFERENTIAL EXTENSOR STRENGTHENING; and it works because you SELECTIVELY HYPERTROPHY the extensor muscles of the spine to keep the discs in an extended configuration at rest.** "Hypertrophying" means to strengthen the muscles to the point that they become larger and stronger than they would otherwise be in the unaltered state. So doing makes it more difficult for the discs to inadvertently enter into a flexed configuration. In this way, the same mechanism that causes a weight-lifter's arm to rest in partial flexion when the biceps are over-developed works to the advantage of the back pain sufferer to keep the spine more in an EXTENSION posture at the site of a flexion-damaged disc.

The type of exercise is necessarily dependant upon the site and mechanism of damage; but true exercise should only begin when the disc material is "in." "In," means that the fragments of disc material have been centralized sufficiently by an EXTENSION or a HYPEREXTENSION such that they will not be squeezed or pinched more posteriorly or peripherally. **Until that point is reached, strengthening exercises should not be applied; rather, the back pain sufferer should rely upon the non-exercise MANEUVERS to bring them closer to the time when exercises can be started.**

Notice I didn't say "pain-free" when referring to the time of exercise onset. You still can have some pain and even some mild degree of discomfort in HYPEREXTENSION and slight limitation in WEIGHT-BEARING CIRCUMDUCTION. I say this because the only absolute necessity I see is that no greater harm is done by the exercise. The greater harm can only reasonably come when the disc material is abutting upon the ligamentous capsule and in danger of prolapsing when repetitive muscular contraction forces are applied.

In keeping with this concern, it is best to **strengthen the muscles as soon as possible after you are certain the disc is "in" to give the disc material the least opportunity to migrate posteriorly or peripherally again**; but one needn't instantly become a "spinal" body builder to achieve this end. A simple accommodation in lifestyle can accomplish nearly the same end, by **consciously making an effort to contract those muscles and sustain the contraction for as long as comfortable every time you think about your back pain. Program yourself to MAINTAIN EXTENSION and each time you find yourself in a flexed position that requires an adjustment into EXTENSION, go a little bit further and "punish" yourself for that indiscretion with a short extensor exercise demand.** Either seated in a chair by arching backwards, standing with your back muscles tightened, in bed with an EXTENSION stretch, or on the ground with a push up like action, contract the erector spinae muscles by arching as strongly as possible for as long as comfortably possible in the direction of the pain's site using those extensor muscles of the back in close proximity to the site of the problem disc unit. This should be done as though you were lifting an imaginary weight with your hips. However, before so doing, be certain that the disc is "in" by doing an unweighted DIAGNOSTIC CIRCUMDUCTION MANEUVER to test whether there is any arrested motion so you don't aggravate a crimped piece of disc material. Repeat these contractions a couple times at first and increase the repetitions gradually until the point when it starts to become uncomfortable and then stop. Later in the day, when you commit another flexion transgression and the little twitch of pain motivates you to perform an EXTENSION MANEUVER--add to your total daily exercise quantity by doing another set of extensor contraction exercises. By the end of the day, you will have performed enough "exercises" to have accomplished the equivalent of a traditional work-out.

This strengthening should be done as though you were in weight-lifting training rather than aerobic exercises. The goal is to make the muscle bigger and stronger; not better able to work for a long time without tiring by innumerable contractions over a prolonged period of time. You want to build a weight-lifter's muscle, not a long distance runner-type muscle. The distinction is important because studies have shown that the incidence of low back pain is increased in those persons with weak, atrophic, muscles[11] and that muscle strength and density appear to be correlated with low back pain.[12]

I will admonish the back pain sufferer to **not attempt to get "too strong, too fast"** because that has the potential to result in tendinitis, arthritis, or fasciitis (inflammation of the tissues that separate muscles), especially if you, all of a sudden, start rubbing the edges of vertebral bones together that never have felt that degree of friction.

To PREFERENTIALLY STRENGTHEN THE SPINAL EXTENSORS requires energy but not necessarily excess energy. An exercise program doesn't have to demand that a person devote a set period of time each day to work themselves into a lather. It matters little if you do twenty repetitions of an extension exercise all at once or accomplish the same feat scattered inconspicuously throughout the day. I would make no demand that the reader choose between them but, rather, practice a combination of both.

Once a person can extend without the pinching pain and DIAGNOSTIC CIRCUMDUCTIONS convince one that the back is definitely "in," an effort to strengthen the muscles to keep it "in" can be practiced by repeatedly arching the muscles of extension in close proximity to the injury site. This type of exercise system is similar to the isometric exercise methods popular in the 1950's. The object is to preferentially strengthen and, by so doing, cause the muscle to HYPERTROPHY (make the muscle larger by increasing the size of its cellular elements through exercise). **The exercises, however, are limited to those muscles that work to extend the spine.**

This can be accomplished, as alluded to above, by two basic strategies. One, a person can set aside a time period every day to do multiple repetitions of an exercise that strengthens the spinal extensors (backwards neck arching for the Cervical/Upper Thoracic spine and push-up like efforts with the legs left on the ground for the Lower Thoracic/ Lumbar regions). Or, one can make a habit of consciously contracting the same muscles repeatedly during the day (every time one thinks about it, or every time pain catches you in flexion) while lying in bed, pausing during work, sitting in a car or at the office. Either way, if done enough times, the extensors will get stronger and stronger, thereby keeping the posterior elements of the disc space closed most of the time and ultimately preventing posterior migration of disc material.

MOBILIZATION

Another concept which needs to be treated as a general consideration in applying most of *The O'Connor Technique (tm)* methods is the necessity for mobilizing a disc segment that has been subject to a continuously herniated or prolapsed disc fragment for a prolonged period of time. If an injury occurs and the central components have herniated to a position contiguous with the capsule, there is a good probability that this event was secondary to sufficient trauma to have caused some damage to the ligamentous capsule, not to mention other connective tissue structures associated with the disc unit. When the capsule or other tissues are damaged, they can be expected to become inflamed and subsequently scar down. The capsule also can be expected to undergo a scarring process due to its blood supply contributing granulation tissue to the healing process. This, in concert with other traumatic tissue damage, induces a scarring which, over time, can be expected to reduce joint mobility. The traumatized disc unit has an already decreased mobility due to a tendency not to move any spinal segment that has herniated disc material because people tend to naturally and unconsciously avoid moving segments of the spine that are damaged. Instead, they (often unconsciously) preferentially flex, extend, and laterally bend at higher or lower levels to prevent the pain caused by activating the damaged disc.

Also, the altered mechanics caused by the peripheralized disc fragments make certain movements difficult or impossible. Recall in the section on SELF-DIAGNOSING YOUR DISC, circumduction was arrested in EXTENSION over the site of the herniation. Well, this same mechanical interference prevents the disc unit from CIRCUMDUCTING through its full range of motion whenever any attempt to move that disc through its natural range of motion is made during activity. When the natural range of motion is impeded, joints tend to scar down and "freeze" (as anyone who is familiar with a "frozen" shoulder due to adhesive capsulitis can attest). The scarring is a part of the healing process which ultimately restricts movement.

If this scarring occurs in the presence of displaced disc material, it tends to decrease the ability of the fragments to be potentially re-centralized because of the adherence of scar to the

211

fragments which have come in contact with the blood supplied areas of the ligamentous capsule. This makes it much more difficult for the MANEUVERS to function because the anatomy is literally stuck together and more fixed in its position.

I believe this phenomenon accounts for why a person can have a CT or NMRI demonstrating a disc protrusion; yet the patient can reportedly be not symptomatic. The scarring and lack of mobility have been accommodated for by the body through alternative movements, and the displaced disc material has been scarred in place. The patient has, over time, learned to avoid use of that specific disc and, instead, relied upon other joints and disc units. Too, the injuries probably occurred so long ago that the patient doesn't recall the event or recognize the absence of full mobility for so great a time that it is, for all intents and purposes, "asymptomatic." If that is the case, fine, they are not necessarily in need of any therapy unless it becomes symptomatic again; however, in my clinical experience and with the support of statistical back pain findings--this period of relative painlessness is usually only temporary.

However, for those who have been living months to years with chronic pain and MANEUVERS are not immediately successful, it is often necessary to overcome this lack of mobility by repeated attempts at MOBILIZATION of the affected disc unit. The MOBILIZATION is facilitated by practicing the PRINCIPLES and repeating *The O'Connor Technique (tm)* MANEUVERS correctly, frequently, and persistently over an extended period of time, regardless of whether absolute relief is immediately achieved. It may seem like a "cop-out" because it could appear that I would prefer to blame a patient's lack of success on a person's not doing the MANEUVERS enough times or for long enough a period of time. That might be true if I were getting $35 for every failed effort; however, I arrived at this conclusion from both clinical and personal experience. When I relate this phenomenon, I fully accept that a certain percentage of people who read this book and perform the MANEUVERS correctly will not achieve pain-relief if for no other reason than their simple absence of disc disease and presence of alternative diagnoses.

My conviction that I logically had to have disc disease as the source of my pain persuaded me to persist in the only method I knew of that would stand any chance of working. It took me at least eight months of attempts to get a displaced piece of disc material in Low Cervical/High Thoracic region back into place. This may seem like too long a time to expect a reasonable patient to wait. However, the time it took to experience relief was complicated and prolonged, then, by an incomplete understanding of the mechanics and a less than ideal MANEUVERING method. Fortunately, the reader, as well as myself, now, need not sustain this procedural shortcoming due to the knowledge I have gained by going through the process of successfully replacing the disc material and learning how to do it most efficiently. The reader need not go through a time and labor intensive trial-and-error process to achieve favorable results in a more timely manner because that previously missing knowledge is supplied by this book; yet, patience must expect to be needed and practiced by anyone who has a long-term or complex problem.

The immobility I experienced that could be attributed directly to the injury was also compounded by the inborn anatomical lack of mobility of those segments. As mentioned earlier, the thorax has very little innate anatomical mobility, making it difficult to mechanically manipulate. I could recognize, at the time, that this immobility would not allow me to get a full measure of TRACTION at that area. When the disc went out, I had a pretty good working

212

knowledge of *The O'Connor Technique (tm)* but none of the MANEUVERS I was using seemed to work because I hadn't perfected the techniques (especially FLEXION IN TRACTION and the specific low Cervical techniques) by that juncture. Only after almost daily use of these MANEUVERS over a prolonged period of time as well as applying all the other techniques I advocate for months did I gradually experience an increase in mobility, evidenced by an increasing ability to actually separate the vertebral bodies. It finally popped back into place one day during a MANEUVER. I felt the characteristic warm sensation as the pressure was taken off of the capsule, and the arrested mobility in EXTENSION had likewise instantaneously resolved. It was difficult keeping it "in" for a couple of months, but with DYNAMIC POSITIONING and strict adherence to the principles of *The O'Connor Technique (tm)* my neck is now, for the most part, pain-free. However, I have to be very careful not to flex while weight-bearing with it.

As time goes on, though, with not letting it go out and being very careful not to commit any actions that are likely to put it out again, the frequency with which I get pain is so low that I haven't required a MANEUVER to put it back in for months. Now, I'm letting the scarification process work in my favor in that I have intentionally avoided mobility (especially flexion) of that segment. It is apparently scarring down effectively, since it has almost been a year since it went back "in" without any events of the type of pain with which I had previously been plagued.

I also reasoned that an additional element delaying the ability to re-centralize the disc material was that the inflammation had been allowed to persist so long that scarring had reduced the ability of the disc unit to be manipulated. When the lifting incident occurred, I actually felt the disc material herniate into the capsule, predicted that I would be in pain, and actually experienced the onset of inflammatory pain and its prolongation. The only problem was that I didn't have the knowledge I have now to put it immediately back in--so I suffered. When I did figure out what it took to get the disc material back in, I could feel that it wouldn't go because it was stuck. Repeating the MANEUVERS and the MOBILIZATION TECHNIQUES of DYNAMIC POSITIONING, CHIROTATIONAL TWISTING, INCHWORMING, NARROW-ARC ROCKING, ETC., supplied the flexibility and increased mobility I needed to get the disc material to eventually re-centralize completely.

So, the lack of mobility due to either scarring or anatomical inflexibility can be looked upon as a two-edged sword, sometimes it can work against you by inhibiting the ability to mobilize disc material when you want it to re-centralize; and it can work for you to keep appropriately centralized disc material immobile. Understanding this apparent dichotomy is why I can speak of hope when it comes to back pain, because without hope, I would never have persisted; and I would still be in pain. If you do not persist in an effort to MOBILIZE a disc unit that has become immobile due to the aforementioned influences, you may be sealing your fate.

THE CHIROTATIONAL TWIST

A technique closely allied to increasing mobility that serves to centralize peripheralized disc material is what I have termed the **CHIROTATIONAL TWIST** because I believe this action is what constitutes the majority of the effect attributed to the chiropractor's manipulations, although the true chiropractic mechanism has yet to have been scientifically, anatomically, mechanically, or physiologically explained. **The CHIROTATIONAL TWIST is an effective**

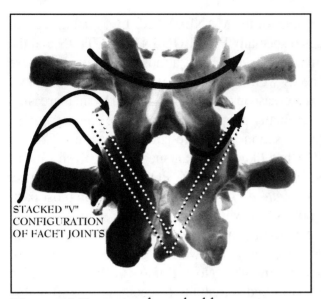

Figure 49 Rotation of vertebral bone causes separation from adjacent bone due to facet configuration

method to assist in maximally tightening the peripheral ligaments that hold the vertebral bodies together by twisting or "wringing" them. Its effectiveness is magnified if accomplished while in TRACTION; but the disc need not necessarily be in TRACTION but should always be UNWEIGHTED and never WEIGHT-BEARING.

Chiropractors seem to help a certain percentage of back pain suffers without the use of intentional TRACTION; and other therapeutic exercise regimens rely upon the beneficial aspects of the rotation phenomenon to relieve spinal pain. When a chiropractor performs the "Low Amplitude/High Velocity Thrust", due to the stacked "V" shaped configuration of the planes of the facet joint's surfaces and alignment of the posterior elements of the vertebral bones, a forceful rotation is implemented that requires the disc unit's vertebral bodies to be separated in order for the rotation to proceed (See Figure 49). As the surface of one facet joint hits the other during the twisting phase, the disc unit is forced to separate because the planes of the surfaces of the facet joints will not allow the rotational force to proceed strictly laterally without the vertebral bones moving away from each other. Something has to give and the consequence is a sort of traction by default. In essence, this constitutes a violent, rapid, separation effect as rotation forces one facet to ride against the other and the only option one vertebral bone has is for it to be separated vertically away from its adjacent vertebral bone.

On the contrary, *The O'Connor Technique's (tm)* **CHIROTATIONAL TWISTING can be looked upon as a gentle, controlled, twisting or rotating of one vertebral bone relative to an adjacent one (usually in an opposite direction).** This technique is best accomplished by twisting one vertebral bone of the painful disc unit attached to that part of the torso that is hanging in TRACTION in one direction then twisting in the opposite direction (or fixing the position of) the other vertebral bone on the opposite surface of the disc unit that is not hanging.

Figure 50 shows one way in which CHIROTATIONAL TWISTING can be executed so that the Lumbar vertebrae are rotated relative to their adjacent vertebrae. Note that the upper torso above the point that hangs over the mattress edge is rotated in one direction while the hips are being rotated in the opposite direction. The same tactic can be applied to any level of the spine. The means, timing, and ideal positions to effect this technique are explained more fully for each level of the spine when the individual MANEUVERS are discussed, so there is no point

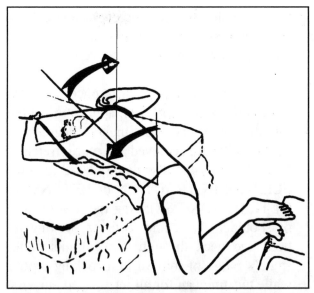

Figure 50 CHIROTATIONAL TWISTING of Lumbar region

in covering them all here.

The operant principle, as I see it, is not as complicated as it may at first seem. If one were to picture the bodies of two vertebral bones with lax peripheral ligamentous structures (as in Figure 51A) attached to the outer rims connecting each, you would see that twisting one vertebral bone in one direction and the other in the opposite direction would tighten the ligaments (See Figure 51B). Tightening the ligaments has the effect of straightening them; and, if there was any material between the vertebral bones contacting the ligaments, it would be "wrung" towards the center. Similarly, if you were only to twist the one vertebral bone while holding the other stationary, the twisting effect would occur as well, however, perhaps less strenuously.

Anatomically, when vertebral bones on either side of a disc are twisted relative to each other, the posterior longitudinal ligament and the peripheral fibro-cartilaginous ligaments that hold the vertebral bodies together are being stretched. When they stretch, they come to their full length. This pushes disc material in contact with the capsular ligaments centrally (See Figure 52). If one is hanging a disc unit in TRACTION, usually the hanging body segment is free to rotate or twist upon the fixed body segment. By twisting the hanging segment relative to the fixed segment, the wringing effect can be

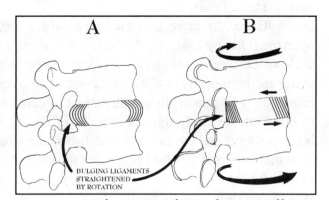

Figure 51 Tightening and straightening effect on peripheral ligamentous structures when vertebral bodies rotate relative to each other

brought to bear upon the disc material in question. This action, if done properly, especially while the disc unit is in FLEXION or EXTENSION IN TRACTION, effectively focuses the wringing action right at the disc in question, magnifying the probability that disc material will be centralized sufficiently to relieve the pain or for other techniques to be able to work.

I am convinced that this wringing action is closely related to the effect caused by the enigmatic "chiropractic manipulation." That's why I termed it CHIROTATION. In essence, the peripheral ligaments are "wrung," by the chiropractor, bringing them rapidly to their maximum length by the twisting action of manipulation. As they are brought to their maximum length, they straighten the bulge and push the disc material centrally. However, since chiropractors do not incorporate intentional TRACTION, they are committed to using the power of their manipulation

215

to open the disc unit. That's how I believe they get into trouble. It is too forceful, and the force is applied without a complete comprehension or assessment of the problem nor a clear understanding of its mechanical ramifications to insure that more damage will not result from the application of such major force.

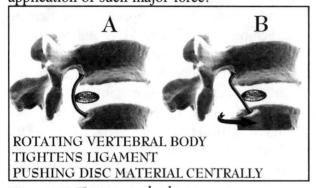

ROTATING VERTEBRAL BODY
TIGHTENS LIGAMENT
PUSHING DISC MATERIAL CENTRALLY

Figure 52 Exaggerated schematic representation of disc material being moved centrally when inferior vertebral body is rotated.

The principle difference in *The O'Connor Technique's (tm)* application of this set of forces is that higher degrees of TRACTION are achieved and more stretching engendered by the disc being placed in either FLEXION IN TRACTION or EXTENSION IN TRACTION. Swinging the legs or arms or shoulders back and forth or twisting the head and neck through to the limits of the spine's range of motion in a rocking motion while twisting can for all intents and purposes surpass in efficacy the thrust of a chiropractic manipulation; however, in *The O'Connor Technique (tm)* it is self-administered and done slowly and carefully.

Gradually increasing the length of the arc of the twisting motion of one vertebral body upon the other by swinging the legs, arms, trunk's, or head's motion slightly more and more with each successive twisting and rocking motion can judiciously apply the equivalent forces of chiropractic manipulation without the fear of exerting too much force too fast, as chiropractors often do. This action allows the patient to control the rate, amplitude, and extent of the rotation of one vertebral body upon another to effect the wringing action. As one carefully adjusts the body position and rocks back and forth, the maximum tolerable amount of tension is placed incrementally and careful upon successive fibers so that regardless of where the herniated disc material is situated, it will be eventually contacted by the peripheral ligamentous structures and moved centrally.

Each vertebral body can rotate a few degrees relative to one another (otherwise you could not rotate your spine). As a person rocks and twists, one is steadily and carefully taking this rotation to its maximum range of motion; and, at the end of the arc of the extremities, head, or twist of the torso, one can advance that range of motion carefully and progressively so as to be certain that it is not overdone or too much too fast. This is what I contend makes *The O'Connor Technique (tm)* far safer than any form of chiropractic or osteopathic manipulation.

CHIROTATIONAL TWISTING is much more effective and efficient than chiropractic manipulations because, by inducing simultaneous TRACTION, a space is created and sustained into which the disc material can travel unobstructed. On a chiropractor's table with the standard manipulation, this is not done; and the ligaments are "wrung," often without anywhere for the disc material to go. Consequently, a protrusion or partial extrusion can go to a full extrusion, pain can be induced in the peripheral ligamentous structures without appreciable gain, or a sequestered herniation can occur if there is a weakening or tear in the capsule.

In contrast, one needn't worry too much about doing damage with the CHIROTATIONAL

216

TWISTING technique. If the disc is extruding through the ligaments, you will not be able to tolerate the MANEUVER because increasing discomfort will stop you at the point when it is obvious you are doing more harm than good. In contradistinction, a chiropractor cannot sense your pain; and, after he initiates his "high velocity, low amplitude thrust," it is too late to stop him once pain is induced. The chiropractor's thrust either works and you get instantaneously better, it doesn't work and you have paid for nothing, or it oversteps its limitations and you get worse. Due to the obligatory commission of rapid chiropractic manipulative force in order to be effective, you won't know whether the wrong action has been taken until it is finished and you are left in greater pain.

Some mild discomfort associated with straightening and twisting of the peripheral ligaments of the annulus fibrosus and posterior longitudinal ligaments can be expected doing the CHIROTATIONAL TWIST since they are usually inflamed and tender when a herniation or protrusion is present. However, the movements described in this book's MANEUVERS are done slowly and cautiously until one is convinced that they can be performed with safety and ease. One can limit any excess pain by re-positioning, reducing the extent of the rotational excursions, or not putting as much TRACTION or tension on the ligaments at any given time by reducing the amount of FLEXION or EXTENSION IN TRACTION. When doing CHIROTATIONAL TWISTING in this fashion, the slower and the more controlled, the better. No fast moves are absolutely necessary.

However, there is another type of fast CHIROTATIONAL TWIST that closely if not identically resembles the "low amplitude/high velocity thrusting" chiropractors accomplish that you can do for yourself if you are frustrated by lack of success and want to accept a similar risk as attending a chiropractor. It amounts to using your hands to assist the twisting component by placing one of them superiorly and the other inferiorly to the problem disc on the body (or visa versa) and pushing them towards each other such that the body part on the superior side of the disc in question is rotated in one direction (counter clock-wise) and the inferior aspect is rotated in the opposite direction (clock-wise), or visa-versa, while TRACTION is maintained.

You can apply this type of CHIROTATIONAL TWISTING during any MANEUVER when your problem disc is in FLEXION IN TRACTION. You can even try using it when the disc is, later, in EXTENSION IN TRACTION; however, it is a little more difficult to get your hands on your hips when in extension. You are basically doing the same thing to the disc unit as in the technique described above; however, your hands are used to add force and speed to the thrust. Each time you apply a twisting force, you carefully, rapidly, but not too forcefully, twist one part of the spine on one side of the problem disc unit, further and further, so that, with the final and most forceful twisting thrust, you slightly exceed the natural limit of the range of motion of the problem disc. This rotating/twisting nearly reproduces the "low amplitude/high velocity thrust" occasioned in the chiropractic manipulation methodology. The difference being, here, that you can control the forcefulness of your thrust and consequently the degree of twisting so as not to be hurt. This forceful "wringing" of the disc unit can be done gently in stages of progressively increased force to be sure that you don't damage anything by intentionally not exceeding your pain tolerance limit. The action of pushing your hands towards each other should be done rapidly and jerkingly, but you don't have to use your maximum safe strength until you have tested the degree of force applied enough times to convince yourself that you are not going to induce pain or damage when you incrementally increase the force.

I find that often an audible "clunk" is generated that results in recognizably immediate pain relief while performing this technique as well as variations of it. I have concluded that this sound is the actual hardened cartilaginous disc material moving against bone or other fibro-cartilaginous material as it is centralized. It could be from some other mechanism; however, I reason it to be equated with the sound made when hard cartilage strikes hard cartilage--similar to when a knuckle "cracks". I would be the first to admit that I have not put a sound transducer accompanied by a fiber-optic camera in the disc space to prove it, but it doesn't really matter so long as the relief is achieved and is reproducible. Repeatedly being successful performing CHIROTATIONAL TWISTING on both myself and my patients has convinced me that I have satisfied both criteria.

HYPERWEIGHTING IN EXTENSION

Once the disc material has been re-centralized enough to eliminate pain, efforts can be made to increase the probability of it staying that way. This understanding now serves as an ideal starting point for introducing the concept of **HYPERWEIGHTING IN EXTENSION. I hesitate to make this as a formal recommendation because you really have to be competent in *The O'Connor Technique (tm)* and be able to absolutely ascertain the near-complete centralized position of your disc material to be able to do this without risk.** However, I feel the need to include it because I do it successfully to more permanently seat my problem discs, and it works for me. Therefore, I include it as an option only for the judiciously intelligent and brave who feel confident in their ability to determine the position of their disc material yet have discs that decentralize too easily, requiring of them constant MANEUVERING to keep it centralized.

Of course, no extension pressures should ever be attempted until the disc is free of any pain when CIRCUMDUCTION IN EXTENSION is accomplished. The old "working through the pain" does not apply in this instance nor does the adage "no pain--no gain." If there is any substantial increase in pain while attempting this or any MANEUVER described in this book, the recommendation is clear--**STOP!** There is no reason why anything done following the instructions in this book should cause a significant increase in pain. The character of the pain might change and usually does. You may feel an activation of the nerves from the area from whence the pain truly originates become recognizable (when referred pain becomes direct pain); however, no quantitative, substantial, increase in pain should occur at any time. If that happens, stop all movement, re-check your procedure to insure that you have followed the directions and carefully re-initiate movement only if such movement can be instituted without additional pain.

Certainly, muscles can spasm involuntarily giving twinges of pain and a serial set of MANEUVERS can give additional soreness due to the stretching of muscles and ligaments that have not been activated for a long time resulting in some increased discomfort; however, I'm referring to substantial pain brought on by any MANEUVER that was not present before beginning the MANEUVERS.

Having satisfactorily prefaced the following, for the confident and clearly knowledgeable disc pain sufferers who want to take the risk of using some force to more permanently seat the disc material in the central position as a means to reduce the frequency

of its going "out," a HYPER WEIGHT-BEARING IN EXTENSION can be tried. Based upon the understanding that disc material is decentralized to the posterior periphery usually because of forceful lifting, the **use of forceful lifting while in extension can be assumed to be able to push disc material anteriorly and centrally when it seems to repeatedly go "out."**

This is done, simply, by first convincing oneself that the disc was centralized enough to not be pinched or squeezed posteriorly by the body's weight through testing it with a WEIGHT-BEARING DIAGNOSTIC CIRCUMDUCTION IN EXTENSION. So long as no pain or arrest in movement occurs, then, one places the spine into extension directly over the area of the fissure and one attempts to lift a heavy weight or its equivalent. This heavy weight borne by the disc serves to force the displaced disc material through any fragmented laminations of the annulus fibrosus that may be restraining it from re-centralizing with just the weight of the body. Of course, this should be a very carefully done process, with only progressively stronger lifting forces so that they can be stopped at the first indication of pain. **Do not proceed if pain ensues**. While the weight is being sustained, gentle adjustments like small one or two degree circumduction-like actions that continue to maintain that segment in extension over the area of herniation should be tried; but always be careful not to be too forceful or use too heavy a weight because you could put other discs at risk for trauma if they are in flexion at the time of the HYPERWEIGHTING of the putative disc in EXTENSION.

Lifting a weight is not necessarily limited to lifting an actual object with mass. It can be simply acting as though you were trying to lift an immovable object such as a door knob, an automobile, or anything with a grip at about hip level that is so heavy it cannot be moved. HYPERWEIGHTING IN EXTENSION can be equivalently accomplished by angling your spine and body backwards while dragging a movable object such as a heavy garbage can or bag of potting soil. Pushing a car with your back in EXTENSION as seen in Figure 25 of this Chapter is also an excellent example. **In any case, the spine at the problem disc should be in extension and the lifting attempt should be such that it is equivalently forceful as an effort capable of pushing out a disc.** By that, I mean that the **degree of force sufficient to put a disc "out" can be applied in the opposite direction to put a disc "in."** If bending forward (anteriorly) in flexion to lift up a trash can is capable of pushing disc material from the center to the periphery of the disc, then bending backwards (posteriorly) in extension and lifting the same trash can should be reasonably able to squeeze that same piece of disc material from the periphery to the center. Of course, in the latter case, it is controlled and can be accompanied by some wriggling and adjustments that predispose the disc to move. It can also be done slowly and stopped instantaneously should discomfort intervene. Nevertheless, it is more than a theoretical consideration, it works for me and my discs; yet I have not, so far, had the opportunity or assurance of safety sufficient to advocate it for enough of my patients to feel secure in advancing it as a generic recommendation on the basis of proven efficacy. My primary hesitancy emanates from not being certain that patients (or readers for that matter) are completely capable of ascertaining the readiness of the disc to accept a forceful stress. I, therefore, leave it as a personal decision; since only the individual performing it can know their level of sophistication and expertise in determining the position of their disc material.

1.   Liira JP, Shannon HS, Chambers LW, Haines TA. Long term back problems and physical work exposures in the 1990 Ontario Health Survey. *Am J Public Health*. 1996;86:387.

2.   Marras WS, Lavender SA, Leurgans SE, et al. Biomechanical risk factors for occupationally related low back disorders. *Ergonomics*.1995;38:377-410.

3.   Bigos SJ, Battie MC. Acute care to prevent back disability: ten years of progress. *Clin Orthop*. 1987;(221):121-30.

4.   Bigos SJ, Spengler DM, Martin NA, et. al., Back injuries in industry; a retrospective study II Injury. *Spine* 1986; 11(3):246-51.

5.   Biering-Sorensen P. Physical measurements as risk indicators for low back trouble over a one year period. *Spine*. 1984;9(2):106-19.

6.   Hansson TH, Roos BO, Nachemson A, et al. Development of osteopenia in the fourth lumbar vertebra during prolonged bed rest after operation for scoliosis. *Acta Orthop Scand* 1975;46(4):621-30

7.   Bigos SJ, Battie MC. Acute care to prevent back disability: ten years of progress. *Clin Orthop*. 1987;(221):121-30.

8.   Bigos SJ, Spengler DM, Martin NA, et. al., Back injuries in industry; a retrospective study II Injury *Spine* 1986; 11(3):246-51.

9.   Wilson TA, Branch CI, Thoracic Disk Herniation, *American Family Physician*, May 1992;45;5:2162-8.

10.   Beurskens AJ, de Vet HC, Koke AJ, et al, Efficacy of traction for non-specific low back pain: A randomized clinical trial, *Lancet* (Dec 16) 1995;346:1596-600.

11.   Parkkola R, Rytokoski R, Kormano M. Magnetic resonance imaging of the disc and trunk muscles in patients with chronic low back pain and in health control subjects. *Spine*. 1993;18:830-836.

12.   Hultman G, Nordin N, Saraste H, et al. Body composition, endurance, strength, cross sectional area, and density of erector spiny muscles in men with and without low back pain. *J Spinal Disord*. 1993;6:114-123.

CHAPTER FIVE: SPINAL PAIN MANEUVERS

In medical practice, there are numerous mechanical actions accomplished with the body for specific desired results. For instance, the Valsalva "maneuver" is performed by closing the mouth, forcefully exhaling, and bearing down to increase intra-pulmonary pressure, the pressure change causing heart murmurs to vary for diagnostic significance.   Since the physical actions to be described in this book cause alterations in the body's mechanics, they, too, are most appropriately defined as "MANEUVERS" rather than "exercises."   Since the techniques described in this book are designed to move spinal anatomical structures, they are best termed "SPINAL PAIN MANEUVERS." By prior reading, the reader has undoubtedly familiarized him or herself with the principles associated with discogenic pain and its resolution; but, up until now, the practical directions for the actual movements have not been described. **The following sections are dedicated to describing** *The O'Connor Technique (tm)* **"SPINAL PAIN MANEUVERS." They are probably the most mechanically and physically important components of this book and comprise, in large part, the fundamental, actively beneficial, constituent of** *The O'Connor Technique (tm).*

The knowledge of these MANEUVERS did not come to me as a result of sitting at a computer with schematic vertebral designs moving through three dimensional, two hundred and fifty six color, cyberspace with a committee of government-granted University level orthopedists and neurosurgeons mulling over the economic intricacies and politically correct wording of proposed guidelines. I sustained at least three major Lumbar, two significant Cervical, and several insignificant Thoracic disc injuries and, out of necessity, in order to remain functional and pain-free, I developed these MANEUVERS to put my own discs back "in." I tried numerous MANEUVER strategies and devices, then narrowed the field down to the options to which you will be exposed below. They may not be perfect, but I tried to make them realistically capable of being done by the majority of people without the additional expense of complicated devices. Believe me, I tried countless other strategies and experimented with numerous alternatives, devices, contraptions, and methods. What you read immediately hereafter is the end product of all that trial and error.

Now, one could say that "these might work on him, but my back is different and unique." Well, I covered that contingency by trying out these MANEUVERS on too-numerous-to-count patients and acquaintances with back pain. I boiled my instructions down to the minimum and limited what I taught to those MANEUVERS that led to seemingly universally successful relief of back pain in the overwhelming majority of patients I identified with a disc problem presumed treatable by physical therapy. I found that, if my instructions were too complex or they could not understand them, they couldn't do them; and the outcome was the same as if I had not done anything--they didn't get better until I communicated the most appropriate instructions to them.

The following directions on how to perform the MANEUVERS is the product of a rather extensive, not unscientific, trial-and-error process as well. In choosing the MANEUVERS to publish, I considered which ones were the easiest to describe and accomplish. They may seem complex and difficult at first; but when confined to written communications, I have no idea whether the reader is understanding every necessary point. So, I have endeavored to be exhaustingly wordy and repetitive in order to get the message across. After reading and attempting a MANEUVER, a reader of average intelligence should readily see how basically simple and easy they are to perform as well as how effective they are at relieving pain in most cases.

In my medical office practice, I can relate one of these same MANEUVER directions with a brief description of the principles underlying the reasoning behind the movements in as little as twenty minutes. However, some patients require several visits to adequately understand enough to get themselves out of pain. Of course, this book is much more exhaustingly detailed because it must cover every reasonably possible contingency, stand as the substitute for actual face-to-face education, and serve as the alternative to a personal encounter with myself. An entire medical library could be devoted to that equivalent. So, that being said, **one must first understand some basic, universal considerations that pertain to all of the MANEUVERS, especially the Lumbar-type.**

First, if repeated attempts using these MANEUVERS over a reasonable period of time result in no relief or increased pain and/or none of the other methodologies described in this book are successful, then it is time to consider the expensive imaging studies and possibly only surgical relief as the last resort. I guess the problem with this statement arises when one asks what is "reasonable." I would probably say a couple of months, by my own experience. If a person's spine isn't very flexible, it may take that long before the MOBILITY is achieved to open the disc space sufficiently to allow anterior migration of the disc material. For a detailed treatise on the theoretical advantages of increased MOBILITY, go to the MOBILIZATION Section in Chapter Four.

These MANEUVERS are not always immediately successful in all patients, quite often they are, but I have honest, personal, as well as clinical, experience to the contrary. However, putting the MANEUVERS into prolonged practice in the absence of immediate relief never substantially or permanently harmed myself or anyone else known to me, there have been no instances of neurological compromise. I found my patients and I could easily tolerate the inconveniences. Above all, there apparently exist no other alternative, equally as effective, self-administered prospects for relief.

In the time it took to achieve personal success, my faith in the veracity of my methods was sometimes sorely tested; however, even then, the existence of the probability that I could remain in perpetual pain motivated me to persist in the face of a lack of success. Quite possibly, had I not been successful, I suspect I would eventually have become frustrated and decided to get an NMRI with the intent of eventually seeking surgical remedy especially if the pain became increasingly intense or aggravatingly unending.

At what point you may be caused to consider a surgical option is as much a function of your individual level of disease as it is your frustration level versus the belief that eventually you will succeed. One thing is for certain, you will probably not succeed if you give up, and I encourage you to keep trying these MANEUVERS until your last and final surgical option needs be exercised. Even right up to the day of surgery.

All the spinal pain MANEUVERS have the same basic goal--to re-centralize disc material that has migrated posteriorly. The *modus operandi* of all the spinal pain MANEUVERS consists of a sequential combination of FLEXION IN TRACTION in a direction away from the area of pain reference, PASSIVELY CIRCUMDUCTING IN TRACTION (rolling the body while one part hangs relaxed) into an EXTENSION IN TRACTION posture directed towards the pain reference area without activating the spinal musculature, and, finally, WEIGHT-BEARING IN HYPEREXTENSION (re-weight-bearing while maintaining an exaggerated extension posture).

After reading and understanding this book's basic PRINCIPLES (CHAPTER FOUR) deemed pertinent to all the following MANEUVERS, it should have become easier for you to appreciate the origin and source of your pain as disc-related; and, if one applies the understandings arrived at concerning CIRCUMDUCTION, FLEXION, TRACTION, AND EXTENSION forces' actions on disc material, some readers may already be competent enough to determine the location of their displaced disc material and re-centralize it. However, it is no simple task to figure out by oneself **how** to employ this understanding in a practical manner. That's where it is helpful to have each MANEUVER described in detail to direct the reader in a step-by-step manner. That way, one can benefit instantly by acquiring the years of experience with trial-and-error that I have accumulated in the development of *The O'Connor Technique (tm)*. If, as you are reading the directions for a MANEUVER, you encounter a term that is singular to *The O'Connor Technique (tm)* it will usually be in all capital letters. The definitions and concepts related to those terms can be found in the table of contents, which one can review at any time.

No reader need suffer as long as I did trying to discover the most effective means to manipulate the spine nor experiment with so many techniques until discovering the most advantageous methods. I have already done most of that work. There are probably an infinite number of alternative means to the same ends; but what follows are what I have found to be routinely successful and universally effective techniques and the easiest to apply for the majority of back pain sufferers. Some variations may be more effective than others for any given individual's spinal problem and situation; so, I have, whenever possible, included several different MANEUVERS for each spinal region in the event one or the other proves inadequate.

The reader will note that there are two thematic distinctions consistently made in the description of the MANEUVERS. They differ in whether the pain has a lateral component (such as to the side of the neck, the shoulders, the lateral chest, the flanks, the hips or one or the other extremities) as opposed to its being found to be experienced largely in the posterior midline of the body, where common sense would seem to dictate where pain of a spinal origin should rationally be located.

This may interject a slight confusion; but I found it necessary to approach the descriptions in that manner rather than to literally double the length of this section of the book to provide a complete separate direction for each condition for each MANEUVER. The difference can basically be equated by the understanding that, in both, you are attempting to direct your actions towards the site of the herniation and along the axis of the fissure. The fissure can be aimed from the center of the disc to the midline posterior resulting in pain localized to the midline posterior region or it can be more laterally aimed such that it appears to be originating in a more lateral structure. MANEUVERS accomplished taking this understanding into account have a higher

223

probability of succeeding, hence the necessity for me to treat them separately. When meeting with descriptions that draw this distinction, either ignore that particular direction or wait to see if you succeed with the other option, if not, go back and try the choice dedicated to the alternative pain-radiating area. It is not that great an issue as you will see once you have gone through a complete MANEUVER. Above all, don't let this minor complexity confuse you, try one MANEUVER and if that works, hurray! If not, try the next one described. No big deal, you are not performing brain surgery and the prospects of you hurting yourself by doing it "wrong" are slim to none if you pay attention to the below-elaborated "ground rules."

It is not necessary for the reader to master, concentrate on, or even read about, all the area-specific MANEUVERS; since, if you don't have pain in one particular spinal region, it is not productive to focus upon that region's MANEUVERS, especially if it comes at the expense of addressing your individual need. So, **if your pain is localized to a specific region of the spine, go to that section and begin your reading**, disregarding any non-pertinent MANEUVER instructions. Learning, doing, or practicing a Cervical pain MANEUVER if you do not have an interest in neck pain is unnecessary, and there is no reason to do any MANEUVER if you do not have a problem with your spine because these MANEUVERS are only designed for discogenic spinal pain. **MANEUVERS are not exercises to strengthen the spine, they are movements designed to move disc material that has been displaced.** If one were to move disc material that has not been displaced, no appropriate purpose is served.

In keeping with this philosophy, while accomplishing these MANEUVERS, **focus your efforts as much as reasonably possible on the painful disc unit, trying not to expose uninvolved discs to traction or flexion forces.** Temper this statement with reasonableness. It is not necessary to obsessively focus on avoiding involvement of other disc units to the extent that it interferes with your concentration on a given MANEUVER or expend a great deal of effort to prevent it. Traction, flexion, or extension forces generated during MANEUVERS most likely won't hurt them, but it is better to not risk the chance of a wrong move that can put a disc "out" that would have otherwise remained "in". This event is unlikely to happen unless there is previous damage to that particular disc; however, no one can recall all the possible past injuries that may have predisposed a particular disc to be susceptible to an unintentional migration of disc material during these MANEUVERS. The most common example of this nature comes when, while trying to manipulate a Lumbar disc, the patient holds their neck or thorax in an awkward WEIGHT-BEARING FLEXION position during postural adjustments. If one adheres to **the standing admonition to not persist in any movement that significantly increases pain and if any sharp increase in pain occurs or if the movement is accompanied by electric shock like pains that go down the leg--you stop at once.** By so doing, you will probably not have any such adverse events regardless of their origination.

Remember, when you induce FLEXION IN TRACTION or EXTENSION IN TRACTION to accomplish a MANEUVER, you do so to cause the disc material to move. If you jerk or alter your position violently in the wrong direction, or rapidly or forcefully induce flexion to one side or to the anterior, there exists the possibility that you could cause a disc (from another old injury site at an adjacent disc on the opposite side) to be moved peripherally and posteriorly. The discs go "out" frequently enough on their own when equivalent forces are applied unintentionally during the course of normal activity; therefore, there is reason to assume that, if you make a forcefully wrong move when the spine is bent to one side during a MANEUVER, you can push the mobile disc material "out" on the other side of a nearby disc space.

Especially during TRACTION, the disc units are necessarily in a position that has the vertebral bodies separated greatly; and a flexion event could cause a displacement of the disc material. Rest assured, it is unlikely that a person would be able to painlessly generate the force necessary to cause a normal, never-damaged disc to herniate simply by the gentle forces applied during these MANEUVERS. I make an issue of this concern mostly for those few people who have other damaged disc units and may inadvertently develop discomfort at other levels while accomplishing MANEUVERS directed towards the level in question.

During the actual practice of this method over the years, I have found that in the unusual patient with multi-level, contiguous, disc disease, **putting stresses on one disc level's damaged disc, during an attempt to effect change at an another level (or visa versa), can be counter-productive and may result in attempting to help one disc unit at the expense of aggravating another**. Wherever possible, I have designed these methods to eliminate that event; however, it is sometimes difficult to secure a completely segregated effect because of the disc unit's inseparable connections and the close proximity of all the structures to each other. Therefore, an attempt should be made, as best as possible, to **determine the precise level at which the disc pain is operant and limit activity to that area**. This is done by DIAGNOSTIC CIRCUMDUCTION as described in the SELF-DIAGNOSING YOUR DISC section of this book. Once identified as the source of pain, that particular disc unit is the area to which you should limit the majority of your effort. However, realistically, this is sometimes a difficult policy to maintain.

In addition, **if a particular MANEUVER is successful, remember the specifically successful MANEUVER and stick with it whenever an identical pain presents itself**. That will eliminate, to a large degree, superfluous MANEUVERS that could create unnecessary difficulties elsewhere, allowing you to focus on the most productive movements.

In light of the foregoing, **understand that pain at the same or an adjacent disc level can even appear to change from one side to the other after a MANEUVER.** This can be seen as a consequence of the reality that one side's extension is the other side's flexion. In complicated disc problems, flexion can occasionally cause a disc to go "out" on the opposite side as the side to which one is flexing by an unintentional weight-bearing or muscular contraction event during a MANEUVER. **In that event, it is necessary to instantly correct the problem. To do so, one should execute an identical MANEUVER following the technique directions for pain radiating to the opposite side as the MANEUVER you were originally doing. Only it should be done <u>without weight-bearing, without contracting any muscles in the immediately affected disc's region, or without moving around any more than is absolutely necessary</u>.** This should centrally re-position any disc material that may have been minimally displaced before it has time to move too far or become seated peripherally. This same practice should apply to the advent of pain anywhere else in the spine that is occasioned by a MANEUVER elsewhere. Once the painful site is identified, a MANEUVER directed towards remedying that new pain should be accomplished before any other movements are made. This movement would be the same as if the pain had originated spontaneously or independently from the MANEUVER you were doing at the time, and you simply apply the most appropriate MANEUVER for that particular disc level and side. A good rule of thumb to prevent any of these eventualities is to **judiciously AVOID WEIGHT-BEARING FLEXION at any and all disc levels during the MANEUVER process**.

Again, in keeping with this consideration, depending upon the vertebral level from which your spinal pain originates, you should, for the most part, **limit your MANEUVERING to that MANEUVER or modification of a MANEUVER that best suits that particular region of the spine and your particular problem.** In that way, you will limit the probability that you will be mobilizing disc material in discs that don't give you trouble. It is not alien to my experience to have patients cause spinal pain at some distant area during a MANEUVER calling for unusual movements to which they are not accustomed. But almost uniformly, upon inquiry or observation, they have committed some error in the MANEUVER that usually can be attributed to an inadvertent, unrecognized, WEIGHT-BEARING FLEXION action at some other spinal region.

Complementing this concern, it is not unusual for someone to think you are clowning around when you are accomplishing a MANEUVER. After all, you may be hanging over the edge of a couch wiggling and squirming and to the uninitiated this may seem like an invitation to play. They may unknowingly jar you or "horse-around" with you causing you to slip your elbow or lose your grip or make a fast flexion move to protect yourself (like your spouse or friend wanting to jump on top of you for emotional fun). Seriously, this could cause damage because when you are in traction and relaxed, your discs are very vulnerable. Your disc spaces are open and material within them is prepared to be moved. If an annulus fibrosus tear or tract exists at another level of the spine (as well as the affected disc) which is exposed to the TRACTION forces during the process of a MANEUVER and some quick or relatively violent forces are applied, they can cause disc material to move in a disadvantageous manner. **If such a probability exists in your situation, make sure anyone who comes near you knows that you are adjusting your spine and not to fool around while you are doing a MANEUVER.** Earthquakes are so rare as not to be described here as an additional cause for concern.

As a final legitimate disclaimer and valid warning, emanating from a concern for the readers' total well-being yet not to be construed as a justification to be immobilized by fear, ALWAYS PROTECT YOUR SPINE WHEN IT IS RELAXED or IN TRACTION. NEVER TRY TO GET UP FAST BY A WEIGHT-BEARING FLEXION ACTIVITY SUCH AS USING FLEXION TO SIT UP IN THE MIDDLE OF AN ABORTED MANEUVER. WHILE IN THE MANEUVERING POSITIONS YOU SHOULD ALWAYS MAKE CONTROLLED MOVES AND MAKE NO FAST OR UNINTENTIONAL MOVES THAT WOULD CAUSE A DISC UNIT TO BE UNCONTROLLABLY FLEXED, CAUSE YOU TO FALL, OR CAUSE YOU TO BE RAPIDLY JERKED. NO ONE WHO IS HORSING AROUND (ESPECIALLY CHILDREN) OR WHO COULD POSSIBLY CAUSE YOU TO HAVE TO MOVE RAPIDLY SHOULD BE ALLOWED THE OPPORTUNITY TO INTERFERE WITH YOUR MANEUVERS. THEY MAY ASSIST, BUT IT MUST BE IN SOBER EARNEST AND CAREFULLY DONE.

LUMBAR (LOW BACK) PAIN MANEUVERS

When most people think of "back pain" as an entity, they usually are referring to low back or Lumbar pain. It is by far and away the spine's most commonly painful site. Anatomically, it endures the most weight-bearing flexion of any mobile segment and, therefore, is subjected to the most damaging movements and forces. As elaborated in detail earlier, these forces create injury and most of the time it is due to flexion forces. Understandably, these forces act mostly on that disc unit that carries the most weight and commits the most flexion, as it happens, the L5-S1 disc sustains the most injuries. Consequently, it suffers the most pain. Statistically, the most frequently herniated disc is the L5-S1 disc; and, if you have low back pain, more likely than not, this is the disc that gives you the problem. The following MANEUVERS take that into consideration and are designed to centralize this disc preferentially; however, the basic MANEUVERS can be modified to work at any Lumbar or Low Thoracic disc level. The Lumbar region, because the discs are structurally so similar, is herein treated as a separate entity to be distinguished from the Thoracic or Cervical spine regions. So, consequently, it has its own particular MANEUVERS that are best employed in this region. The basic principles remain the same throughout the spine; however, the specific positions and postures are necessarily different from other more distant regions of the spine because the actual as well as attached anatomy is different.

THE BED-BASED LUMBAR PAIN MANEUVER
OR
"THE HIP-HANG"

Advance Preparation

Before you begin the HIP-HANG MANEUVER, **you need to find a comfortable platform (a <u>bed</u> is best, or a couch or a padded table), at least two bed-pillows or (better) one or two large, firm, <u>couch-cushion/pillows</u> to give you greater elevation to generate greater FLEXION IN TRACTION. You also need <u>a chair</u> upon which to rest your feet as well as <u>a rope or its strap-like equivalent</u> such as a mover's strap.**

The pillows are not always absolutely necessary; however, when used, they should be positioned at the edge of the mattress so that they are available to be laid upon when the MANEUVER starts. The pillows are used to increase the amount of FLEXION and EXTENSION achieved during the MANEUVERS. For this reason, they should not be easily compressible and their bulk should be enough to support your weight about a foot off of the surface of the mattress or platform. Ideally, they should be long enough to allow you to roll over on them. For this reason, the long couch-back cushions are excellent choices. Even couch seat cushions are okay, but you have to balance on top of them. Regular pillows are sometimes sufficient, but they really don't get the elevation if you need it unless you crowd them beneath your abdomen; and you have to frequently adjust them as you progress through the MANEUVER.

You also need to acquire a platform upon which you can rest your feet. It can be any kind of kitchen-type chair or chair equivalent such as a foot stool, box, or anything solid so that you can move it easily and support the weight of your legs, so long as it is stable with a wide base and about the height of a dining table-type chair if your bed is an average height off of the floor.

The surface of the chair should be parallel to and about the same height as the bottom surface of your mattress. If you are using another type of platform, the foot rest/chair-equivalent should be about a foot lower than the platform upon which you lie. The chair is positioned with its seat closest to the end of the bed (or table) close enough that when you are lying with your hips at the edge of the bed, on its surface, you can reach the chair with your feet. See Figure 2 for the position and distance from the edge of the platform.

Since part of you will be hanging off the edge of the bed, you need some assistance to prevent your sliding off. A human assistant can suffice; but the best effect is garnered with a rope-type device. Directions on how this is managed can be found in Chapter Four's ROPE-ASSISTED TRACTION Section. This set-up is usually necessary to accomplish this MANEUVER so that when your hips hang over the edge to produce traction, you do not automatically slide to the floor. It also frees up your arms; and, since you do not have to use your arm musculature to hold onto the sheets or the mattress, the rope makes it more likely that you will be able to totally relax your spine to accomplish the MANEUVERS.

You must be careful not to put yourself in a position that could cause your legs to fall off the bed or result in your slipping off the bed and landing forcefully on your buttocks. Having someone there to assist you is recommended, regardless, until you become comfortable with and proficient in the MANEUVER.

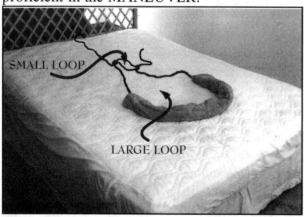

Figure 1 Rope in ideal position with small knotted loop and larger loop with blanket rolled

The rope-type apparatus should be made adjustable; so tie a small (6-12 inch) loop such that it is situated about a couple feet from the head of the bed. You then make a large loop with the other end of the rope leaving sufficient extra rope to be able to adjust the size of the loop when holding it in your hand. Figure 1 shows the ideal rope positioning so that you can let out rope as you hang further and further off the edge. You then slip your head and arms through the large loop of rope, placing it around your back so that it travels anteriorly through your arm pits (See Figure 2 & 3). Adjusting the end of the rope that has been passed through the knotted loop will let the large loop slide and lengthen so you can move your body more inferiorly or superiorly on the bed to arrive at the proper hanging position relative to the end of the bed. For a more intricate rope-related description, the reader is referred back to Chapter Four's FLEXION IN TRACTION Section which describes Rope-Assisted Traction.

The HIP-HANG MANEUVER begins with a FLEXION IN TRACTION positioning.

This position, as in other FLEXION IN TRACTION positions, allows for the posterior longitudinal ligaments and the peripheral fibro-cartilaginous ligaments to be stretched and recruited into pushing the disc material centrally. By stretching these ligaments, the posterior longitudinal ligament puts inward pressure on the disc and the peripheralized, solidified, portion of the nucleus pulposus either directly (if it has bulged) or indirectly (through the distorted annulus fibrosus) can be expected to travel centrally.

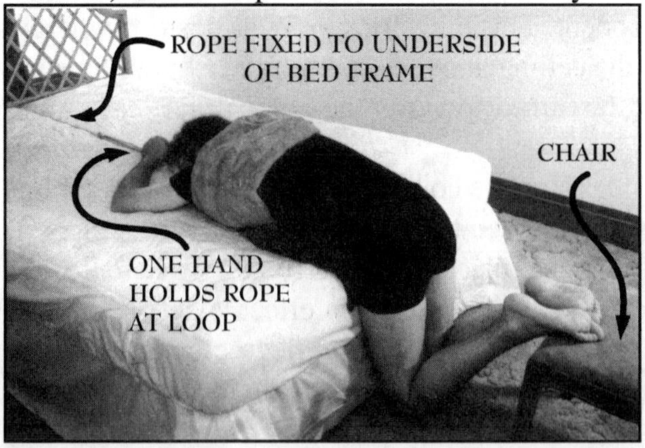

Figure 2 Starting position for Lumbar disc pain radiating to midline posterior

This extra nudge of pressure often is necessary to push the disc material inward enough to allow for the remainder of the MANEUVER to be successful. A sensation of discomfort as the character of the pain changes is not unusual at this point, but it is usually not intolerable. Depending upon how medially or laterally the disc material is protruding determines how efficient this portion of the MANEUVER is going to be. By slowly gyrating the hips (ACTIVE THERAPEUTIC CIRCUMDUCTION), NARROW-ARC ROCKING, or rolling from side to side (PASSIVE THERAPEUTIC CIRCUMDUCTION), the disc material can be coaxed somewhat to move back along the path it exited from the center. In fact, any of the assistive actions and MOBILIZATION techniques such as RELAXATIONAL BREATHING, INCH-WORMING, CHIROTATIONAL TWISTING, and maximizing FLEXION IN TRACTION by configuring the body into a "jack-knife" like position are helpful. **It is understandable that the more significantly herniated the disc material, the greater degrees of FLEXION IN TRACTION are required. In the severely protruded discs, the more FLEXION that can be created while in TRACTION, the better; but, go slowly and gradually increase the FLEXION or TRACTION only depending upon the need to do so.**

For a pain that radiates to the midline posterior it is started by lying face-down on the abdomen identical to Figure 2. The pillow(s), if used, should be placed directly under your lower abdomen at the level of the disc unit you will be manipulating.

If the pain radiates more to one side, the MANEUVER is initiated by sitting upright on the edge of the mattress at the foot of the bed, swinging your legs towards the side opposite the pain until the lateral aspect of your leg on the side opposite to the pain touches the end of the mattress while your feet are still on the ground; then, you lie down on your non-painful side which places the painful site aimed at the

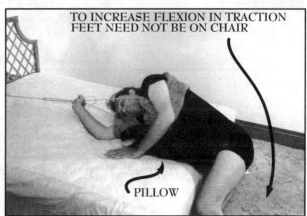

Figure 3 Starting position for Lumbar disc pain radiating to Left side.

229

ceiling so that you drape your spine over the pillows at the end of the bed in such a manner that the pillow(s) are positioned directly under the painful disc, letting your hips hang over the edge of the mattress (See Figure 3) .

Try to arrange your body so that the spot that is most painful is at the very top of the "mountain" created by your body hanging over the pillows. To get your spine into a greater degree of flexion, you may need to use extra pillows and your feet may need to come off of the chair during the FLEXION IN TRACTION component. This may bring you to a position wherein your lateral, up-side, hip is not aimed directly at the ceiling above you but, rather, more towards the walls. The painful site, nevertheless, should be aimed towards the ceiling and placed into maximum FLEXION IN TRACTION.

If your knees hit the floor, or if having the legs stretched out is uncomfortable or awkward, your feet may be rested on the chair so long as well-weighted traction produced by the weight of the legs continues to be present. Your thighs provide the majority of the TRACTION force; so, if your legs are too much supported by the seat of the chair, the traction effect is defeated. You can kick the chair away or pull it closer with your feet to get the ideal degree of traction and comfort. Or, for maximum FLEXION IN TRACTION, you can let your feet touch the floor or the bed and try to tuck your knees as close to your chest as possible, so long as your thighs still induce the TRACTION. **After you are lying down, you must position yourself superiorly or inferiorly on the bed (that is further up or down on the bed) to locate the exact position that most stretches the disc unit originating the pain.** This can be done just about any way you want to, but there is a very effective way that insures that maximum traction and effort to centralize material is produced.

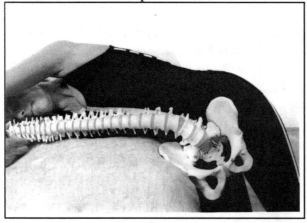

Figure 4 Hip position demonstrating maximum FLEXION IN TRACTION at L3-L4 for pain radiating to Left

First, position your entire hip on the bed so it is supported several inches in from the edge of the bed and on the pillows. Then, you use the "INCHWORM" technique by lifting your pelvis upwards (toward the ceiling) and while it is up move your body inferiorly on the bed a few centimeters. Next, let the rim of the hip (lateral iliac crest) fall back down to the surface of the mattress, plant it, and relax, letting the legs fall. The weight of the legs falling pulls the up-side of the hips away from the upper torso and stretches the spine putting the desired disc (See Figure 4) in FLEXION IN TRACTION. You can keep repeating this "ratchet"-like or "jack"-like movement to approximate the movement of an INCH-WORM until you reach the point where the maximum amount of traction is placed on the problem disc unit.

I use the term "jack"-like because, essentially, you are working your hip nearly identical to the principle functioning of an automobile jack used to lift a heavy weight, only your legs are the handle of the jack and the weight you are lifting is in essence the traction exerted on the disc unit. When you relax you will notice that the down side part of your hip is becoming a fulcrum and the weight of your legs is balancing on your hips so as to put a lever action on your spine causing it to stretch at the specific location of the pain. Keep doing it until the exact site of your disc pain is stretched in this manner. I have found that for the L5-S1 disc unit (the disc most likely to herniate) the maximum traction can be reached when the area between the rim of the pelvic bone (lateral iliac crest) and the hip bone (the greater trochanter) is positioned right on the edge of the mattress (where the top surface meets the end's surface).

As mentioned earlier, you should know you are stretching the putative disc unit when the character of the pain changes. Often the pain that has been radiating to the buttock or the thigh changes; and it suddenly becomes obvious that it originates in the spinal disc because the referred pain becomes direct disc-associated ligament pain when stretch receptors are being maximally activated at the site of the herniation.

Once you have found the ideal positioning for FLEXION IN TRACTION, you can adjust the tightness of the rope so it keeps you at that level on the bed. By grasping the rope as it passes through the small loop, only the muscle of one hand need be activated to sustain the TRACTION. This positioning can be considered an approach to the concept of DYNAMIC POSITIONING. Of course, it might be a bit uncomfortable to attempt to stay in this position for any great length of time; however, once you have arrived at this position and the problem disc unit is definitely placed in FLEXION IN TRACTION, it is an excellent posture to remain in until you are convinced some disc material movement towards the center has occurred. I don't think it reasonable to actually sleep in this position, but remaining in it for a length of time that is comfortable is certainly within your purview of best interests. When you have come to the conclusion that this DYNAMIC POSITION has served its purpose for the short term, then you can continue with the remainder of the MANEUVER.

Returning to the positioning choice for those whose back pain is felt directly to the posterior in the midline rather than to one side or the other, you should begin the entire MANEUVER by simply lying flat on the bed (with the pillows, if they are used, at the edge so that they are placed under your abdomen superior to the hips and directly under the problem disc). In the face down position, the anterior pelvic rims (anterior iliac crests) are planted on the edge of the mattress so that the posterior aspect of the disc space is opened by the FLEXION IN TRACTION. You will note, by comparing Figure 4 with Figure 5, that as the hips go further off the edge of the bed, traction is placed more superiorly on the Lumbar spine.

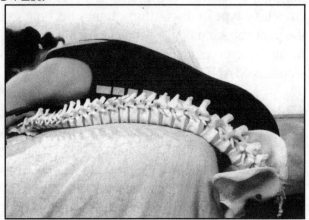

Figure 5 Position for midline posterior pain with maximum FLEXION IN TRACTION placed on L1-L2

With your upper body held by your assistant or the rope you let your hips slide off the edge of the bed in the direction of the waiting chair which is positioned so as to give you a place

231

for your feet when later you will go into a hanging EXTENSION and to support your upper body as you eventually get to the standing position.

To continue the MANEUVER, you then gradually move yourself with snake-like, or "INCH-WORM" movements of the Lumbar spine until your hips are hanging off the bed and the pillows have flexed your Lumbar spine to its maximum. To get to this position, you should have had to, in some way, manage the rope. Either you had to have let out slack on the free end of the rope to move inferiorly or you tightened the large loop by pulling on the free end of the rope to move superiorly. Doing so allows you to maintain TRACTION supplied by the weight of your legs while your upper body's position was altered by the change in the size of the large rope loop.

When you have attained the ideal position with respect to the degree with which you are hanging over the bed, you can wrap the rope around the loop a number of times so that just light gripping pressure by one hand can keep the rope's length fixed. You can also tie a knot that fixes the size of the loop, insuring that you will be kept in the ideal position for the maximum mobility and traction at the specific problem disc site, leaving your hands free to assist in other techniques. Using the rope to fix the position of your upper body in this manner is much more effective than any other alternative because you **do not need to activate any muscle groups if you aren't exerting energy trying to hold on to the bed or the rope.**

Greater degrees of FLEXION IN TRACTION can be supplied by the additional pillows or they can be used for comfort on the edges of a table or couch. You, can continually adjust yourself by repositioning the pillows or changing the length of the large rope loop to constantly feel the maximum amount of traction and stretching of the problem disc unit that you can tolerate.

As mentioned above, stretching the exact problem disc unit should cause the character of the pain to change. Often, it is described as a loss of the wedge-type pain converting to a stretching type of discomfort. It may become somewhat uncomfortable; but it should not increase the pain substantially or send electrical shocks or numbness down your legs. If it does, that may mean some entrapment of the nerve or a spinal stenosis--so you should proceed with caution or stop this MANEUVER in that case.

Now, regardless of the site of pain, at this juncture you should be in FLEXION IN TRACTION. To help re-centralize the disc material, you can begin to gently rock from side to side with your painful site continuing to be aimed at the ceiling. This is the NARROW-ARC ROCKING described previously. By "side-to-side", if you are dealing with a lateralized herniation pain and the painful side is aimed upwards, I mean it is as if you were almost trying to roll to your abdomen and, then, alternating by starting to roll onto your back; but the full roll is never completed. You only rock back and forth though a narrow arc that preferentially tightens the ligaments as the arc of tightness traverses over the exact herniation site. As this technique is executed, anatomically speaking, the posterior longitudinal ligament and the peripheral fibro-cartilaginous ligaments that hold the vertebral bodies together are being preferentially stretched. When they stretch, they come to their full length. This pushes adjacent disc material centrally. As you rock back and forth, the maximum amount of tension is placed upon successive fibers so that regardless of where the protruded disc material happens to be located, in all probability it will be contacted and moved centrally.

This traction effect can also be assisted by RELAXATIONAL BREATHING and

232

prolonged exhaling to achieve the maximum amount of relaxation and, hence, traction. Also, gentle "hula"-like THERAPEUTIC CIRCUMDUCTION can be performed here as well. In fact, THERAPEUTIC CIRCUMDUCTIONS can be performed at any juncture during the MANEUVERS to free up the difficult to mobilize disc material. Just as in any mechanical part being fitted into another, jiggling it makes it go easier. You are encouraged to wiggle, gyrate, "INCH-WORM," or fish-tail the hips so long as, after each, you relax and let TRACTION return before proceeding to the next step in the MANEUVER.

When the disc unit is in FLEXION IN TRACTION, as it is at this point, it is an excellent time to perform an assisted type of CHIROTATIONAL TWIST. For the Lumbar spine, especially in the presence of pain that radiates to one side, the wringing action can be accentuated by assistance from the hands. You may have to do some adjusting of the rope or tie a knot to secure the large loop's size (so you can use both hands) or your leg's position to get the disc unit into as much of a CHIROTATIONALLY TWISTED configuration as possible before you actually do the thrusting, but this is not too difficult. Simply let your legs rotate fully clockwise if you are going to be pushing your hip clockwise before you initiate the actual thrust. The thrust can be done by placing the up-side hand on the up-side hip and pushing it anteriorly (towards the abdominal side) while at the same time the down-side hand is placed on the abdomen/chest wall area and pushed posteriorly (towards the back) while traction is maintained. The directions that the hands push can then be reversed to push each segment of the torso in the opposite direction for the full effect.

For instance, for a left-sided pain, you would be lying on your right side, the up-side hand would be on the up-side hip, the legs would be rotated as far to the right (clockwise) as comfortably possible, and you would then push the hip further clockwise while rotating the inferior/anterior chest wall to the left or counterclockwise (Refer to Chapter Four's Section on THE CHIROTATIONAL TWIST since those diagrams closely approximate the position without showing the hand action). This creates the "wringing" effect that often successfully centralizes disc material. If unsuccessful, you can rotate your legs as far as they will go to the opposite direction while still maintaining FLEXION IN TRACTION, and this time pull on the hip with the upside

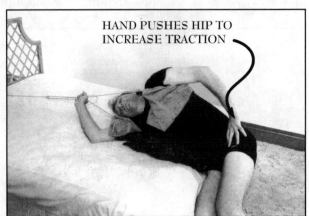

HAND PUSHES HIP TO INCREASE TRACTION

Figure 6 Using hand to push hip inferiorly to increase FLEXION IN TRACTION while exhaling to maximize relaxation of paraspinous musculature

hand to get it to go in the counterclockwise direction while you pull on the inferior posterior chest wall to get it to go clockwise. One of these two should get the desired result if the disc material is going to centralize with this action. If not, persist with the other MOBILIZATION techniques.

You can apply this type of CHIROTATIONAL TWISTING during any MANEUVER when your problem disc is in FLEXION IN TRACTION, and you can even try using it when the disc is, later, in EXTENSION IN TRACTION; however, it is a little more difficult to get your hands on your hips when in EXTENSION.

To increase the probability of centralizing disc material enough to make the remainder of the MANEUVER effective, you can combine RELAXATIONAL BREATHING with ACTIVE TRACTION by physically pushing the hips away from the trunk with your up-side arm. Your hand can be placed on the lateral iliac crest and in combination with a long exhalation you can maximally separate the designated disc unit (See Figure 6).

To get maximum FLEXION, your abdominal region should be supported by the pillow(s) so that you are in maximum FLEXION IN TRACTION; and your painful disc should maintain the same position relative to the end of the bed so that it is receiving the maximum amount of stretching. If you want to increase the degree and strength of the flexion you can flex at the hips as though you were "kneeing" the underside of the mattress. When lying on your side, it is as if you were trying to touch your knee(s) to your chest. First do it lightly and slowly with one leg, then the other, then both.

If your pain is in the midline posterior, you can increase the effectiveness of this quirky little dance by rolling to one side or the other while maximizing the knees' movement superiorly towards your chest. If the pain radiates to one side, put that side up towards the ceiling while flexing at the waist by rolling onto the side opposite to the pain. The more the pain is to the lateral aspect of the disc, the more you want to roll to the opposite side. For midline pain, you also would want to lay flat on your abdomen and use both legs at once. Of course, the bed gets in the way; however, just making the attempt puts the necessary tension on the posterior longitudinal ligaments while the disc unit is in FLEXION IN TRACTION and that's the important consideration. You can increase the FLEXION by putting more pillows under the hips.

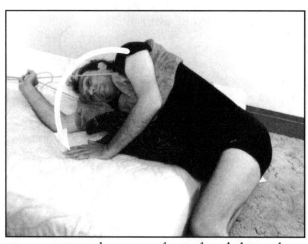

Figure 7 Initial position for Left-sided Lumbar pain in preparation for rolling PASSIVE THERAPEUTIC CIRCUMDUCTION

You might find that this action causes you to hit the floor with your knees because your legs are too long for the height of the bed. This is where the chair comes in handy. Sometimes you can't perform this because your knees and legs hitting the ground destroys the TRACTION effect. So, if the tops of the feet are put on the chair's seat with the chair moved closer to the bed, you can use the chair as a pivot point allowing the knees to clear the floor. The feet should not be so supported by the chair as to defeat the TRACTION effect. The feet and lower legs can be rested in any comfortable position just so long as the leg's weight is still producing a TRACTION effect.

At this juncture, it is usually necessary to adjust the pillow(s) under your abdominal area. If they do not seem to be elevating your hips to affect significant FLEXION IN TRACTION (which is often the reason for difficult discs not to centralize the herniated material), find more pillows or crowd the ones you have more underneath you to give your torso more altitude.

Now, while maintaining TRACTION supplied by gravity's action on the legs/hips, you do some final **THERAPEUTIC CIRCUMDUCTIONS, RELAXATIONAL BREATHING, and consciously work to achieve the highest degree of TRACTION, FLEXION, CHIROTATIONAL TWISTING, and mobility possible. Then, relax and let the FLEXION IN TRACTION function, again, to bring all the ligamentous and muscular elements to full length.** This may take a while, so relax, read something (like this book), and be prepared to spend some time in this posture as a DYNAMIC POSITION if your disc is difficult to manipulate.

Now comes the most critical and unique movement of this particular MANEUVER. **You must roll towards the side of pain until you are 180 degrees rotated from your original position, all the while maintaining TRACTION at the problem disc unit.** The manner in which this is done is demonstrated in Figures 7-10. At the end of the roll, **you want to have the painful site that was originally <u>up</u> eventually placed in the <u>down</u> position.** If your left side was up during FLEXION IN TRACTION, you should roll to your abdomen-down position and continue the roll until the left side is down. The rolling should leave you with that side (the left side in this example) down but the hips still hanging. Only now, the disc unit should be hanging in EXTENSION IN TRACTION.

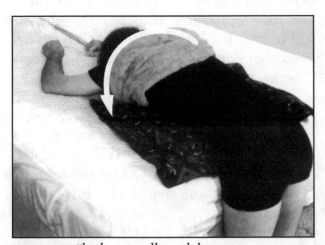

Figure 8 Clockwise roll to abdomen

In the case of an exactly midline, posterior pain, it may not much matter which way you roll. Try each way to see which seems to work the best and repeat that direction in the future if it is successful. Regardless of the direction, you would eventually want to end the roll so that the anterior aspect of the body is in the up position (therefore, flat on your back facing up) as in Figure 10.

In either case, **the affected disc unit should be caused to go from FLEXION IN TRACTION to EXTENSION IN TRACTION via a PASSIVE THERAPEUTIC CIRCUMDUCTION (rolling).** By passive, I mean that the muscles acting on that disc unit should not be activated or contracted. The disc unit musculature should stay in the most relaxed and stretched-by-gravity condition as possible. The strength and muscle activity responsible for the movements necessary to effect the roll should come from the arms, legs, and adjustments of the torso.

By frequently adjusting your position

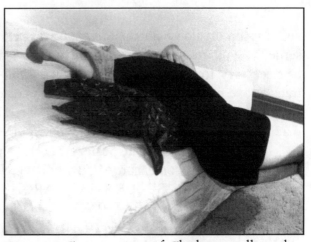

Figure 9 Continuation of Clockwise roll until left side becomes the down side

relative to the edge of the surface you are lying on, the maximum amount of flexion at the onset and extension at the end should be kept at the problem disc level where the pain originates. For this reason, anticipating where you eventually want to end up in maximum EXTENSION IN TRACTION should dictate to what degree you are hanging over the edge of the bed or surface upon which you are rotating. Too, if you think about it, you don't want to roll off the side of the bed when you complete your roll. So, before you roll, position yourself on the bed and the pillows so that you have an area on the bed to roll onto so you won't end up half way through the roll without bed space or pillows upon which you can come to rest. **It is essential to maintain TRACTION during the entire roll; however, you do not need to change position relative to the left or right side of the bed. You can roll in place (as depicted above) by careful adjustments of your torso so long as with each movement you re-establish TRACTION before proceeding with the roll. Sometimes you may find rolling in place more effective because it allows you to better keep the disc unit in question at the ideal TRACTION site. Rolling in place, by virtue of the necessarily repeated postural adjustments, fortuitously incorporates a sort of rolling "INCH-WORM" action that benefits the MANEUVER.**

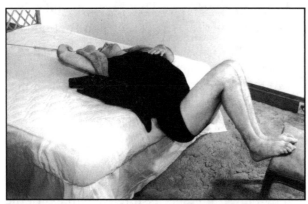

Figure 10 Clockwise roll in TRACTION terminating in EXTENSION IN TRACTION for Lumbar region disc

Then, after resting with your painful site down so as to re-establish maximal TRACTION IN EXTENSION and doing a few "hula"-like THERAPEUTIC CIRCUMDUCTIONS, you breathe to relax. **At this point, you should have the putative disc unit in an extension and the full EXTENSION IN TRACTION should be occurring directly over the painful site**

It is very important to try your best to maintain traction during the rolling. Sometimes it is hard because you need to adjust your hips or torso, or use your arms, and that results in a disturbance of relaxation because you need to contract some muscles and it is almost impossible not to contract ones acting on the disc unit. If this happens and you sense that you are not in traction, stop and re-establish traction before you continue. It may even be necessary to re-adjust your position on the bed by "jacking" your hips again to get more traction and extension at the exact site of the disc. Do this at any point you feel you have moved such that the exact problematic disc level is not being stretched. At the end on the roll, while in maximum EXTENSION IN TRACTION, your bending should be directly over the herniation site.

Whether for midline posterior pain or pain that is lateralized to one side or the other, after you have done some more MOBILIZING with CHIROTATIONAL TWISTING, NARROW-ARC ROCKING, SEQUENTIAL ARCHING THERAPEUTIC CIRCUMDUCTIONS, RELAXATIONAL BREATHING, in-place "INCH-WORMING," THERAPEUTIC CIRCUMDUCTIONS WHILE IN TRACTION, and generalized wriggling, **return to the face up position with your hips hanging so that your posterior is facing down. Your hips should still be hanging, only this time you are face up** (See Figure 11) and ready to proceed with the

236

MANEUVER.

At this juncture the opportunity presents itself to apply DYNAMIC POSITIONING. If you are not certain that you were successful in moving the disc material centrally during the progress of the MANEUVER, maintaining your Lumbar spine in the most ideal position to facilitate centralization exists as an alternative, potentially successful strategy. The degree of both TRACTION as well as EXTENSION can be reduced and made to conform to a comfortable and tolerable

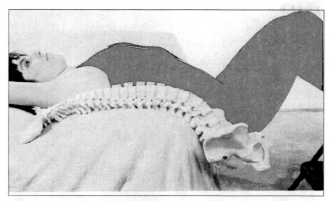

Figure 11 EXTENSION IN TRACTION showing configuration of Lumbar spine.

level. Relaxing for a time in this configuration insures that all the soft tissues come to full length. I doubt that you would want to sleep in this position; however, the longer you stay in it, the greater the probability you will move disc material centrally. Be reasonable and sensitive to the realities of your back, and don't persist in this position longer than is comfortably tolerable. It is not unreasonable to experiment with progressively longer times until you reach the point of diminishing returns.

Once you are face up with your hips hanging and your feet on the chair so that their arches are on the edge closest to the bed, relax. You can carefully pull yourself back onto the bed while keeping your hips relaxed so that you are able to rest in extension without the absolute necessity of using the rope. Here, again, after every adjustment in position, "hula"-type ACTIVE THERAPEUTIC CIRCUMDUCTIONS can be highly effective.

At this point, your disc material may have centralized enough to complete the MANEUVER; however, quite frequently this is not the case. **If it has not centralized, you may experience a pinching or crimping sensation that prevents you from going comfortably into the full EXTENSION IN TRACTION.** This is the same type of pain described in the pain section of the book caused by the disc material creating a fulcrum effect or an actual crimping of protruding disc material. This pinching indicates that the peripheralized disc material still is producing an obstruction to the full range of motion of the joint. In order to meet with this problem you have to do some more mobilizing before continuing with the MANEUVER. What follows are some strategies to use in order to get difficult disc material to go "in."

On the other hand, if there is little or no discomfort associated with this position of EXTENSION IN TRACTION and you feel that the roll was sufficient to centralize your disc material, you can go directly to the last part of the MANEUVER (described below) and ignore these extras.

First, you must consider that the reason why the disc material is not re-centralizing could be because you did not generate enough FLEXION during the first part of the MANEUVER. So long as TRACTION is maintained (here is where tying off the loop of rope to prevent it from elongating helps free up your hands), using your hands to bring one leg at a time as close to the chest as possible can again induce a FLEXION IN TRACTION without weight-bearing that can immediately be converted into an EXTENSION IN TRACTION when you let your legs down and hips hang again. It is this action that can "pump" or "milk" the disc material anteriorly.

The painful side's leg should be tried first by grasping it at the knee with the same side hand and pulling it towards the chest. The lifted leg's ankle can also be positioned across the other chair-supported leg and moved along its anterior surface towards the body until the lower part of the leg being lifted can be grasped to get more leverage. More FLEXION at the Lumbar region can be garnered if the thigh is allowed to fall to the side in external (away from the body) rotation, letting you grasp the lower leg near the ankle like half of a yoga-type sitting posture. An additional degree of FLEXION IN TRACTION can be achieved here by doing something very much akin to a sit-up as if you were trying to touch your feet to your forehead. Only babies and contortionists can really do this, but making the motions like you are trying to do it, as much as you reasonably can, is sufficient for most purposes. Flexion, even somewhat forceful, is allowed here because you should still be in a totally unweighted (in traction) position due to the hip still hanging. So long as you are in traction or at least non-weight-bearing, the de-centralized disc material has some place to move into as the posterior ligamentous elements are tightened.

The other leg can be done the same way, and it should be tried if it hasn't appeared that the disc material has moved.

Sometimes, the reason the disc will not re-centralize is because not enough TRACTION has been achieved. Additional traction can be garnered by another means while in this position, especially if you have noted no evidence of disc movement thus far. You lie backwards in full EXTENSION on the bed while keeping the hips hanging, totally relax but keep your feet on the chair, and place your hands on the anterior aspects of the upper thighs as close to the hips as possible. The thigh bone can be grasped between the index and thumb (almost as if you had your hands in your pockets with the thumbs outside of your pockets pointing to the midline of your body) or you can put your thumbs in your belt and push the thighs away from the torso by extending at the elbows. It may take some adjusting so that the rope through your armpits will allow your hands to get down that far; or you may have to move up on the bed to reduce some of the HIP-HANGING so as to make these other moves feasible.

The force of your arms pushing the thighs away from the body should separate the upper torso away from the hips which are still hanging over the edge of the bed. While the legs are on the chair, you can push the thighs away, which, because they are connected to the hips, will pull the sacrum away from the Lumbar spine. This induces as much ACTIVE TRACTION as your arms can generate if you can keep the hips and Lumbar region relaxed. Some "hula"-type THERAPEUTIC CIRCUMDUCTIONS simultaneously coordinated with RELAXATIONAL BREATHING exhalations gives extra mobility in TRACTION.

I have found that thin people's legs do not always supply enough weight to sufficiently tract the disc unit. In that event, some source of traction other than the weight of the legs has to be found. The arms work well for this purpose. If you feel brave, an assistant can gently provide additional force by using their own weight to help push or pull your hips away from your torso.

While the ACTIVE TRACTION is applied, try CIRCUMDUCTING in both clockwise and counterclockwise directions to try to move "stuck" disc material. Again, keep adjusting your position on the bed, if necessary, so that the problem disc keeps the most TRACTION available applied to it.

238

You can also slide off of the bed so much that your Lumbar spine assumes an almost vertical alignment while you rest on your elbows, letting the Lumbar spine straighten by pushing it away with your hands and then alternating this several times with arching it into HYPEREXTENSION to again try to "milk" the disc material "in" after it has been exposed to TRACTION magnified by the strength of the arms.

Also, this technique can be combined with an EXTENSION INCH-WORMING in which your pushing on the thighs restrains the hips from moving superiorly as you perform the spinal extensions (by contracting the erector spinae muscles) and you attempt to pull the posterior aspect of your hips closer to the posterior aspect of your shoulders (just like a real inch worm only on its back). The problem disc should start in passive extension in a HIP-HANG during the traction phase, and this action keeps the disc in maximum traction until the extension contractions cause the disc unit to close posteriorly first. This ACTIVE HYPEREXTENSION serves to squeeze disc material more anteriorly and centrally.

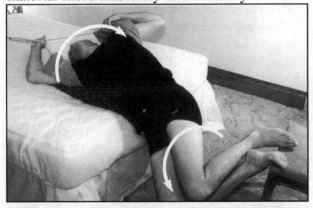

Figure 12 CHIROTATIONAL TWISTING of Lumbar region while in hip-hang with legs fully clockwise and shoulders counterclockwise.

Combining this type of action with a SEQUENTIAL ARCHING THERAPEUTIC CIRCUMDUCTION described earlier in the book is particularly useful at mobilizing difficult disc problems. By sequentially moving through all the possible areas where the disc material may be peripheralized you are less likely to miss the precise location that would lead to a movement of disc material centrally back along the fissure axis.

As an aside, this type of movement need not be restricted to a HIP-HANG, it can be used in a supine position with the Lumbar spine supported in extension with pillows or a towel. It is extremely effective if you repeat it in a rhythmic manner that involves pushing away with the arms while exhaling; then, just as the disc unit is in maximum active traction, you contract the erector spinae muscles into an ACTIVE HYPEREXTENSION with strong muscular contraction. As this series of actions is repeated you can effectively milk the disc material centrally. The beauty of this "sub-MANEUVER" is that it can be done without going through the rigmarole of an entire HIP-HANGING MANEUVER anytime it has been shown to work successfully. It can be done in bed simply when lying down with a Lumbar support as a morning stretching activity to centralize disc material that may have spontaneously migrated during the night's sleep. I f A C T I V E   T R A C T I O N   o r HYPEREXTENSION doesn't result in an obvious relief of pain, to assist centralization of disc material, **you can perform CHIROTATIONAL TWISTING while in a hip-hanging position**. It is simple enough to effect by holding your upper back and Thorax relatively stationary and allowing your legs to fall as far to one side and then to the other as they will go. The falling legs will lift the opposite side's chest off of the mattress. That is, as the legs fall to the left (See Figure 13), the right chest comes off the mattress due to the weight of the legs twisting the spine into its maximum range of rotatory motion, attempting to exceed this range of motion causes the chest and shoulder to raise up. You can push the limits of the rotatory range of motion of the spine if you twist the upper thorax in the opposite direction. That is, force the lifted shoulder to go back down into the mattress by extending the arm of the shoulder that is being lifted. The arm's weight or grabbing on to the mattress edge to hold it down really cranks the spine into a twisted configuration. By doing this in a quick rapid moves like a "crack the whip" effect, you are

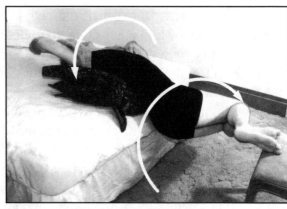

Figure 13 CHIROTATIONAL TWISTING of Lumbar region in HIP-HANG with legs fully counterclockwise and shoulders clockwise

performing CHIROTATIONAL TWISTING at its best. If it works, give yourself $30 because you have basically done what a Chiropractor does.

Sometimes it helps if you get as vertical as possible while in a HIP HANG while you do CHIROTATIONAL TWISTING. This involves letting out as much rope as necessary to bring your Lumbar spine to the near vertical axis. This puts as much gravitational force on the discs to tract them without any interference from the bed. You can take your legs off of the chair at this point and pivot on your toes to get your legs to move together as a unit as they swing from side to side, twisting the Lumbar region while in traction. You may have to keep your heels directly under your buttocks to do it, but the idea here as with other CHIROTATIONAL TWISTING is to maximize the ligamentous twisting effect. This can be done by gradually increasing the size of the arc through which they move. If you do it faster and faster, the momentum of the joined legs continues to move the legs and causes them not to stop immediately upon reaching the usual, natural, range of their rotatory motion. It causes the natural range to be exceeded instantaneously, especially if your give your upper body a twist in the opposite direction at the same instant. This physically approximates what a Chiropractor accomplishes when you are on his table. By pulling yourself back onto the bed, in increments, while continuing this motion, you can successively put any disc unit through its rotatory range of motion. If the disc is normal, this should cause no problem. If the disc is herniated, it should assist the centralization process by tightening the peripheral ligamentous structures through a

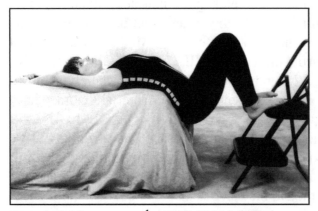

Figure 14 Initiating the HIP-HANGING EXTENSION IN TRACTION Lumbar CASCADE when pain is at midline/posterior

240

wringing action.

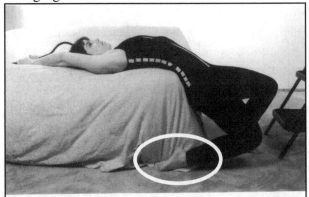

Figure 15 Feet being positioned for CASCADE while maintaining EXTENSION

Now, you are ready to proceed with the remainder of the entire MANEUVER which amounts to sliding off of the bed in a very specific, controlled manner which I term a HIP-HANGING LUMBAR CASCADE. Anatomically, what you are accomplishing with the CASCADE element of this MANEUVER is a successive HYPEREXTENSION IN RELAXATION AND TRACTION of every individual disk unit, such that each, as it falls off the edge of the bed, is allowed to achieve the highest degree of TRACTION IN EXTENSION that proceeds automatically into a WEIGHT-BEARING EXTENSION. This gives the performer as much EXTENSION IN TRACTION as possible without the aid of some device (such as an inversion/traction machine) or clinical (chiropractic) assistance.

In preparation for this you bring yourself back onto the bed, put your feet on the chair, and let yourself get completely relaxed so that your hips are barely hanging over the edge, letting the bed support the majority of your body's weight. Your hips need only be slightly hanging **(See Figure 14)**. By now, most people are pain-free while resting in this position. If not pain-free, the pain is usually significantly reduced by the wedge-like component no longer being present. If you are not sure, **you can test whether your disc material is "in" or not by gently rolling your entire body from one side to the other.** Since your hips are hanging and as long as you don't activate the muscles at the problem disc level, bending the spine while rolling essentially constitutes performing a PASSIVE DIAGNOSTIC CIRCUMDUCTION. This rolling will tell you whether there is any arrest in motion as you put the problem disc level through a non-weight-bearing circumduction. As you roll, the hips should still be hanging in such a position that your

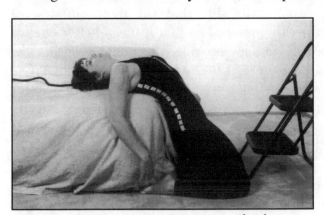

Figure 16 CASCADING to rest on heels in WEIGHT-BEARING EXTENSION

problem disc should be in extension when the site to which the pain usually radiates comes to a downwards facing configuration. If there is any disc material impeding the circumduction, it should become apparent as you roll onto it and compress that portion of the disc in extension. **If there is no impedance to a DIAGNOSTIC CIRCUMDUCTION, no wedge-like pain, or pain-arrested mobility, it is safe to assume that the disc material has migrated sufficiently to allow for the next step-- WEIGHT-BEARING in EXTENSION .**

This stage of the MANEUVER begins

241

by resting most of your body weight and relaxing on the bed with your hips slightly hanging. This posture eliminates the necessity for the rope; so you can remove it from around your body but continue to hold onto it so you can control your rate of sliding off the bed when the time comes. Your upper body should be supported by the bed enough so you don't slide off the edge just yet. This position allows you to free up your feet so you can push the chair away to give yourself some more room.

Then, you put your toes on the ground in preparation for the slide off of the bed. **You must put the top (anterior) surface of your feet and toes (the part that you see when you look down, not the bottom, plantar surface) on the floor.** (See Figure 15) This hyper-extends the ankle, and to do it without discomfort you must move your feet closer to the bed and well under your buttocks. This positioning has very little to do with the ankle and a lot to do with the ability to slide off the bed and still keep your back in EXTENSION. Without this pre-positioning of the feet, it is impossible to keep the back in the degree of HYPEREXTENSION necessary to properly complete the MANEUVER.

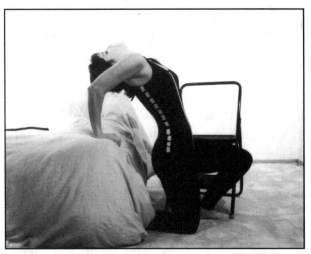

Figure 17 Keeping spine in EXTENSION while coming to standing

Now, you slide your hips off the edge and CASCADE (like a waterfall) off of the bed. The best way I can describe this is to place your feet, top side down, one at a time, as far as possible underneath you. You may have to do a little tip-toe-walking backwards, as you are cascading, to manage this. Then, keeping the back relaxed, you slowly CASCADE off the bed so that eventually you land on your knees just like a Japanese person traditionally sits on their heels (See Figure 16).

It helps to CASCADE while bending the spine at the affected disc, extended, and leaning towards the side that has the most pain (the side that the pain radiates to) because this helps to "capture" and squeeze the disc material so that it has a better chance of being moved centrally. The farther pain is felt to the side when tested during the DIAGNOSTIC CIRCUMDUCTION test in the section on "SELF-DIAGNOSING YOUR DISC", the more leaning to that same side should be done when you CASCADE off the edge of the bed. Here, you are performing a "pincer-type" effect to capture the disc material by extending directly over the herniation to cause it to move centrally. **During the entire process of getting off the bed and onto your feet, you should remain in EXTENSION and, by all means, DO NOT FLEX ANY PART OF THE SPINE.** You might note that even the neck is kept in EXTENSION. This insures that during the time you are later getting to your feet that you do not mistakenly or unintentionally flex any part of the spine.

The rate of your CASCADE can be controlled by retaining the rope and gradually releasing or increasing your grip. You can, in this manner, stop the CASCADE at any painful

242

point and do some "hula"-type THERAPEUTIC CIRCUMDUCTIONS to jiggle any reluctant disc material free. If, as you are circumducting, the same wedge-type pain returns, that means you have not freed up the disc material sufficiently for it to move centrally. If so, go back and repeat the whole MANEUVER again starting with the FLEXION IN TRACTION component until you can sustain full EXTENSION without this wedge-like, pinching pain. It may take several attempts. You might have to get accustomed to and comfortable with the MANEUVER enough to convince yourself that it isn't going to hurt you and that you can trust yourself to do it correctly and painlessly. You might have to practice the MANEUVER so that you can do it in, smooth, successive steps. Don't dismay, if you don't think a particular component of the MANEUVER is successful, re-read the description and make sure you aren't violating any principles. One really must obey the general sequence of FLEXION IN TRACTION, rolling to EXTENSION IN TRACTION without tightening any of the disc unit's muscle groups, then WEIGHT-BEARING IN EXTENSION; however, any particular posture or action can be prolonged or varied depending upon need.

If at any time you begin WEIGHT-BEARING, a crimping or pinching pain is felt, this signals that the disc material has been previously herniated or protruded so far beyond the circumferential periphery of the disc unit that it will not allow for WEIGHT-BEARING EXTENSION without pain. In essence, the disc material is being trapped like an inner-tube

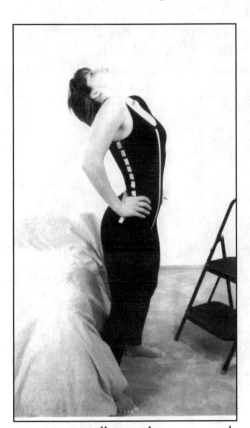

Figure 18 Fully standing in partial WEIGHT-BEARING EXTENSION

sticking through a slashed tire. If you cannot sustain the weight of your body on the disc in question while in EXTENSION because too much pain ensues, that means the extruded disc material has not been centralized adequately. In that event, relax the degree of EXTENSION, pull yourself back onto the bed, repeat the entire MANEUVER, or get up in what ever manner results in the least amount of pain and go on about your business until you want to try another MANEUVER.

If no wedge-like, pinching, or crimping pain is felt, you can then come to a standing position. This is done carefully by using the bed and the chair for support as you judiciously keep your entire spine in as much EXTENSION as your comfort will allow. **You must get to your feet by first bringing, to a flat-on-the-floor stance, the foot on the opposite side as the side to which the pain radiates most.** Coming to standing using that leg first keeps the opposite side that has the disc herniation in the most WEIGHT-BEARING EXTENSION, trapping the disc material, and preventing it from moving peripherally.

Once standing, the final "seating" of the disc material can take place. You put both your hands on your hips and push inferiorly. (See Figure 18) This slightly unweights your Lumbar spine so you can CIRCUMDUCT IN EXTENSION back and forth several times. The pressure your hands are exerting inferiorly can be gradually decreased making the CIRCUMDUCTION progressively more WEIGHT-BEARING so that you do not suddenly put too much pressure too rapidly in the event that the disc material is still too far peripherally to properly centralize. To do so might be unnecessarily painful. Also, you should not FLEX at all during this stage of the MANEUVER. The entire process of CIRCUMDUCTION should be done while kept in EXTENSION. This requires that you limit the arc of your CIRCUMDUCTION to the 3:00-to-6:00-to-9:00 range. It probably will be uncomfortable to do otherwise, anyway.

The action that your hips and Lumbar spine goes through in this final action should resemble something akin to a "Bump and Grind" with your pelvis pushed as far anteriorly as possible to HYPEREXTEND (See Figure 19) the Lumbar spine so as to move any residual disc material with what, in essence, constitutes a THERAPEUTIC AND DIAGNOSTIC ACTIVE CIRCUMDUCTION. It is THERAPEUTIC in the sense that if everything goes right, this final gesture will seat the disc material back into the most central position it can occupy. It is DIAGNOSTIC in the sense that if any disc material is still peripheralized, the CIRCUMDUCTION will disclose its presence and position, indicating that you may need to repeat the entire MANEUVER or try again at some future time.

Usually, if this MANEUVER is unsuccessful the problem rests in not obtaining enough centralized movement of the disc material because it is still too peripherally herniated or protruded. This means that you should focus more on the FLEXION IN TRACTION component of the MANEUVER until you feel the wedge-like obstructing pain is resolved. For difficult discs, it may take a lot of trials with MOBILIZATION TECHNIQUES and THERAPEUTIC CIRCUMDUCTIONS (clockwise or counterclockwise) especially during the EXTENSION components of the MANEUVERS. You may have a disc like that portrayed in Figure 42 in Chapter Four, requiring that you play the "'BB-in-the-Maze Game" with SEQUENTIAL ARCHING THERAPEUTIC CIRCUMDUCTIONS; however, getting this complicated a disc "in" calls for some ingenuity based upon a careful study of the PRINCIPLES of *The O'Connor Technique (tm)* not a visit to a surgeon or chiropractor.

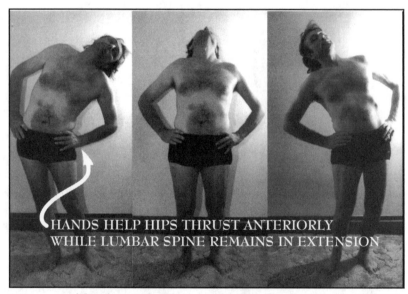

HANDS HELP HIPS THRUST ANTERIORLY WHILE LUMBAR SPINE REMAINS IN EXTENSION

Figure 19 THERAPEUTIC AND DIAGNOSTIC ACTIVE CIRCUMDUCTION as upper torso swings through an arc in EXTENSION.

FLOOR-BASED/PILLOW-ASSISTED LUMBAR TRACTION ROLL
OR
"THE LUMBAR PILLOW-ROLL"

Sometimes, if you don't have immediate access to a bed or are overweight and rolling roped around on the edge of a bed with couch cushions is exceptionally difficult, another method can be successful, especially if the disc herniation is not very severe. For want of a better term, I call this method FLOOR-BASED/PILLOW-ASSISTED LUMBAR TRACTION ROLL or THE LUMBAR PILLOW-ROLL. It is another, oftentimes effective, means of accomplishing FLEXION IN TRACTION with a rolling THERAPEUTIC CIRCUMDUCTION into an EXTENSION IN TRACTION. It is all-in-all probably less effective than a HIP-HANGING MANEUVER because neither the degree of TRACTION nor EXTENSION is as great as in THE HIP-HANG; but it's convenience makes it especially useful. Nevertheless, its use is not mutually exclusive with any other MANEUVER. **That is, it can be used in conjunction with other MANEUVERS and need not be looked upon as something that must be used to the exclusion of other techniques or MANEUVERS.** I would encourage the reader to try them all.

Advance Preparation

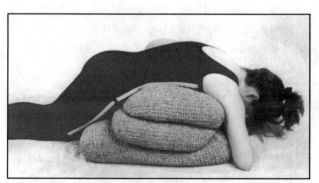

Figure 1 FLEXION IN TRACTION with pillows for midline High Lumbar/Low Thoracic discs

This MANEUVER requires that the pain sufferer **build a small mound of firm pillows or couch cushions on the floor** to allow for FLEXION IN TRACTION in a recumbent position. It is better to acquire the largest and widest pillows available; and a couch cushion seems to be the most readily available pillow to most households, however, sleeping bags, rolled-up foam rubber mats, or any stacked objects covered with padding will suffice so long as it is comfortable and capable of resisting movement along the surface of the floor by virtue of its mass and friction. The pillows are arranged so as to be in the shape of a small ridge on a carpeted floor with the widest and longest pillow being at the bottom. The wider the pillow the better because during the MANEUVER, a rolling of the body needs to take place and the person **must be able to remain supported by the pillow while rolling in place from one side to the other.**

The MANEUVER begins with a FLEXION IN TRACTION activity by lying with the painful side up on the mound of pillows so that the spine's problem disc segment is supported in a flexed position with the pillows directly beneath the site of pain (See Figures 1 & 2). This places the area of the spine in question into a gently flexed position to one side (if the disc material is herniated to one side) or flat on the abdomen (if the disc is herniated directly to the posterior). If the pain radiates to one side, then that side should be made the high side, aiming the pain towards the ceiling.

It is essential that one never flex unless unweighted and this MANEUVER allows for the necessary support to sustain such a flexed position without increasing direct prolapsing pressure. Remember, all of these motions are to be accomplished gently; and, **if any sharp increase in pain occurs or if the movement is accompanied by electric shock like pains that go down the leg, then stop this at once.**

The next step involves bringing the peri-vertebral musculature at the problem disc site to the maximum level of relaxation. This is done by the RELAXATIONAL BREATHING

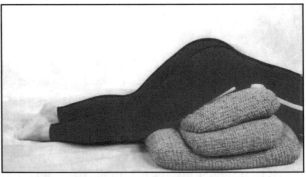

Figure 2 FLEXION IN TRACTION with pillows for midline Low Lumbar discs

technique (described in Chapter Four) combined with a constant effort to not attempt to move any part of the body that is attached muscularly to the portion of the spine being worked on.

Some people have difficulty relaxing the back muscles. For those who do, a particularly effective RELAXATIONAL BREATHING exercise can be tried when using pillows beneath the abdomen for Lumbar disc problems. First, the abdominal muscles are contracted as though one were sucking in their abdomen at the end of a large inhalation. Then, as the air is exhaled, you push your abdominal contents into the pillows (as though you are sticking out your abdomen to make it as protuberant as possible). Then, the abdominal muscles are relaxed along with the back muscles and the whole area associated with the abnormal disc is allowed to totally relax and hang. This relaxation should be sustained and no attempt to activate any muscle group in the areas adjacent to the painful area should be allowed once that they have been relaxed.

Now, TRACTION is being applied by the height of the pillows and the draping of the involved segment over them to separate the vertebral bodies so as to allow the disc material a space to move into and to take advantage of the plunger-like suction effect that centrally originating negative pressure has on the disc material's movement to the center where it belongs. This can be accentuated by using the down side elbow(s) planted into one of the pillows as a rocking platform upon which to pull the upper body away from the lower body. The elbows act with a fulcrum-balancing-effect or a pole-vault-like-effect to pull the upper body away from the hips which are impeded in their superior movement by the pillows. Then, the elbow is leaned into so that progressively more of the weight of the flexed and relaxed head and neck acts to pull the rest of the body after it. As the shoulder(s) fall superiorly the elbow(s) and the upper arm(s) get positioned closer to the body and more inferiorly along the axis of the body so that, as they are incrementally leaned into, the upper torso is rocked forward. The portion of the spine below the painful area is restrained by the pillows and not allowed to be pulled superiorly when the elbow-balanced upper torso is caused to rock forward by the ideal positioning of the elbows under the chest. This generates TRACTION on the lumbar spine as one "teeter-totters" so that the problem disc unit is using the pillows' peak as the point directly upon which it rests as it is being pulled superiorly by the weight of the body superior to it.

The fingers can be dovetailed so that the hands are clasped together beneath the abdomen at the level of the belly-button and the down side elbow(s) are used again like a pole to vault the torso forward away from the hips which should be dragged to a point where the pillow arrests their forward progress. This arrest of forward progress holds the hips from moving superiorly and discs superior to the hips can be put in an intensity of TRACTION greater than gravity alone could develop. For this reason, the pillows should be weighty enough to insure that they are capable of stopping the hips from moving forward as the upper torso is pulled by leaning into the arms.

Once the TRACTION generated by this action is felt on the Lumbar spine, the upper arms are placed slightly more superiorly along the axis of the body in a more vertical position so that their axis runs more perpendicular to the plane of the body. The body is then rocked forward so that the angle formed by the torso and the upper arms is reduced. This action, if the elbows are kept stationary on the superior side of the pillows, and the hip's forward movement is prevented by the pillows, causes the lumbar spine to be placed in greater traction which can be maintained without the exertion of energy or muscle use if the balancing is done properly.

Then, gentle movements of the upper torso are made while concentrating on the sensations generated in the back so as to apply the maximum amount of TRACTION to the effected disc space while FLEXION of the disc unit is applied by an on-and-off sort of rocking movement. This action, also used of the Cervical spine is similarly portrayed in the PILLOW-ASSISTED CERVICAL (NECK) MANEUVER Section's Figures 4,5, & 6. However, for the Lumbar region, the pillows are more directly beneath the Lumbar spine. Nevertheless, the balancing use of the elbow(s) functions identically to pull the inferior torso superiorily simply by managing the gravitational pull on the upper torso and head.

By adjusting your position superiorly and inferiorly relative to the pillow mound, the correct area to be put in FLEXION IN TRACTION is identified by a change in the character of the discomfort. Quite often, just doing this takes away the pain that was felt in the hips or legs and causes it to be localized at its true origin in the lumbar spine. Intermittently putting more or less traction on at that site and paying attention to the effect should convince one that they are applying traction with flexion at the correct site.

Rolling the portion of the body above the painful disc as far into its range of motion onto one side and then the other while rolling the portion of the body below the painful disc in the opposite direction can produce CHIROTATIONAL TWISTING nearly identical to that which chiropractors practice to "wring" the peripheral fibro-cartilaginous ligaments to maximum length forcing prolapsed disc material centrally. This can be done by rolling onto one side (preferably with the painful side up) and flexing the up-side leg at the hips which positions the thigh perpendicular to the axis of the spine while its knee is flexed. The weight of the knee at a distance from the axis of the spine anchors the lower torso into a slightly counter-clockwise twist relative to the disc you are stretching. Keeping the down-side leg extended allows the upper torso to be twisted clockwise in the opposite direction as a means to effect this MANEUVER in one direction. Then, the roles of the upper and lower torso are reversed, in that the upper torso is twisted to its maximum counter-clockwise limit while the flexed up-side knee is swung in a clockwise arc to twist the hips below the level of the painful disc.

Bringing the knees closer to the chest and against the pillow while the affected segment of the spine is kept high on the pillow's center can maximize the traction and twisting on that one

247

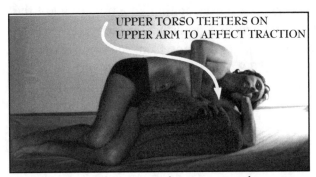

Figure 3 Initial position for Low Lumbar pain to Right

side. A similar position with the other knee for pain when it is on the other side can do the same. As the twisting is accomplished near the end of the range of motion, a fast, jerking, kind of twist using the momentum of the swinging leg will extend the range of motion. If this is repeated many times, with each twist rotating the spine through an ever so slightly wider arc, you can insure that no excessive, potentially damaging movement is made.

Pinioning the upper torso to the floor in its full clockwise range of motion and letting flexed knee travel through an arc that twists the spine of the lower torso is another method.

The back muscles should remain relaxed during both because any muscle activity will interfere with the maintenance of traction and will prevent the vertebrae from separating along their axis and will limit the range of motion attained.

After this portion of the MANEUVER, the TRACTION is then re-established by the rocker-arm action of the upper arms pivoting on the elbow(s). If the back muscles are in spasm due to acute pain, then it may take a while to draw them out to their full length. Any time spasm prevents relaxation, hold off on the MANEUVERS and wait until the spasm is relieved. This can only be done with sustained, persistent traction and purposeful relaxation of the back musculature. The back can't, by definition, relax if it is in spasm. This is an excellent opportunity to put DYNAMIC POSITIONING into effect. Doing so will provide the necessary time for the spasm to be relieved by a sustained stretching that brings the connective tissues their optimal, full, length.

Once this TRACTION is sustained, the Lumbar spine is kept in TRACTION and relaxation while a series of gentle torso adjustments using the extremities accomplish a **rolling in place in the direction towards the side of most pain. This is the PASSIVE THERAPEUTIC CIRCUMDUCTION component of the MANEUVER. You continue the rolling until you are lying such that the side that was up is, at the completion of the roll, facing down (See Figures 3,4, & 5).** If the pain is in the midline, you will necessarily be on your back facing up after the roll. The rolling is done by using the arms or legs depending upon which ones are farthest from the area of the spine that

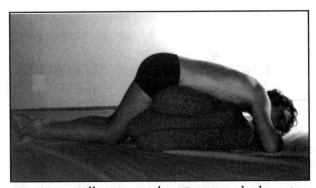

Figure 4 Rolling to Right (Counter clockwise) for Right sided low Lumbar pain

is painful. That way, the least amount of muscular activity is generated close to the lesion. This helps maintain as much relaxation as possible.

It is realistically impossible when performing a THERAPEUTIC CIRCUMDUCTION to

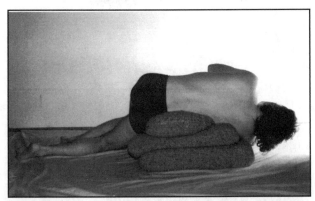

Figure 5 Continued Counter clockwise roll (circumduction) until painful Right side is now down

simply roll because very few pillows are that long to allow a person to roll in one continuous movement. Therefore, it usually requires a series of postural adjustments in which the feet and shoulders are simultaneously planted and the arms are used to raise the torso at a distance from the damaged disc. This lets the problem disc area remain relaxed and to be moved passively by first rolling the half of the body above the disc unit, then relaxing and moving the half of the body below the disc in question. Done carefully and in small increments of movement, the body can remain directly over the pillows; and "roll" in place.

Picturing in the mind what is happening as the body rolls towards the side of pain, the vertebral bodies are separated and circumducted in such a manner that what was once FLEXION is PASSIVELY CIRCUMDUCTED into EXTENSION (without the activation of muscles acting upon those affected vertebrae). The vertebral bodies are kept optimally separated by sustained traction created by the weight of the body on either side of the problem disc. This action allows the off-center disc material to be coaxed centrally by forces progressively moving from the anterior aspect of the periphery of the disc to the posterior.

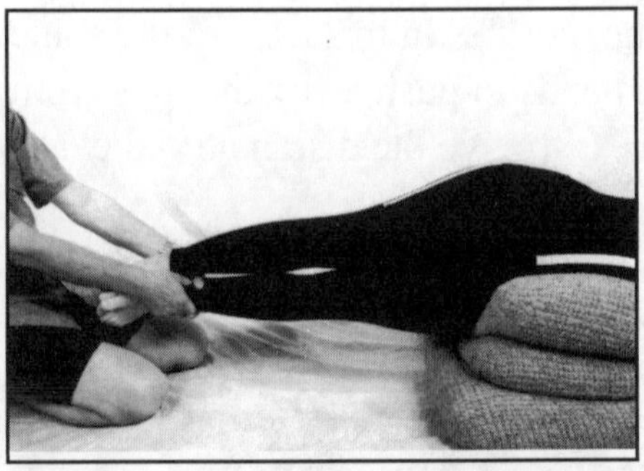

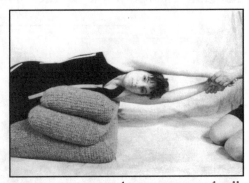

Figure 6 Terminal component of roll with traction assistance for a left sided pain (ant. facing camera)

The most important consideration here is to maintain the TRACTION during the time the spine is taken from FLEXION to EXTENSION through the rolling action. For

without the traction, pressures and disc components existing centrally can offer no space for the solidified disc material to migrate into. Regardless of the level of the disc, the "mountain" of pillows should have its peak directly beneath the site of pain or slightly superior to it so that the weight of the hips produces the traction.

This rolling action can be also coordinated with SEQUENTIAL ARCHING THERAPEUTIC CIRCUMDUCTION movements. Since this is adequately covered previously, the reader is directed to that section for its proper execution and justification.

If the rolling is unsuccessful when accomplished first in the direction towards the side of most pain, try

Figure 7 Terminal component of roll with arm- pulling TRACTION assistance for High Lumbar Left-sided pain

rolling to the opposite direction. It is better to keep the hips off of the ground during this whole MANEUVER by letting them slightly hang from the pillows. It is, in large part, the weight of the hips draped over the pillows that helps maintains the necessary traction. If maintaining traction is difficult, another individual can assist in this MANEUVER by gently pulling on the arms or legs during the roll part of the action (See Figures 6,7,& 8).

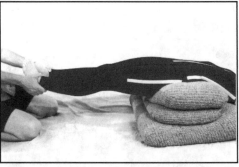

Figure 8 Terminal component of roll with assistance for midline posterior pain

Once the body is in mild EXTENSION IN TRACTION at the completion of the roll, rest in that position for a few minutes and, if necessary, use disc material MOBILIZATION techniques such as SEQUENTIAL ARCHING THERAPEUTIC CIRCUMDUCTION, "INCH-WORMING," CHIROTATIONAL TWISTING, and knee-chest FLEXION IN TRACTION.

Now, if you are not in the face up position, roll to that position so that you are EXTENSION IN TRACTION (See Figure 9). Then, with the knees comfortably flexed and the hips still not touching the floor, gently contract and relax all the muscles in that area of the spine while intermittently remaining relaxed long enough to use the hands to push away the hips from the torso to assist a TRACTION WHILE IN EXTENSION so as to give the disc material every opportunity to move centrally. This position is ideal for more mobilizing actions that can be accomplished while the arms push the hips away to give ACTIVE TRACTION IN EXTENSION. This activity can be likened to a "hula dance/bump and grind" while lying in the supine position pushing your hips away in the same manner as described above.

Then adjust your position in a hip-hanging configuration so the pillows are

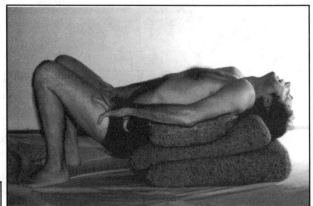

Figure 9 Using hands to push away hips to increase EXTENSION IN TRACTION

directly under the problem disc, supporting it in EXTENSION IN TRACTION (See Figure 10)

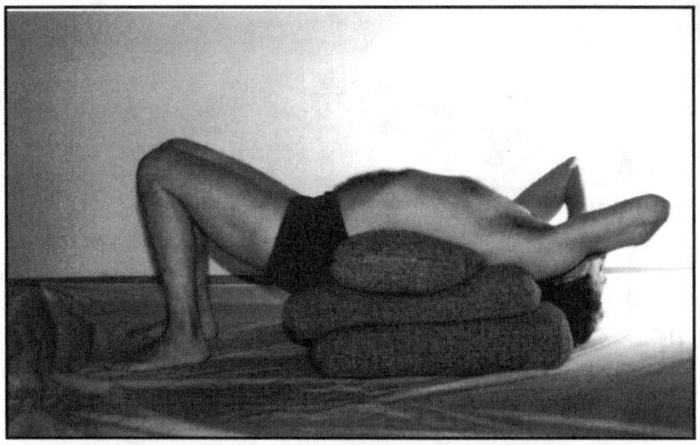

Figure 10 EXTENSION IN TRACTION with pillows directly beneath problem disc

Next, comes the unique component of this MANEUVER. **Keeping your back locked in EXTENSION, you roll again as if you were rolling onto your abdomen (See Figure 11)** as much towards the painful site as possible. This time, however, **as you are rolling, you change your position by moving your whole body inferiorly on the pillow mountain so that the peak of the pillow mountain that supports your weight lies**

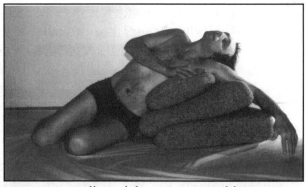

Figure 11 Roll to abdomen initiated keeping back in EXTENSION towards site of pain

about a foot superior to the area of the painful disc (See Figure 12).

The roll should be planned so that, as you complete your roll and you are beginning to enter the face down position, the pillows are there to support the weight of the chest; however, at the same time you

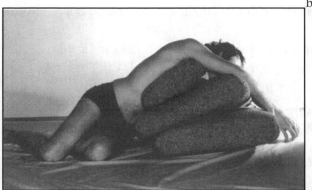

Figure 12 Roll continues as you slide inferiorly off pillows while maintaining EXTENSION

are rolling to the full prone (face down) position, you come off the pillows, using your hands and arms (especially the down-side arm) to lift your upper body off the pillows (See Figure 13).

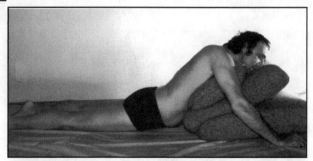

Figure 13 Using arms to bring upper body off of pillows

Your hips should stay on the floor as you catch yourself in a push-up exercise-like posture being fully extended at the elbows. **This puts the problem disc into a PASSIVE WEIGHT-BEARING HYPEREXTENSION (See Figure 14).** Ideally, the spine should be put into a maximum amount of EXTENSION directed directly over the site of pain so as to trap the aberrant disc material in a pincer-like effect without using any muscles of EXTENSION that would tend to pull the disc space closed. The same consideration holds that if your pain is to one side, you should finish your roll resting so that the painful site is facing up when your roll is finished.

You must maintain your Lumbar spine locked in EXTENSION while coming to a standing position. This keeps the posterior disc space closed and prevents the disc material from escaping to the posterior. This can be achieved by simply bringing your knees under your torso into an "on all fours" position and walking your hands up the cushions to raise your upper body into an upright posture.

As you come to an upright posture, if their is a pinching-type pain, this indicates that the disc material has not moved and you may need to repeat the MANEUVER or relax the EXTENSION and resort to going about your business with the disc out until some other MANEUVER is successful. It often helps to try all of the other types of MANEUVERS because one is often more effective than another in a particular individual. An excellent one to attempt at this point would be the MOSLEM PRAYER.

Of course, once up, a THERAPEUTIC CIRCUMDUCTION-type "bump and grind" should be done to seat any slightly off-center disc material. See the previous Section's Figure 19 for this.

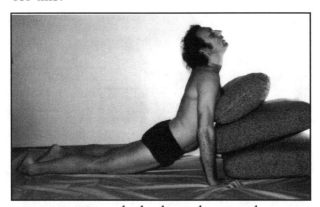

Figure 14 Upper body elevated so Lumbar spine in full PASSIVE HYPEREXTENSION

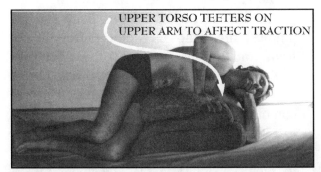

Figure 1 FLEXION IN TRACTION for Right sided Lumbar pain

Named after the Sea-Lion due to the similarity in movements, this variant technique of the **LUMBAR PILLOW ROLL starts by following the previous PILLOW ROLL MANEUVER instructions to the point where you are generating a FLEXION IN TRACTION with the painful site facing the ceiling, supported by pillows (See Figure 1).**

The same disc material MOBILIZING methods and TRACTION generating mechanisms are to apply up to the part where you are prepared to roll over in the THERAPEUTIC CIRCUMDUCTION phase.   In this MANEUVER, **you do not roll**. Instead, **you slide your body inferiorly off of the pillows which changes a FLEXION IN TRACTION to an EXTENSION IN TRACTION and on to a WEIGHT-BEARING EXTENSION (See Figure 2).**   As the chest slides inferiorly off of the pillows, you will note that the problem disc unit that was at the top of the pillow peak slides smoothly towards the ground, without any contraction of back musculature, into a hanging EXTENSION (you are essentially hanging your hips in extension when your chest is held higher than your hips) IN TRACTION. Then, as the sliding continues, the disc unit begins to bear the weight of the upper torso, turning it into a WEIGHT-BEARING EXTENSION. Instead of using the arms to maintain TRACTION while rolling onto the back as in the previous maneuver, **a person simply raises their upper torso off of the ground with their arms as the torso above the problem disc unit slides inferiorly off of the pillows,** forcing the Lumbar spine into EXTENSION without having to contract any disc-associated muscles.

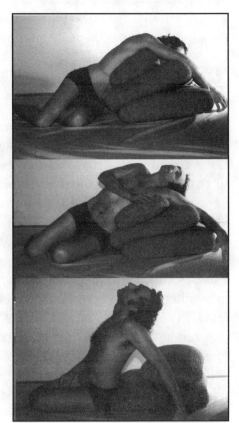

Figure 2 Body slides off pillows into a WEIGHT-BEARING EXTENSION towards the Right for Right-sided pain

For a midline herniation, this is done by starting in a face down position of FLEXION IN TRACTION draped over the pillows (See Figure 3) followed by **a backwards hand-walking type of action with the hands placed under the pillows positioned like a sea lion with the fingers**

aimed in towards each other. With both of the hands directly under the chest like a frog and elbows flexed (similar to that position adopted when preparing to do a push-up with the fingers pointed towards each other); **the hips should simply be allowed to slide to the ground.**

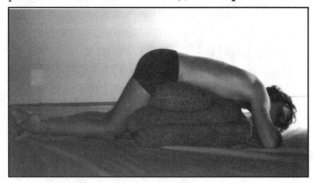

Figure 3 FLEXION IN TRACTION initiating a move of the body inferiorly when Lumbar pain is midline.

Instead of the elbows being on the pillows, **the hands are placed flat on the floor and the elbows are winged forward slightly** (See Figure 4). This posture causes the weight of the head and neck in combination with an extension of the elbows to pull forward (superiorly) that part of the body inferior to the shoulders. It is to be done in such a manner so that the upper torso's weight is balanced upon the arms. The center of gravity of the upper torso is then shifted towards the head so that the weight of the upper torso shifts anterior to the shoulders and the Lumbar region is dragged superiorly.

This creates a TRACTION effect.

To properly complete this move, one needs to treat the body inferior to the problem disc as though it were completely paralyzed or as if your task was to drag yourself forward without using your legs, very much like a SEA LION moves forward. It is almost as if you were acting like you were trying to push the ground underneath your hands towards your hips. This also requires the shoulders to be leaned into, bringing the upper torso's weight extending superiorly over the shoulders to maintain traction. Since the weight of the legs needs to be dragged and the pillows are underneath impeding the hips' forward motion, TRACTION is generated. **As this TRACTION is continuously being applied, the**

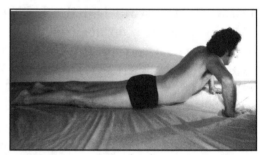

Figure 4 Position for leaning upper body superiorly into shoulders with frog-like arms to induce TRACTION by dragging the legs (pillows not shown)

elbows should be further extended and the upper torso raised higher and higher off of the floor while making tadpole-like motions with your upper body, allowing the lower body to passively wriggle.

Little if any use should be made of the back muscles to lift the upper torso, the means by which the upper body reaches its maximum height off of the floor should be by an extension of the elbows (See Figure 5). If this is found to be difficult due to arm weakness or too much weight of the upper body, a pillow can be crowded closer and closer to the hips to assist in the bearing of the upper torso's weight. At best, the back muscles are judiciously not contracted at all and should remain completely relaxed as the putative disc unit is hung in an EXTENSION IN TRACTION.

The arms are eventually straightened out maximally as though they were raising the

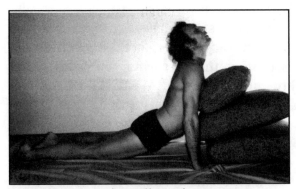

Figure 5 Extending elbows brings upper body to full height and Lumbar disc into WEIGHT-BEARING HYPEREXTENSION

upper body to the highest part of a push-up; but the hips are not allowed to be lifted off the floor. As the area of the shoulders is rising off of the ground, moving the head from side to side while at the same time alternately leaning one shoulder further forward than the other again and again causes the spine to move in a sea lion-like movement. **This action, if coordinated properly, has the spine passively bending into EXTENSION IN TRACTION; and, at the same time, a snake-like movement can help "wiggle" the disc material back into its proper, centrally located, place.**

If the pain radiates more laterally and, therefore, the herniation is more lateral, the same basic movement can be accomplished, only it is done by starting while aiming the painful site more towards the ceiling. It looks a lot like one is doing a half-hearted, one-handed push-up while leaning on their side (that is, they are leaning on the non-painful side). This sounds difficult, but the other arm can assist, and the leaning into and on the outstretched arm makes it less of a push-up, and more of a simple positioning effort. No matter how out-of-shape a person is, they still could raise themselves up over one outstretched arm for a short time and support themselves for less than a minute with the elbow locked. You don't have to be a Marine drill sergeant to do these maneuvers because the pillows are always there to help carry the weight if you push them closer and closer to the hips as you raise the superior torso. Also, you can maneuver the elbow onto the pillow and use the height of the pillow(s) to increase the height of the upper torso as you rest on the elbow which is elevated by the cushions..

If you find that you cannot get enough TRACTION because every time you drag your upper torso superiorly your legs come with it, find some way of securing your legs, either with a rope or by hooking your heels under the bottom edge of a sofa. Another person can assist you by holding onto or pulling on the legs during the TRACTION part of the maneuver especially while you are leaning over your elbows. Additionally, while in TRACTION and as the upper torso goes to the maximally vertical posture, the assistant can gently rock the hips with the legs to assist in mobilizing the disc material through a twisting of the Lumbar spine (See Figure 6). Also, to achieve fuller EXTENSION, an assistant can gently lift your legs off of the ground.

EXTENSION is then progressively increased to the extent that the torso is maximally angled (hyper-extended), by the assistant or your outstretched arms, to its maximum height. At some point, during this HYPEREXTENSION, the weight of the upper torso begins to come to bear on the disc unit. **When the torso approaches the near vertical position, the lumbar discs should automatically experience a WEIGHT-BEARING HYPEREXTENSION.** Immediately before this is felt, some more tadpole-like wriggling of the hips and Lumbar spine can be done to help MOBILIZE the disc material to better insure that the disc material will move centrally.

Before you have reached the point of maximum HYPEREXTENSION, your disc material

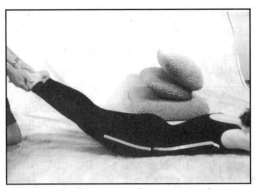

Figure 6 Assistant elevating and putting TRACTION on the legs immediately before and during the extension component of the maneuver.

may have centralized enough to consider the MANEUVER successful; however, **if it has not centralized, you may experience a pinching or crimping sensation that prevents you from going comfortably into the full WEIGHT-BEARING HYPEREXTENSION.** This is the same type of pain described in the pain section of the book caused by the disc material creating a fulcrum effect or an actual crimping of protruding disc material. This pinching indicates that the peripheralized disc material still is producing an obstruction to the full range of motion of the joint. If this type of pain occurs, do not force it. In order continue, you have to do some more MOBILIZING (with more INCH-WORMING, NARROW-ARC ROCKING, THERAPEUTIC CIRCUMDUCTIONS, SEQUENTIAL ARCHING THERAPEUTIC CIRCUMDUCTIONS, DYNAMIC POSITIONING, and/or CHIROTATIONAL TWISTING before continuing with the MANEUVER or go back to the FLEXION IN TRACTION position and start over, now, or at some later time, or try a different MANEUVER.

Finally, as the terminating action of all the pillow-based MANEUVERS, you can get up to the standing position in any convenient manner so long as the problem disc is remaining in HYPEREXTENSION.

If you find it easier to get up by bringing your legs underneath your abdomen and going to an "all fours" intermediate stance, you should use the arms as much as possible to bring oneself to an upright position as though you were getting up from a push-up exercise.

You can also roll back onto the pillows again into a more relaxed EXTENSION position draped over the pillows face up, get your legs beneath your hips, keep arched without much energy expenditure, and lock the Lumbar spine into a maximally extended posture over the disc herniation site by contracting the back muscles into a fully actively extended position aimed directly at the site of pain. Keep the entire spine extended and especially **keep the problem disc unit HYPEREXTENDED in an arched position until coming to fully standing**. If easier, you can use another person, or your arms and any stable object to help you up if necessary (See Figure 7), but don't allow the back to leave the arched, fully extended position. Again, if a pinching sensation or sharp pain intervenes at any time during EXTENSION, assume that the disc is not centralized enough and continue attempts to re-seat it, later, until you can get up in EXTENSION without any significant pain.

Any successful combination of these movements is fair game so long as the pain is not increased. If it is, then stop the maneuver instantly. Also, it is important to be in EXTENSION if any time a re-weighting of the disc occurs after TRACTION is

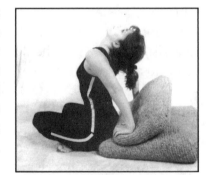

Figure 7 Getting to standing with spine locked in extension using pillow for support

accomplished. **Do not flex the spine while it is bearing weight such as in a sit-up position nor end these maneuvers by getting up without the back in an extended position. If you do, you may have wasted your entire previous effort by committing a WEIGHT-BEARING FLEXION which puts the disc "out" again or forces the disc material further peripherally.**

After you have reached the standing position, a similar final "seating" of the disc should be accomplished as described in the preceding HIP-HANG MANEUVER directions. See the final component of those instructions referenced around Figure 18 in that Section for details.

Any of the positions described in this MANEUVER can be remained in for a prolonged time to effect a DYNAMIC POSITIONING. The actions undertaken can be delayed in favor of resting in any given posture until the desired effect is achieved. What is done in this MANEUVER is almost identical to the **movements** described in the DYNAMIC POSITIONING Section, SELECTING THE IDEAL POSITION. Although the bulk of the above instructions were dedicated to a midline posterior painful disc where the presumed herniation is directly posterior and in the midline, the basic same actions can be accomplished when rolled onto one side so that the painful side is caused to go through the same machinations. By now, the reader should have sufficient mastery of the principles to be able to improvise intelligently no matter where the painful disc unit is located or to which site the pain radiates.

As an additional MANEUVER strategy when it appears that the previous techniques have not been successful, especially if rolling into an EXTENSION IN TRACTION does not appear to result in a WEIGHT-BEARING IN EXTENSION that is pain-free and without arrest in CIRCUMDUCTION, **a couch can be used as the platform** upon which you operate. **INSTEAD OF PLACING THE PILLOWS ON THE FLOOR, THEY CAN BE PLACED UPON THE TOP OF THE BACK OF A COUCH.** This method is described and portrayed in reference to Cervical discs later in the book. You can put your arms and superior torso on the seat portion of the couch, letting your legs drape over the couch's back, or kneel on the couch's seat, draping your arms and superior torso over the back of the couch. Either way, an extreme degree of FLEXION IN TRACTION can be achieved for the Lumbar discs. A chair can be placed behind the back of the couch for added support and balance; however, until you are accustomed to this balancing act and certain it is safe, **you should have an assistant standing by to help you** if you need it. Always be certain that the couch will support your weight and not tip over. If the assistant sits on the couch to keep the front from rising off of the floor, be certain that he/she knows that getting up might cause you to tip over. **The extreme danger attendant in doing this MANEUVER causes me to warn the practitioner that it should only be utilized when absolutely necessary and with the greatest of care.** However, I envision a subset of back pain sufferers who need that degree of FLEXION IN TRACTION to tighten the posterior or lateral intervertebral ligaments; and I cannot think of any other readily available platform that will suffice. Rather than to deny relief to those unfortunates, I include it here as an option with the understanding that you re-read the DISCLAIMER. If you need two assistants, find two. **If you are at all uncertain of your capabilities, don't do it.** Above all, try the other less problematic MANEUVERS a sufficient number of times to insure that you have no other option before attempting this strategy.

257

STANDING TRACTION/EXTENSION MANEUVER

One of the *caveats* of *The O'Connor Technique (tm)* is to use MANEUVERS or their equivalent as soon as possible after the onset of pain. Often, immediately following the onset of spinal pain, it is difficult to manage a MANEUVER that requires lying down in the prone position. At public events, at the office, at work, outdoors, etc. it is hard to find a place that one can lie down with a pillow or even just lie down without evoking the stares or commentary of persons around you. Nevertheless, back pain often comes at these times, especially when caused to sit for long periods of time in situations and environments that have no regard for the reality of back pain and without the advantage of a pillow or equivalent object to support the spine. For these times, the use of **a standing MANEUVER that starts with FLEXION IN TRACTION, progresses to an EXTENSION IN TRACTION, and ends in a WEIGHT-BEARING HYPEREXTENSION can often provide rapid relief without the need to find a place to lie down, especially if accomplished as soon as the pain is recognized and before the disc material migrates too far off-center**.

This MANEUVER, although located in the LUMBAR Section, can be used for any level of the spine below the shoulders. It involves first finding a suitable platform or structure approximately as high as the top of your hips that will support safely the full weight of your body. A table, a desk, a hand rail, the tailgate of a truck, the fender of a car, or any similar level structure that will allow you to bring your body directly in contact with it and have sufficient room above and below it to allow your upper body and legs room to navigate will

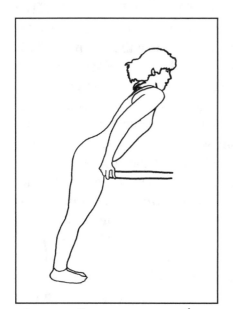

Figure 1 Starting position for STANDING MANEUVER

suffice. Ideally, if you can lean on it and get your legs under it (a table is best) so that your upper body can hang over, resting on the edge and you can be draped over it at the abdomen, you can start by inducing a FLEXION IN TRACTION for the most optimal results.

To begin, one approaches the surface of the structure with hands hung directly below the shoulders and palms facing away from the body towards the structure. **The pads of the palms rest, externally rotated so that they are aimed away from the body, on the top surface of the structure, so that the fingers can be used to grip the structure, providing extra ability to hold on.** The hips are then brought into contact with the edge of the structure (See Figure 1). The hands should be firmly positioned so that they will be able to support the weight of the body, when the elbows are eventually locked into a rigid, straight, extended position.

Now, if the structure allows it, the upper body is rested so as to recline in the prone (face down) position on the surface of the support or hang over the other side. You then relax letting the hips hang in as much FLEXION IN TRACTION as the support will allow. If the support structure allows for it, you can let your legs walk forward, forcing your Lumbar spine into greater flexion. Rest for a minute in this position to allow relaxation to bring the Lumbar ligamentous structures and muscles to full length. Without activating the erector spinae muscles, you can stretch the problem disc more effectively by rolling such that the side with the most pain is aimed towards the ceiling. This is also an ideal time to practice RELAXATIONAL BREATHING and use the MOBILIZATION techniques such as NARROW-ARC ROCKING, THERAPEUTIC CIRCUMDUCTIONS, and modifications of CHIROTATIONAL TWISTING. In fact, at any juncture in this MANEUVER, these methods can be brought to bear to help centralize disc material.

Then, without activating the para-spinal muscles, **the upper body should be raised up by extending and locking the elbows to the point that it is only slightly leaned forward so that, in concert with the arms, a tripod effect is achieved with the torso that will allow the hips to hang freely when the support offered by the legs is removed.** (See Figure 2) Adjusting one's arms and body to acquire the most comfortable position can be done on an experimental basis until one is certain that the weight of the body can be supported without the use of the legs. This position can put every vertebrae that hangs inferior to the shoulders in nearly vertical TRACTION depending upon how you adjust your position relative to the table support. To get higher levels in preferentially more TRACTION, you can lower yourself to your elbows; however, for the Lumbar spine, the straight arm configuration seems best.

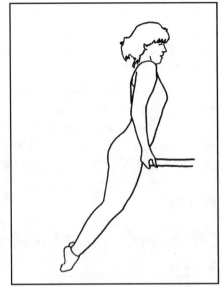

Figure 2 Putting TRACTION on Lumbar spine by carrying weight with arms

The knees are then flexed (bent) so that the feet can be lifted up such that little or no weight-bearing is accomplished by them. The minimal weight left for the feet to bear can be accommodated by using the toes to help balance and retain some stabilization for the legs. The act of flexing the knees causes the weight of the hips to no longer be supported from below by the legs but rather from above by hanging from the spine. This is how the spine is put into maximal TRACTION.

Once the spine is in a TRACTION configuration, the muscles are allowed to relax by the RELAXATIONAL BREATHING method earlier described. An accentuated relaxation, MOBILIZATION, and maximum TRACTION efficiency can be assisted by gently doing a "Hula dance"-like THERAPEUTIC CIRCUMDUCTION of the hips combined with sucking the abdomen in and pushing it out. **Then, the upper body is leaned farther forward with the hips being restrained by the weight of the legs contacting the edge of the platform's surface.** This action should elicit a stretching sensation at the affected segment of the Lumbar spine recognizable as the correct segment by a reproduction of mild discomfort at the origination site of the back pain discomfort. If it does not, then adjustments in posture, forward or sidelong lean, leg position, or hip configuration should be made until you can feel that you are at the right segment of the spine and exerting maximum TRACTION at the affected disc. If the problem disc is at the high Lumbar or Thoracic region, this same MANEUVER can be accomplished by resting on the elbows with your hands clasped for greater support. This reduces you flexibility, but relieves some of the stress on the arm muscles so they don't have to sustain the body's weight as it hangs in TRACTION. In this configuration, simply leaning forward will produce FLEXION IN TRACTION, and leaning backward produces EXTENSION IN TRACTION.

Oftentimes, this action or the previous FLEXION IN TRACTION is enough to change the character of the pain from the radiating or referred type that feels as though the hip or leg was painful to a direct, distinct, Lumbar spine pain or discomfort. Most probably this happens because the TRACTION action moves the solid disc material centrally, and it no longer is applying pressure on the posterior longitudinal ligaments, leaving behind only the inflammatory component which, in combination with the TRACTION induced stimulation of stretch receptors in the ligaments that, when present, allows the mind to localize the pain correctly. Too, FLEXION IN TRACTION itself frequently pushes the disc material centrally enough to relieve pressure on the peripheral ligamentous portion of the annulus fibrosus, and the pain is markedly reduced even before the extension component is completed.

At the point that the TRACTION is maximized the Lumbar spine should then be positioned in EXTENSION IN TRACTION (See Figure 3) so that eventually a WEIGHT-BEARING EXTENSION can be used to exert stronger forces to move the disc centrally. This is done by **arching the back into full EXTENSION while still in un-weighted TRACTION.**

This is an ideal opportunity to practice SEQUENTIAL ARCHING THERAPEUTIC CIRCUMDUCTIONS. Arching EXTENSIONS should be especially aimed directly along the same axis as the source of pain. If the pain is located more to the right than directly in the midline, then arch as much to the right as necessary to be aimed directly over the site of pain. If the pain centers to the midline, then arch directly backwards.

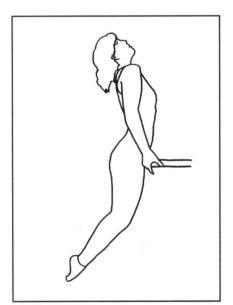

Figure 3 Lumbar spine is arched into EXTENSION while still IN TRACTION

After these techniques are utilized a couple of times, you will probably be able to rapidly determine exactly at what spinal level and in what direction the pain exists in relation to the midline and be able to direct your TRACTION and EXTENSION in such a manner as to most efficiently apply the forces necessary to get the disc material back into the center of the disc.

Now comes the final ARCHING EXTENSION. The arching should be done as much as possible without activating the muscles at the level of the painful disc. While still arching, the legs must be positioned under one's center of gravity in preparation for the upcoming WEIGHT-BEARING EXTENSION. This is done at the same time that the arching is being completed because the arching action can only go so far backwards without the support of the feet and legs. One will fall backwards if the legs are not put down to catch you as you fully extend enough to be effective. When the arching begins to cause you to feel as though you may fall backwards, the feet are brought under the center of gravity. If one is arching more to one side, the opposite side's leg should be flexed (at both the hip and knee) and brought forward so the weight is on the heel, and the other leg (the one on the side to which you are arching) should be allowed to extend behind, nearly straight, with the weight on the bent toes. The straight leg behind the body will first bear the most weight to prevent the body from falling backwards; however, later, the forward leg is used to bear the most weight, later, when you eventually straighten up.

The best analogy to this position that I can think of is like when a baseball outfielder prepares to catch a high fly ball that is coming straight down to him, and he has time to fix his position to the one that still allows him some forward and backward upper body adjustment and the stability that comes from a broad base of support with the legs. In this position you are best ready to stand upright for the next part of the MANEUVER (See Figure 4).

In case you are confused about which leg to put forward when the pain is midline posterior, either leg forward will suffice. Use which ever feels the most comfortable and remember which one works best.

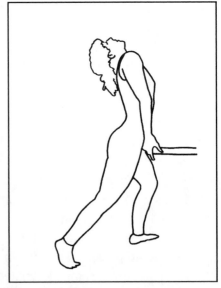

Figure 4 Leg positioning in preparation for WEIGHT-BEARING IN EXTENSION

All this positioning is necessary for the next step which is the most critical. It involves a coordinated arching with simultaneous weight-bearing. **Remember, at this point, although your legs are positioned under you, they are not yet bearing weight.** They are prepared to bear weight, but have not done so because the arms are still supporting a majority of the weight. The arching into EXTENSION that will come will be done in a smooth manner until the hands can no longer be relied upon to carry the weight and the legs must come into play (which they do). As they do, they will lift the hips up to again carry the weight of the upper torso. This is the RE-WEIGHT-BEARING IN EXTENSION.

In order to properly execute a **RE-WEIGHT-BEARING IN EXTENSION, you first EXTEND the entire spine as much as the muscles will comfortably allow then smoothly return to WEIGHT-BEARING while maintaining a full EXTENSION of the entire spine (See Figure 5).** The weight-bearing is accomplished specifically by a coordinated move **putting your weight on the forward leg, bringing the other leg forward until both are brought close enough together, and simultaneously standing-up while maintaining extension as much as comfortably possible towards the direction of**

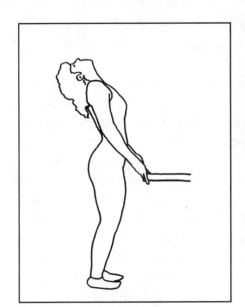

Figure 5 RE-WEIGHT BEARING IN EXTENSION for a midline posterior Lumbar pain

261

the painful site. The leg that you previously had brought forward by flexing at the knee should bear most, if not all, of the body's weight as you go to standing. It is the forward leg you are in effect standing-up on, by straightening (extending) it at the knee. The other leg, is simply dragged forward for balance so that both of your legs are below your center of gravity when you are standing straight up. At the same time, you should be extending as much as possible towards the side opposite the forward leg side except if the pain is in the midline. In that case, the extension should be aimed directly posteriorly.

At the time of weight-bearing, often a sensation is felt like a knuckle cracking deep in the Lumbar spine. This is the sound and sensation that disc material makes when it contacts and courses between the cartilaginous laminations and the frayed remnants of the annulus fibrosus as it actually repositions centrally through the herniation fissure. This feeling that something moved in the back should not be accompanied by pain since there are no pain receptors in the annulus fibrosus. If sharp pain does come at this point or, for that matter, at any point during the MANEUVER, it could mean that the disc has prolapsed or herniated completely through to reach the ligamentous capsule of the annulus fibrosus or the posterior longitudinal ligament.

Too, severe pain associated with this MANEUVER can indicate that the disc material has migrated laterally through a circumferential tear and is trapped within the outermost peripheral layer of ligamentous bands and the rest of the annulus fibrosus. If this is the case, go back into the TRACTION by re-UNWEIGHTING the spine with your arms and do some gentle FLEXION IN TRACTION by again leaning forward over the platform, then again try some THERAPEUTIC CIRCUMDUCTIONS IN FLEXION by letting your hips and arms support your upper body's weight and angle your upper body almost as if you were rolling back and forth on your shoulder opposite to the site of pain. This will supply as much FLEXION IN TRACTION as you reasonably can generate given your positioning limitations.

Then, raise back upright while still keeping the disc unit in TRACTION by supporting your weight with your arms into a more erect posture and try CIRCUMDUCTIONS IN EXTENSION to attempt to move the disc material anteriorly. As you recall, THERAPEUTIC CIRCUMDUCTIONS IN EXTENSION progressively change the point where maximum extension forces (pincer effect by the edges of the vertebral bodies) are applied and can be extremely helpful in this MANEUVER. **This is accomplished by EXTENSION IN TRACTION through an arc while performing a CIRCUMDUCTION, first in one direction (from anterior to the painful site in a direction towards the midline) then, if unsuccessful, in the opposite direction from anterior to the other side of the painful site back towards the midline.** The extensions should be carried back and forth through the area of the painful site. To elaborate on this action: If your pain is more on the left, you should start the EXTENSION laterally as far to the left of the midline as possible. You would then CIRCUMDUCT the lower torso counterclockwise (bending initially towards the left lateral and CIRCUMDUCTING in the direction the posterior midline) while MAINTAINING THE EXTENSION so that each point on the vertebral bodies where the maximum EXTENSION force is applied moves progressively closer to the midline.

You may find that it is difficult to support your weight continuously on your extended arms. In that event, you can drop down to your elbows and support your weight with them. Or, you can even roll onto your back and sort of drape the Lumbar spine over the edge of the platform you are using if it is stable and strong enough to safely allow it.

262

Alternatively, **to more forcefully achieve the same end, you can arch (arching being an active extension accomplished by contracting muscles) and relax, arch and relax, all the while circumducting along an arc parallel to the posterior rim of the vertebral bodies, each time closer to the midline than the arch before.** I have earlier described this action as SEQUENTIAL ARCHING CIRCUMDUCTION because each time you arch, you follow by relaxing the arch and restarting the arching again, only the next time closer to the midline, by an incrementally small CIRCUMDUCTIONAL movement. That is, **with each increment you arch, you move the point where the vertebral bodies pinch together a little more along the periphery of the disc, and then arch again. This sequential arching that moves along points on the periphery of the disc can gently force and move the disc material circumferentially between layers of ligamentous tissue as well as centrally along a radial tear.** For this reason, I find it highly effective.

If doing this in one direction isn't helpful, try arching first laterally on the other side and progressively direct the force towards the midline or start at the midline and progressively direct the arch to one side or the other. If your disc is degenerated significantly, you could be playing the "BB" in-the-maze game" described earlier in Chapter 4's THERAPEUTIC CIRCUMDUCTION Section. So be aware of this consideration if your disc material is difficult to centralize or the pain is not ablated with the "easy" MANEUVERS.

This technique is very similar to the PASSIVE THERAPEUTIC CIRCUMDUCTION method accomplished during the rolling MANEUVERS in the recline; but, now, it is combined with arching that allows a certain measure of force to be applied. Yet, it is not really supposed to be a weight-bearing force at this time. It is only to be the force that your back muscles can generate. If any pain were to intervene, you can instantaneously stop the contraction of muscles to unload the vertebrae by returning to simple hanging TRACTION a lot easier than UNWEIGHTING after letting the weight of your body come to rest.

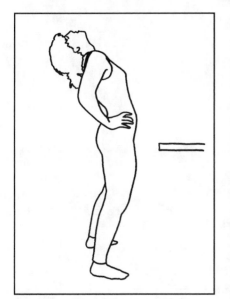

Figure 6 Final seating of disc material by partial weight-bearing HYPEREXTENSION

Repeating sequences and incorporating combinations of MOBILIZING movements are as much fair game in this MANEUVER as the others, but the **basic principle of terminating the procedure with arching before returning to weight-bearing shouldn't be violated.** Re-weight bearing while in flexion is taboo, but WEIGHT-BEARING IN EXTENSION is not--it is the intention! Feel free to experiment, so long as nothing induces pain that shoots down the legs or increases its severity. Make an effort to remember which ever seems to result in favorable disc movement or relief of pain so you can reproduce the same series of movements again in the future.

To finally seat the disc material, as in the other MANEUVERS, you do a standing, partially weight-bearing, THERAPEUTIC CIRCUMDUCTION and hip thrust/bump and grind to finally seat the disc centrally (See Figures 6 & 7). Another sometimes helpful little

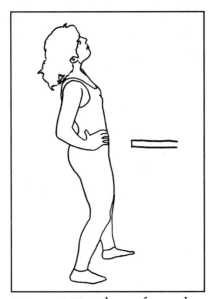

Figure 7 Hip-thrust forward while circumducting clock-wise in HYPEREXTENSION

quirky movement aids in this final seating. With your arms still in the akimbo position, you put one hand on your hip and the other on the lateral abdomen of the other side. Then you push the hands as though trying to make them touch each other in the center of your body while at the same time pushing down with the arms to lift the upper torso off of the hips. This is a standing CHIROTATIONAL TWIST, serving to rotate one vertebral body relative to the adjacent one in the problem disc unit.

Doing some little THERAPEUTIC CIRCUMDUCTIONAL movements at this point can finally centrally seat disc material that otherwise wouldn't be totally centralized by any other action. If one way doesn't do it, then reverse the position of the hands and try again. I only recommend doing one or two of these; and, if they have no obvious beneficial effect, don't persist because it is in a WEIGHT-BEARING position and disc material that still is positioned away from the center doesn't have much ability to go anywhere even if it were to move.

FLOOR-BASED MANEUVER or "THE MOSLEM PRAYER"

Sometimes, there are no beds, pillows, or platforms available with which to elevate the torso to get sufficient FLEXION or EXTENSION IN TRACTION; or, the other maneuvers may be unsuccessful due to a particularly unique set of forces that must be applied in order to move Lumbar disc material. In either case, there is another maneuver which is rather difficult to describe but easy to perform once it is understood. It often succeeds when other attempts fail especially at the L5-S1 disc. It doesn't have to be done on a floor, which can be hard on the knees. It can be done on a bed or with pillows under the knees on the floor or beneath the abdomen for additional support; however, it is not necessary to use any other appurtenance than the ground.

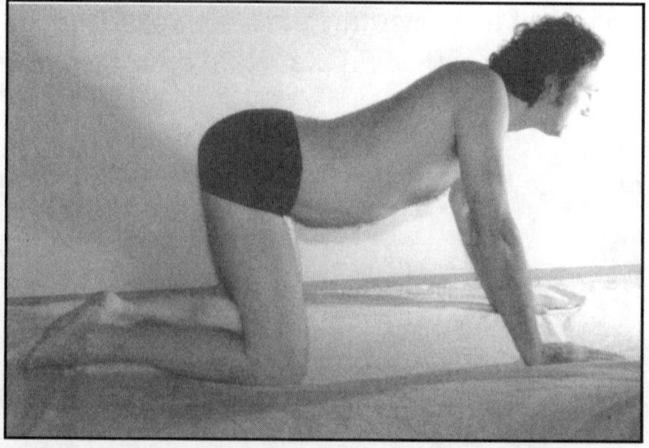

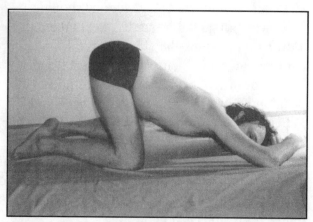

Figure 1 Initial position for "Moslem Prayer" with Lumbar spine in EXTENSION

The maneuver starts by your **sitting on your heels with your knees spread as far apart as possible.** You then **let your hands catch you as you fall forward and end up supporting yourself on all fours. With a combination of CIRCUMDUCTIONAL wiggling and relaxed swaying of the back, you let your abdomen hang down towards the floor as much as your physique will allow (See Figure 1).** This position puts the Lumbar spine in a hanging EXTENSION with the hips being vertically elevated, by the thighs, to their unaided maximum.

Then, **you collapse your arms so that your face is resting at the level of your hands and arms** (See Figure 2), increasing the EXTENSION of the Lumbar spine because you keep your thighs vertical. This causes you to look somewhat like a Moslem praying. The difference is that you are literally hanging your Lumbar spine from your hips which should be kept as high off of the ground

Figure 2 Hanging in EXTENSION from elevated hips

as possible. The knees, however, are kept wide apart so as to give your abdomen a place to go as you make every effort to get the Lumbar spine to hang in maximum EXTENSION from the hips. To accentuate this extension, you can let your thighs leave the vertical by bringing the knees closer to the chest.

Now comes the complicated part. **You rest your upper body's weight on one of your shoulders and face so that your hands are free. (See Figure 3)** The shoulder you choose should

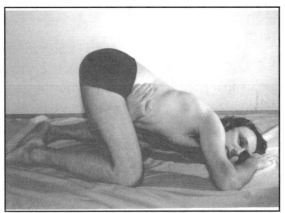

Figure 3 Magnifying EXTENSION with hand for Right sided Lumbar pain

be the one on the opposite side of your back pain. That is, if your pain radiates to the right hip or leg, you should start by resting on your left shoulder and left face. One hand, preferably the one on the opposite side of the pain, reaches under the abdomen to grasp the flank and side of the Lumbar region. By pulling down (ideally with the bare hand on the bare skin of the back), the extension at the lower discs of the Lumbar spine is increased. The traction can be increased by using the other hand to push the pelvis at the junction of the upper thigh and hip away from the abdominal area (See Figure 4). Making these two

motions simultaneously in a quick jerking movement, a CHIROTATIONAL-type twisting can be actively induced to centralize disc material because when you pull down on one side this slightly rotates the torso while keeping the hips fixed.

This maneuver necessarily results in an awkward positioning of the face and shoulder. The face is first, and primarily, kept aimed in a direction towards the side that the Lumbar pain radiates to, then, later, turned to the other side when you alternate to do the same positioning and twisting to the opposite side.

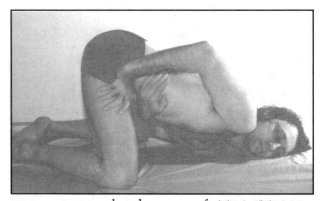

Figure 4 Using hand to magnify TRACTION with Right-sided Lumbar pain

When you try the same motions to the other side, the arrangement of the hands, too, is reversed in both position and function. Performing the same actions to the other side increases the probability that the disc material will centralize, especially if the pain does not definitively localize to one side or the other. It may be very difficult to know in advance which side, towards which the maneuver is directed, will be successful; so, **to reduce the probability of failure, doing both sides is a good idea.**

Once you have demonstrated which side works best for your particular disc, you needn't do both sides every time. You are welcome to work with this position, as well, with ACTIVE CIRCUMDUCTION, RELAXATIONAL BREATHING, weight shifting, and resting in a DYNAMIC POSITION such that varying forces (except WEIGHT-BEARING FLEXION) are applied to encourage centralization of disc material.

After this maneuver is accomplished, keep your back in EXTENSION until WEIGHT-BEARING in the upright standing position again. While on the floor, you can add to the probability of success by maintaining extension and going to a flat, prone, position by letting the upper torso slide superiorly and following with a, seal-like, HYPEREXTENSION arrived at in

266

concert with a sea lion-like wriggling action at the hips (See Figure 5).

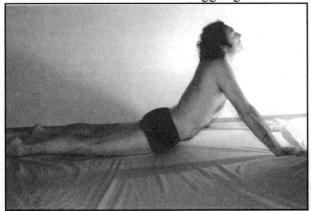

Figure 5 Sea Lion-like HYPEREXTENSION position for Lumbar pain.

If this MANEUVER is done on a bed, the EXTENSION can be converted to a "hip-hang" by rolling. One would then get to standing by the most convenient means appropriate for keeping the Lumbar region in EXTENSION until WEIGHT-BEARING. **To re-iterate, if a pinching sensation occurs when in extension as weight-bearing proceeds, then stop and return to the previous pain-free posture and get to standing in any way that does not produce increased pain.**

Lastly, as previously described, seat the disc with a standing "bump-and-grind" type, ACTIVE CIRCUMDUCTION with the hands on the hips pushing down with the arms to partially unweight the spine (as described and portrayed at the end of Chapter 5's "HIP-HANG" Section), then gradually increase weight-bearing to insure that no pain is produced. If the disc material has centered properly, you should have no pain and a full range of motion in DIAGNOSTIC CIRCUMDUCTION.

SEATED LUMBAR MANEUVERS

It is always good to know a Lumbar MANEUVER that can be practiced from a seated position If you are in acute back pain and wish to convert the simple action of leaving a seated position into an actual Lumbar back pain relieving MANEUVER you can employ THE SEATED LUMBAR MANEUVER. Besides being a MANEUVER, it serves as an excellent method to safely rise from almost any seated position that has room enough in front of the seat to perform it, such as a cushioned, living-room chair or a couch, especially if no other platform is available.

Too, a heavy chair or couch can be used to perform the seated equivalent of the previously described HIP-HANGING and CASCADING action employed at the end of the PLATFORM-BASED LUMBAR PAIN MANEUVER. In this event, you would just slide off of the front of the couch or chair similar to Figure 2. Although not shown in the figures, one can usually reach above the head and use one arm holding onto the other wrist to serve in place of a rope. Hanging by the arm that grasps the top of the chair or couch's back allows one to hang in TRACTION for a prolonged period or even accomplish a roll for FLEXION IN TRACTION efforts. Using this one-handed technique makes it easier to keep the back's muscles relaxed.

Inevitably, you will find yourself slouching in a seated position and will be reminded that this is counterproductive by the onset of back pain. This can occur at work, in the classroom, on an airplane, or anywhere you find yourself seated while in WEIGHT-BEARING FLEXION. If you haven't figured it out by now, this posture is contraindicated. However, it cannot be realistically avoided. No matter how often you tell yourself not to do it, old habits are hard to break; and you, all too frequently, will find yourself in pain and unaware that you had drifted into a slouching posture.

One's first impulse is to simply lean forward to either get up by the usual method or simply sit up straight by adjusting one's position. Either way, you have just increased the posteriorly directed deformational forces acting on the Lumbar discs. Instead of committing these infractions, **the best way of getting out of a seated WEIGHT-BEARING FLEXION without causing more pain is to consciously prevent yourself from flexing the Lumbar spine and immediately find a means to accomplish a simple EXTENSION IN TRACTION MANEUVER before you attempt any other movement. If you have a disc problem, anytime you find yourself in WEIGHT-BEARING FLEXION while seated, you should not initiate any change in position until you use your arms to UNWEIGHT your Lumbar spine. Then, you must literally lift your upper torso off the seat enough to unweight your buttocks so that you may follow with an EXTENSION IN TRACTION effort.**

For this MANEUVER, you start by putting the Lumbar spine in TRACTION with your arms. Whether you use the seat of the chair or its arms as a platform upon which to place your hands, arms, or elbows is immaterial so long as your Lumbar spine is put in TRACTION by lifting the torso off of the chair's seat (See Figure 1 top). You may have to make some slight postural adjustments depending upon your degree of slouch, the height of the chair's arms, etc.; but, **you must judiciously eliminate further WEIGHT-BEARING FLEXION before you adjust to a position wherein your Lumbar spine is in the neutral or extension posture.** As you extend at your elbows to lift your upper body off of the chair, the discs become UNWEIGHTED so that an EXTENSION can occur with no weight on the discs. Whenever possible, hang over or lean backwards with the head or neck resting on top of the chair-back such that singularly contracting your neck extensors helps to lift the body. This action provides additional TRACTION/UNWEIGHTING. Too, the top of the chair's back acts as a fixed surface against which you can press the occiput to increase the strength and degree of your EXTENSION.

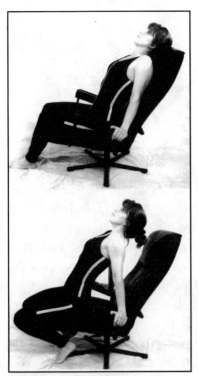

Figure 1 UNWEIGHTING the Lumbar spine with the arms (top) and getting to standing in EXTENSION (bottom).

While you are in TRACTION and EXTENSION, if you gently wiggle, circumduct at the hips, and contract the spinal extensors in an on-and-off manner using the SEQUENTIAL ARCHING CIRCUMDUCTION actions as you are hanging from your arms, any discs that were in the process of migrating "out" can be caused to return to a more centralized position when you arch the back by contracting the muscles that extend the spine. If the pain is more to one side, while you are unweighted, you should extend in the direction of the pain by arching your head backwards against the chair's back, rolling slightly to the side of pain, and gently contracting the same side's erector spinae muscles. To assist this extension, try to keep your face aimed at the ceiling as you press your head against the chair back.

Then, while continuing to contract the erector spinae muscles, you bear weight again by relaxing your arms and return to a more upright seated position only, now, you are in EXTENSION rather than FLEXION. This action, if you are adept at it, in and of itself may eliminate the pain; and you can remain seated if that is your intent.

If you want to get to standing, you have two choices at this point. With the first option, you may lock your Lumbar spine, again, in EXTENSION and carefully get up from the seated position using your arms (Figure 1 bottom) so long as you maintain EXTENSION because you have made a reasonable effort to give the disc material that was inducing the pain an opportunity to go back into the proper position. If the disc is still painful, then sit back down carefully and exercise the second option.

To exercise your second option, **THE SEATED CASCADING DISMOUNT (as illustrated by Figure 2), you again unweight your Lumbar spine with your arms and slide your hips anteriorly off of the edge of the chair.** As you do so, you **relax your posterior extension and allow your hips to hang as you CASCADE off the edge of the chair**. At the point when your hips begin to fall over the seat's front edge, you should pause and allow an EXTENSION IN TRACTION to separate vertebral bodies at the painful disc site. **Letting the hips hang over the edge for a slightly prolonged period as a DYNAMIC POSITION is an excellent opportunity to centralize disc material.** As in any MANEUVER, you can employ all the MOBILIZATION techniques, THERAPEUTIC CIRCUMDUCTIONS, NARROW-ARC ROCKING, SEQUENTIAL ARCHING CIRCUMDUCTIONS with EXTENSIONS at the site of pain, and CHIROTATIONAL TWISTING movements while your Lumbar spine is hanging from a point superior to the painful disc.

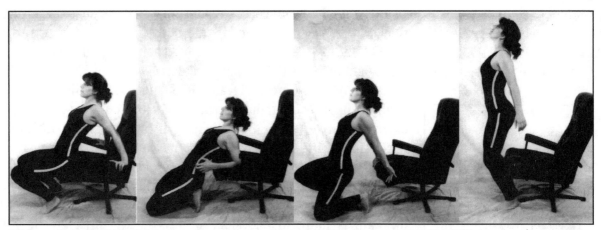

Figure 2 CASCADING dismount during SEATED Lumbar MANEUVER

In order to maintain a sufficient degree of EXTENSION, it is necessary to **tuck and bend your toes underneath** you so that you eventually come to rest sitting on your heels. When you are CASCADING to come to rest on your heels, before you bear weight, you can, and should, aim your EXTENSION, as much as feasible, in the direction of the pain to trap the disc material in a "pincer" effect. In order to facilitate this, your legs can be pivoted over your heels towards the same side that you are leaning, letting the chair edge bear most of your weight.

To complete the MANEUVER, you must get to standing while keeping your Lumbar spine in EXTENSION over the site of the disc pain. This can be a little difficult because **you should ideally keep your face aimed towards the ceiling** if you want to insure that your back stays in the maximum degree of EXTENSION while you jockey yourself into the standing position. So, go slowly, **raise the knee on the opposite side of the painful side to get that foot flat on the ground. Then, using the chair or some other object behind you to assist you in keeping your balance, come to a complete standing position all the while keeping your Lumbar spine in maximum EXTENSION.** This constitutes the WEIGHT-BEARING EXTENSION component of the MANEUVER. The action is terminated like the other MANEUVERS with a standing THERAPEUTIC CIRCUMDUCTION like that described at the end of the HIP-HANG Section.

The principle of AVOIDING WEIGHT-BEARING FLEXION holds true when rising from sitting as well as any other situation. Usually, all you manage to do by getting up from a seated position in WEIGHT-BEARING FLEXION is induce pain that would otherwise not have occurred had you honored that understanding. If you had not done one of these MANEUVERS; and simply yanked yourself to a standing position by flexing forward (as in Chapter 4's Figure 21), there is a good chance you would have induced more back pain; or, had you done it with sufficient force (such as simultaneously trying to lift a weight like a child or even a heavy book held at a distance), you could have advanced a disc herniation to a protrusion because the pain you experienced in the slouching position was the signal that the disc material had migrated to the periphery and was already in a very precarious position at the posterior periphery of the disc space or sitting wouldn't have been uncomfortable.

DRIVING AND THE VEHICULAR EXIT MANEUVER

One of the most painful situations in which back pain sufferers can find themselves is driving for long periods of time. If you watch people getting out of their cars at freeway rest stops, almost uniformly, the first thing they do is put their hands on their hips and arch their backs. They do this because it makes them feel better. What they unknowingly are doing is a partially UNWEIGHTED EXTENSION MANEUVER which is often sufficient for slight degrees of disc material migration. The arms induce a mild form of TRACTION, and they are able to give the disc material a place to move into when EXTENDING and RE-WEIGHTBEARING.

Sitting in a motor vehicle's seat is almost always an uncomfortable proposition for a person with a history of back injury or pain. Prolonging that position quite often leads to back pain because, in essence, it constitutes prolonged WEIGHT-BEARING FLEXION of the cervical and lumbar spine (especially L5-S1) complicated by the constant jarring of the road that increases the stresses applied to the discs (See Chapter 4's Driving Section). Being seated in WEIGHT-BEARING FLEXION is bad enough, but to have the gravitational forces felt by the lumbar spine intermittently increased every time you hit a bump combined with the vibration of the automobile, one can only expect the disc to migrate posteriorly and cause pain.

This MANEUVER is mechanically similar to the previous MANEUVERS in that it can be practiced while accomplishing an action that is necessary anyway. Here again, two ends are achieved. You are able to exit a vehicle and centralize disc material at the same time. Of course, you may not want to or need to do it every time you exit a vehicle; however, when you feel that your disc has migrated to the point of pain while driving--this MANEUVER has the potential to end that pain as you exit the vehicle.

The VEHICULAR EXIT MANEUVER starts by the seated traveler swinging both of the legs out the door frame and placing them on the ground. Once they are on the ground, the hips are made to slide over the side of the vehicle's seat until the hips hang with the problematic Lumbar disc placed in a relaxed, EXTENSION IN TRACTION. Depending upon your level of comfort, you can lie backwards onto the seat or hold onto the top of the door frame with your hands. This starts a slight HIP-HANG that can be prolonged and combined with THERAPEUTIC CIRCUMDUCTIONS, INCH-WORMING, MOBILIZATION,

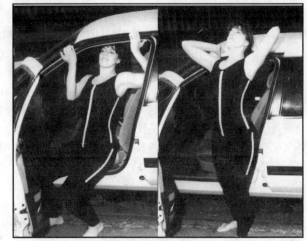

Figure 1 VEHICULAR EXIT MANEUVER

CHIROTATIONAL TWISTING, and RELAXATIONAL BREATHING to free up the disc material identically to the other HIP-HANGING MANEUVERS described above. How long you remain in EXTENSION IN TRACTION depends upon how painful your back is or how easy the disc centralizes. Like the other MANEUVERS, it shouldn't be rushed because the ligaments and muscles still need time to come to full length even if you are in a hurry and the position appears

271

awkward.

Next, you must UNWEIGHT the painful disc unit to induce maximum traction and maintain it while getting to the weight-bearing erect stance. In a vehicle with your legs hanging out the door, it is extremely difficult to get your hands positioned at your sides like in the other, previously mentioned, seated maneuvers. **So, reaching up for some strong hand-hold supplies an equivalent function.** Actually, it is better, except that you must use the muscles of your upper torso to hold on and this can influence your ability to relax your low back muscles. If there is no installed hand-hold, you can use the top of the door frame/roof to satisfy that need (See Figure 1). This allows you to arch into full UNWEIGHTED EXTENSION while you get your feet underneath you. This may take more arm strength than you have to perform it exactly like the figures in this book; however, you may modify it as necessary to accommodate your particular physique. It is best to use just the hands to hold onto the door frame without activating the muscles of the upper arms or back until you can get your Lumbar spine in EXTENSION, then use the upper arms' muscles to raise your upper body enough to get your legs underneath you to support your weight.

For truckers, I would recommend that they make modifications to their cabs and do what ever is necessary to be able to generate a NON-WEIGHT BEARING EXTENSION before coming to a standing posture upon exiting their livelihoods. That may be something as complex as adding a hand-hold bar or simply a rope tied to something in the cab.

For automobile drivers, using the installed hand-holds above the doors or on the door posts can function as an excellent site to anchor the hand. That way, you only need to use the muscles of your hands to hang on with, eliminating some of the effort of the upper body muscles that could influence your ability to totally relax the spine.

Also, even if you are not exiting the car after driving, **the seat itself can be reclined backwards and used as a platform to perform UNWEIGHTING AND EXTENSIONS.** In those cars that allow the seat to recline backwards, the car's seat can be used as an additional platform in your armamentarium of MANEUVER-assistance devices you can use to put your back "in." By reaching backwards and grabbing the hand-holds, holding onto the head-rests, or angling the upper arms over the top of the back of the seat while lying on your side, a TRACTION or UNWEIGHTING can be facilitated sufficiently to perform a PLATFORM BASED LUMBAR MANEUVER similar to that described in the so named Section of this Chapter.

Besides all the other techniques that are usually put to use during a MANEUVER, a CHIROTATIONAL TWISTING action while in this configuration is especially effective in re-centralizing disc material. A pillow-type back support that should be in the car anyway to MAINTAIN EXTENSION can function as a device to keep the Lumbar spine in PASSIVE EXTENSION while the MANEUVER is in process. While the seat is in the nearly horizontal recline, it can function as a tilted "bed." With the addition of a small pillow, **most of the concepts that were elaborated in the HIP-HANG and PILLOW-ROLL Sections can be employed, with modifications, to create an especially effective technique to re-centralize disc material using the automobile seat as the platform upon which one works.**

LUMBAR DYNAMIC POSITIONING
with
MAINTENANCE OF EXTENSION

The normal, neutral, configuration of the Lumbar spine has a smooth, EXTENSION-type, Lordotic, curvature that, notwithstanding criticisms to the contrary, represents an elegant design to accommodate the mechanical forces placed on the human body. Were it not so, humans would not have been, evolutionarily, so successful. This curve, when normal, is basically the same for all humans; but the degree of concavity, length, strength, and flexibility can differ from individual to individual. The maintenance of this curve is essential to the proper and painless functioning of the lumbar spine whether normal or damaged. When a disc unit has been damaged, it is essential to maintain it in EXTENSION whenever possible. This MAINTENANCE OF EXTENSION constitutes the primary, long-term, constituent of DYNAMIC POSITIONING for the Lumbar spine.

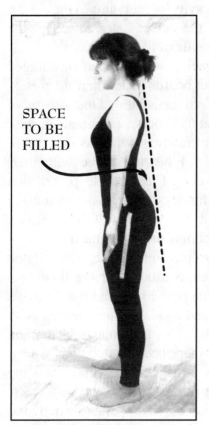

SPACE TO BE FILLED

Figure 1 Lumbar curvature in neutral standing posture

If one considers what percentage of actual time is spent in positions that compete with this curvature, it becomes obvious that behavior plays a large role in maintaining the integrity of the structural design. A classic example is the process of sleeping which, as a single entity, occupies nearly a third of one's life. Beds are usually flat surfaced. The hips and shoulders are the most prominent lateral and posterior features of the anatomy causing the body to be supported by them in nearly all positions of repose (excepting the prone position in persons with large abdomens). In the supine position, for instance, nearly all the weight of the torso is placed on the shoulders and the hips, causing the Lumbar spine to hang like a structural cable on a suspension bridge. Thus, the Lumbar spine's natural curve must flatten with time spent in this position, especially if one is lying on a uniformly soft surface such as a large mattress or foam rubber "futon" bed. **Therefore, the weight of the abdomen forces the Lumbar spine into flexion and opens the posterior elements, allowing for posterior disc migration.** That, in case you haven't been convinced by now, is detrimental.

In order to appreciate the degree of Lumbar curvature of your own back, stand with your heels against a wall so that your buttocks, shoulder blades, and head are pressed firmly against the wall. By taking your hand and placing it over the Lumbar region of the spine between your body and the wall, you can feel the distance to the wall and gain an appreciation of the amount of concavity or bowing of your Lumbar region (See Figure 1). This measurement is important to understand because on a pain-free day, that distance represents the ideal distance from a flat surface that your individual spine needs to support it in the neutral position. I qualify this statement with "on a pain-free day" because, if you are in pain when you try to measure it, spasm or guarding may interfere with a assessment of the ideal distance. **The space created by the concavity that you feel in the erect position is important because it is the ideal size of any Lumbar support structure that is necessary to keep your Lumbar spine in the configuration that provides the exact amount of support necessary to bring your Lumbar spine to the neutral position or slightly extended in traction when lying on a flat surface.** Depending upon whether or not your back is "in" or "out," determines the degree of EXTENSION and/or TRACTION. If it is "in" and there is no necessity to move disc material centrally, a neutral position is sufficient. If your discs are repeatedly going "out" or obviously "out" then the more EXTENSION IN TRACTION would be necessary to DYNAMICALLY POSITION it centrally.

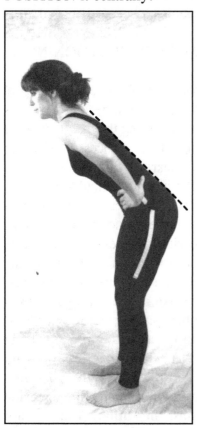

Figure 2 Degree of Flexion required to straighten spine

As you flex the neck and thorax while keeping your heels and buttocks against the wall, you will feel this space decrease and you can appreciate the degree to which flexion alters the mechanical configuration of the Lumbar spine by actually flattening or reducing this concavity or curvature (Figure 2). This should convince you that the act of "straightening" the Lumbar spine actually constitutes flexion.

For years, people with back pain have been encouraged to purchase firm mattresses or put boards under their mattresses to keep the back as "straight" as possible. One survey of orthopedic surgeons revealed that 68% believe that patients with back pain should sleep on a firm mattress whereas only 0.8% recommended a soft mattress.[1] I heartily agree with their rejection of soft mattresses; however, I feel that the proposition for a firm mattress doesn't go far enough unless it includes a recommendation to include LUMBAR SUPPORT because simply straightening the back accomplishes the same mechanical disadvantage as flexing. Most people don't realize it, but if one were to lie on a flat surface such as a board or the floor or a truly firm mattress, the points where the hips and the Thoracic spine meet the surface are fixed and rigid, causing the concavity of the Lumbar spine to disappear. This is identical to stooping forward. The same discomfort experienced by stooping forward for a long time is reproduced by a mattress that straightens the Lumbar spine without providing Lumbar support.

In the past, this existed as a satisfactory recommendation because those persons who found relief with a hard mattress or a board under their mattress did so because, without the straight surface, their weight applied to an exceptionally soft mattress would change a simply flattened Lumbar spine into becoming substantially flexed during the many hours that they slept in the supine position (flat on their backs).

To visualize these differences and the often unrecognized degree of flexion imposed upon the Lumbar spine by sleeping on a soft mattress, please observe Figure 3. By comparing this reclining posture with the equivalent standing posture (Figure 1) and the forwards flexed posture (Figure 2) in the context of how much true flexion away from the neutral lordotic is occasioned when the spine is straightened, you should see that the Lumbar spine is experiencing a flexion event when it is straightened. During sleep in the reclining posture, you will see that when sleeping on a soft mattress's surface, the Lumbar spine is configured the same as if the Lumbar spine was standing and flexed an additional 15-20 degrees. Reclining in a soft mattress that allows a person to sink deep into the plane of the bed, this degree of flexion is an extreme that, when reproduced in a standing position, would most certainly be painful if prolonged since, when standing, the flexion is combined with the additional weight of the upper body pressing down on the flexed vertebrae.

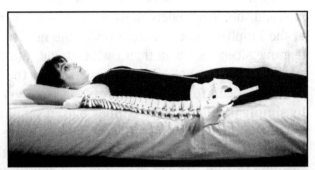

Figure 3 Lumbar curvature flattening with soft mattress

It is not often appreciated, but this degree of flexion imposed upon the Lumbar spine over a prolonged period of sleep (when all the muscles that keep the spine erect and protected to some degree) are in their most relaxed (and vulnerable) state is the less-WEIGHT-BEARING equivalent to stooping over 15-20 degrees for an equal period of time, of course, minus the extra gravitational forces contributed by the upper body's weight in the upright posture. Nonetheless, even without the added pressure applied by the weight of the upper body, this positioning allows for posterior migration of disc material. Anyone who doubts that even small amounts of flexion prolonged for an extended period of time can become painful, I would challenge them to wait until their next event of back pain then stand against a wall with the heels and buttocks touching yet keep the shoulders and Thoracic spine a mere 10 inches away from the wall. After several minutes, pain will probably prove my point; however, I leave this experiment to the most stubborn amongst you who has to prove to themselves the reality of another's finding. For those of you who are willing to conduct the same experiment in your mind and forgo the painful proof, I commend your discretion and credit you with at least some common sense in having the latitude to accept some trivial aspects of life on faith in order to spare yourself the pain of personal experience even if it comes at the expense of the scientific process.

So what practical benefit can be gained from this information? Well, just as you can take away the pain caused when stooping over by simply standing erect, **you can become more comfortable and maintain that comfort by maintaining your Lumbar spine in its most mechanically neutral, extended, position during any time when it would otherwise be placed in reclining flexion.**

There are many ways a person can accomplish the goal of keeping the Lumbar spine in the mildly extended or neutral position. My first recommendation is to buy a good mattress with many individual small coils as support. If it is just a hard flat mattress with conventional wide-spring design, the whole surface bows when your weight hits it. If there are multiple support structures, each one individually compresses while the remainder, adjacent springs, still provide support. This failing of conventional mattresses explains why sleeping on a firm new mattress, like those found in expensive hotels, is often uncomfortable. Your own bed (so long as the mattress is not too worn out or soft) can conform to the shape of your body so long as you sleep in roughly the same place over a long period. On a good mattress that you have worn in, your hips and shoulders indent those areas of the mattress that they impact, leaving a rise at the region of the Lumbar spine which provides the needed Lumbar support. It is not purely psychological that one sleeps better in their own bed and, often, on their "own" side of the bed.

If you cannot afford the mattresses that provide the best support, you are away from your own, comfortable, mattress, or your mattress isn't comfortable, you can compensate by simply placing a foam rubber pad, a small flat pillow, or a soft bath towel folded in such a way that it comfortably fills the space between the Lumbar spine and the bed surface. This way, the Lumbar spine can be supported in slight extension during the hours of unrecognized sleeping flexion. The ideal degree of support is achieved by folding the towel in layers or cutting the foam rubber so that the height of the layers and the positioning of the folds can most closely approximate the identical contour of your individual Lumbar curvature. A shallow pillow is often just as effective. Again, the way one can define their own particular contour and concavity is by standing against a wall with heels, buttocks, shoulders and head against the wall and feeling with the hand the space formed by the Lumbar curve as described above. The pillow, the folds of the towel or the foam rubber can be made so as to profile the varying distances from the deepest segment of the curvature to the least (as it tapers into the Thoracic spine).

One must take into account the degree to which one sinks into the mattress as well as the degree to which the material of the support compresses when deciding what the ideal height to make the Lumbar support device. A very heavy person would necessarily need more layering because they indent the mattress more than a thin person. Similarly, a person with a very old, soft mattress whose springs are worn will sink deeper (creating more flexion) and require a Lumbar support

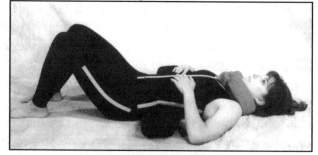

Figure 4 Close-up of foam rubber Lumbar and Cervical support devices.

structure with greater height than a person with a firm mattress that is almost flat-surfaced despite the weight of a body on it. **In any event, the height of the support should be such that the Lumbar spine is kept in its natural curve or a slight, comfortable, amount of extension. It is important to insure that it is not uncomfortable.**

If a foam rubber support (or towel) is used, it should be cut (or folded) so that its long axis can be perpendicular to the body, and it intersects with the plane of the body right at the Lumbar curve. (See Figure 4). In this way, when a person lies on their sides, the anatomical indention formed by the lateral aspects (at the sides of the body) between the hips and rib cage will be serendipitously supported; and the back will be more likely to be kept in a neutral position with regard to lateral curvatures (the convexity formed when the spine bows due to gravity between the support of the hips and rib cage when a person lies on their side) as well.

Many of my patients who claim that they only sleep on their sides do not realize that they may fall asleep on their sides and wake on their sides; but, during the night, they spend significant proportions of their sleep time on their backs and visa versa. Time lapse photography would show these people that a night time of sleep compressed into a few minutes of real time footage can make the soundest of sleepers look like a cross between an epileptic and a break dancer. The proper design and positioning of the support device gives some reassurance that every time the sleeper returns to sleeping on his back the support is there.

If one finds this method too uncomfortable when lying on the sides due to anatomical adiposity or other reasons, experimenting by folding a soft towel sufficiently to insure the right size and height can be productive. Once the ideal dimensions are arrived at, one can trim out a piece of towel and incorporate it into a permanent Lumbar support. A piece of foam rubber equivalently designed to provide the same degree of support when compressed in the reclining position can be used. Once the dimensions of the cut towel or foam rubber are arrived at such that the entire width of the back is accommodated, a long piece of comfortable material can be sewn onto it with enough length to be tied or Velcro attached around to the front of the abdomen. This allows the support to stay in position throughout even the most torso-tossed episode of slow-motion nocturnal squirm-dancing.

I must stress that whichever option you choose, too much elevation of the Lumbar spine in the supine (reclining) position can be uncomfortable. Too much support can actually hyper-extend (bend backwards) the Lumbar spine and result in a painful crimping of the posterior edges of the vertebral bodies or the facet joints. This will lead to discomfort and must be avoided.

The role of waterbeds in the management of back pain is uncertain as far as I am concerned. I have slept on them and found no real relief; however, I have heard of those who do get relief. I suspect that certain persons with the right dimensions, weight distribution, and body shape for a particular water bed will achieve a comfortable sleeping position by the way in which their particular waterbed supports their particular spine. If it happens that the bed supplies the correct amount of Lumbar support, then the pain will be relieved. On the other hand, if one sinks into the waterbed like any other bed such that the spine is left in flexion for hours on end, the result will be continued discomfort.

My recommendation for those with waterbeds is to experiment with a towel as above to see if the neutral position of Lumbar curvature can be achieved. If you don't have a waterbed and you wish to see if one can help, lying on different ones in the showroom may be a successful way of determining whether or not it is effective in reducing back pain or if it can be made to do so with varying degrees of Lumbar support. Unfortunately, a water bed nearly precludes the bed-based Lumbar pain maneuvers, so I really can't recommend them.

The continuous MAINTENANCE of the neutral Lumbar curvature IN EXTENSION is especially important in the period immediately after a flexion-type back injury or accidental trauma wherein traumatic flexion of the spine occurs. It is imperative to maintain the Lumbar spine in its neutral, slightly extended position while it heals. If it is allowed to heal in a semi-flexed position, then the scar which replaces any damaged ligaments will be flaccid in the neutral position. The formation of a scar in flexion almost guarantees less of a return to normal integrity of the spine. Any ligamentous injury that causes a tearing of ligamentous structures can never be expected to return to the same degree of tensile strength that existed in the pre-injury period due to the reality that scar tissue is never as strong as an original ligament. However, if allowed to heal in the position that most closely approximates the neutral Lumbar curve, the scar that is laid down will do so with minimal amount of stretching of the original ligament and the maximal amount of strength obtained by approximating the torn edges of the ligament fibers while they heal. This is especially important because the peripheral posterior ligamentous portions of the annulus fibrosus forming the capsule sustain the most pertinent damage during flexion injuries. By not healing tightly, they predispose the disc to move posteriorly and protrude or herniate more readily.

A person with a "bad back" should always be cognizant of the position of the Lumbar spine and its support when sitting. Many people "slouch" in chairs. This puts the Lumbar spine in FLEXION for a prolonged period of time while WEIGHT-BEARING. This causes the discs to migrate posteriorly (towards the back) and results in pain. A person can be seated on a soft couch, a chair, or especially an automobile, not realizing that the back is in flexion until the onset of pain. The pain causes them to try to get up; and they flex the abdominal musculature to bring themselves to an upright position. This increases the probability that the disc will migrate to the painful position. **So the lesson to be learned here is to not sit without a Lumbar support.** A small firm pillow carried in the automobile that can be placed in the Lumbar area satisfies the problem while driving. If you are a woman, your purse can be tucked in behind your back if necessary. A number of small pillows scattered throughout the house on the couches or chairs can be easily tucked in the small of the back for comfortable sitting.

When sitting in chairs that will accommodate such a posture, sitting such that the head's weight is not felt on the neck and shoulders via a head rest is more comfortable for the entire spine. Also, chair designs that allow the shoulder blades to carry a lot of the upper body's weight can allow a person to relieve some of the pressure of the upper body from bearing down on the problem discs at a lower level. One means of UNWEIGHTING the Lumbar and lower thoracic spine while seated is to rock back on the chair you are seated. By rocking backwards so that even a ridged kitchen type chair becomes more like a recliner, the upper spine's weight is felt against the back of the chair rather than the vertebrae of the lower spine. Of course, be certain that when you rock backwards in a chair that it is both capable of sustaining the weight on the two chair legs and that the back of the chair has a solid object to lean against or your mother's admonition not to rock on your chair will prove prophetic when you fall backwards into a flexion injury.

1.   Anon, For Your Information, *Modern Medicine.* Vol 64 May 1996:27.

CERVICAL (NECK) PAIN MANEUVERS

Neck pain is "a pain in the neck." This age-old analogy has attained classic vernacular status because it is so universally understood and accepted as an exceptionally irritating phenomenon. It is particularly aggravating because, seemingly for no reason, your neck or upper shoulders can begin to hurt, you mysteriously can't look over your shoulder, you can't sleep without discomfort, you can't bend your head forward, and you can be made generally miserable through no discernable fault of your own. It is a pain that seemingly no one can help you with, and modern medicine is obviously only palliative (treatment rendered only to reduce symptoms but not designed to eliminate the source). It can occur at any age. It can be punctuated by furious bouts of nightmarish aching which, usually, with time, get spontaneously better; but sometimes it never leaves. Instead, it persists like background noise on a cheap tape recorder. It's always there waiting; and when you focus on it, it obviously can be recognized as a perpetually antagonizing presence.

I have often described the pain to patients by asking if the feeling is as though someone has been hitting them with a hammer from the base of the neck all the way down to their shoulder and up to their head. They look at me as if I could read their minds or I knew exactly what they were experiencing without them telling me. I do.

Often, it occurs immediately after obvious injuries while that particular segment of the spine is in flexion, but it can just as easily "happen" upon waking from a non-traumatic sleep, leaving you to conclude that you have slept "wrong." Fortunately, at long last, through the proper maneuver, there is an opportunity, now, to make it immediately "right" by a series of careful movements. These are called CERVICAL PAIN MANEUVERS; but, before this understanding can come, there is a need to cover some general considerations.

First, I found it necessary to **treat the different regions of the neck differently** and have designed differences into the MANEUVERS to compensate for the functional and anatomical differences of various levels of the cervical spine. I have drawn a distinction between the upper, middle and lower level neck pain because the **maneuver techniques for upper level pain may not work on lower level pain despite the categorization of both as "neck" pain**. To simply lump the whole structure together as a "neck" is anatomically naive to the detriment of realistic therapy. The neck is a very complex mechanical mechanism whose components are designed to perform differently dependent upon the level of the disc unit being considered. To expect every level to respond equivalently to a single applied mechanical force denies this anatomical and physiological reality. **For that reason, you probably should familiarize yourself with all of the MANEUVER directions, even to the extent of reading and trying those MANEUVERS designed for adjacent Cervical levels (if unsuccessful with the maneuver you think would be most appropriate) for the region of the Cervical spine from which you perceive your pain to be originating. Practicing all the MANEUVERS will increase your understanding of the principles, not to mention giving you multiple methods that may work to relieve neck pain where it is difficult to determine the precise level from which the disc problem actually originates.** Additionally, due to the close proximity of one disc to another, it can sometimes be difficult to differentiate between the origin of pain at one level or another because the Cervical spine is so relatively short and the segment with the highest density of vertebral bones per linear measure.

By way of prefacing this section, *The O'Connor Technique's* neck pain "discoveries" did not just come as the product of intellectual thought processes. I have sustained and largely recovered from at least two chronic neck pain mis-adventures. An upper level disc went out years ago, and I successfully managed it by a technique similar to the one that proved successful on my Lumbar region. Recalling the severity of this Upper Cervical disc lesion, it was so unstable that I had to install a higher shower head because simply flexing my neck in the morning would induce the pain due to a decentralization event. Now, it rarely, if at all, bothers me. However, when I attempted to apply the upper region maneuvers to an injury in the lower region (C7-T1), they did not work. So, I had to put my mind to the task of figuring out why they were unsuccessful before I felt myself competent to write on the subject. Therein, the recognition that I couldn't fix my own disc delayed the writing of this book for a substantial period, since I reasoned that if the method didn't work at all regions of the spine, it may have worked at the other areas simply by luck, and therefore wasn't necessarily reproducible and definitely not universal. Persistence paid off, however, and resulted in a higher understanding of the basic concepts, which I share below.

The Lower Cervical disc went out lifting a table out of the back of a station wagon. When I injured the lower level disc, I was judiciously protecting my Lumbar spine but ignoring my Upper Thoracic and Lower Cervical region. My Lumbar spine was appropriately locked in EXTENSION; however, my Upper Thoracic region was forced into flexion by the weight of the table, and my neck was in a great degree of flexion in order to bend into the back of the car. I was using my strongest arm, my right; and I was slightly twisted to the right and flexing my neck to the right. I felt the disc herniation event as a "squishy-crunch." I immediately recognized the loss of mobility in circumduction to the left, and the pain started within minutes. It was not so bad at first; however, within a couple of hours, it was obvious that I had sustained a very significant herniation.

It took me at least eight months to figure out the ideal process, techniques, and maneuvers to get that disc material back into place. Prior to this injury, I was largely applying techniques that were only appropriate for midline posterior herniations. I learned from this episode just how laterally displaced a disc in the Upper Thoracic and Lower Cervical region can be as well as how **the FLEXION IN TRACTION and EXTENSION IN TRACTION maneuvers sometimes must be aimed at a site far more laterally than posteriorly**. I was later able to account for this phenomenon by coming to an understanding about the effect that the anatomical widening of the posterior longitudinal ligament has on providing extra midline strength in that region, making midline posterior herniations less likely.

The bulk of the following described neck-oriented techniques are a direct product of my own injuries and efforts to remedy them which were, afterwards, tested and re-tested on patients with the same lesions. A lot of my time was spent getting the relatively immobile lower region of my Cervical spine sufficiently MOBILIZED with FLEXION IN TRACTION and other mobilization techniques to allow the EXTENSION IN TRACTION MANEUVERS to be successful. Now, keeping the disc material centralized, by applying DYNAMIC POSITIONING, is becoming easier and the frequency with which it goes "out" has recognizably decreased dramatically; and it never goes out as far as it originally did at the time of the injury. The jury is still out as to whether it will get completely back to the way it was before the injury or whether it will heal as well as the first neck problem at the higher level; however, at this writing, I am at the stage where, when the pain comes, I can at least stop it instantly by putting the disc material back into the central position with a maneuver. The degree to which it is not going "out" as often or as far tells me that it is healing in such a way as to interfere with the posterior and lateral migration of the formerly displaced disc material. (Correction, at the time of this final revision and editing, for at least 20 months, I have had no noteworthy recurrence of pain.)

I attribute my improvement with these injuries only to the success of my methods, and the following described MANEUVERS are the principle means by which that success was achieved, and now I am sharing it with the rest of humanity.

Oddly enough, I was injured by trying to lift a table-like device out of my car to attempt to fix a physician friend's neck problem who happens to work as an orthopedist. His neck problem, nearly identical to mine, is still present because I have, as yet, not completed this book for him to read; and he cannot gain consistent relief despite free access to state-of-the-art orthopedics techniques.

In the process of making that portion of my spine better, I arrived at the understanding that one of the most essential components of the maneuvering process was achieving sufficient FLEXION IN TRACTION and that passive TRACTION is not sufficient--**one can, and must, actively maximize neck TRACTION and FLEXION.** The best means to achieve the TRACTION comes from the use of a rope at the ankle so that the head and arms can produce sufficient FLEXION as you hang over the edge of a comfortable bed long enough to be successful.

There are two main ways that one can concretely produce the magnitude of neck TRACTION necessary to be effective. One, **you can use the muscles of your hands and arms to push your head and neck off of your shoulders** or, two, **you can use the weight of your arms to fix your head, effectively "pinning" it against something (like the floor, a pillow, a rolled towel, the arm or back of a couch, or, better, the edge of a mattress) and pull your body away from your head by using the muscular strength of your torso and legs.** These options can be used by themselves, alternated during a maneuver, or in combination with the other one depending upon how successful either method is for you. The best method is the one that works for you and with some experimentation you should be able to discover it.

A main point here is that you **learn to use muscle groups distant to the neck to effect TRACTION at the neck** because that will not cause the muscles acting upon the disc unit in question to contract and ruin the effect by inducing muscular contraction at the level of the damaged disc.

To use your arms to push your head and neck off of your shoulders is pretty simple and is described in detail later. In employing the second technique option, you lie parallel to the surface upon which you are resting and **pull yourself using your legs, torso, and hips** (a rope comes in handy here to give a fixed place to pull against with your heels as described in Chapter Four's Section on ROPE-ASSISTED TRACTION) **while the head is intentionally fixed and restrained from being dragged by friction or restraint by an immobile object such as the edge of a bed's mattress.** The weight of the hands and arms bearing down on your neck and head provides the means by which the head is pushed against the surface. The idea here is to place TRACTION on the affected disc so as to give the disc material the opportunity to be moved more centrally by the mechanisms previously elaborated in Chapter 4.

So, to effect this, you **position your hands in such a manner as to be above your body so their weight acts upon a site superior to the area that is painful**. In this way, you can use either the back of your head, your knuckles, or both to serve as the surface

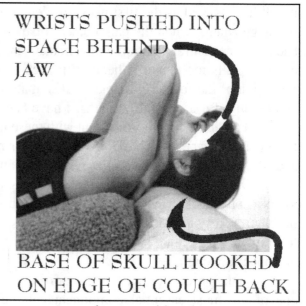

WRISTS PUSHED INTO SPACE BEHIND JAW

BASE OF SKULL HOOKED ON EDGE OF COUCH BACK

Figure 2 Use of arms and hands to grip area above problem disc to restrain its movement inferiorly

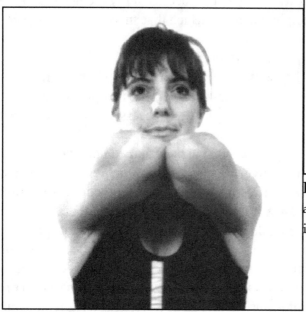

Figure 1 Elbow position to lock neck or head in tight grip

that interfaces with the floor, towel roll, or mattress edge so long as your hands are firmly secured to the head or neck and, thereby, are also secured against an object that doesn't move. The problem in simultaneously satisfying these criteria is that the head tends to be difficult to pinion without employing the muscles of the neck or shoulders. To increase your grip to foster stronger TRACTION, you can use your forearms, hands, and fingers. Your forearms can be squeezed together at the base of the skull so that the wrists are compressing the space behind your jaws on both sides (See Figure 1) and the elbows can be brought so close together that they are as close to touching in front as possible (See Figure 2). These techniques put the head in a vice-grip that requires no neck or shoulder muscular energy to maintain yet adequately make the head or neck able to be fixed against some object by "hooking" parts of the head, hands or arms on the immobile object (i.e. edge of couch, pillow, mattress end, towel roll, etc.).

Once the head and neck's position superior to the area of pain is fixed against the ideal or most convenient surface, you selectively relax the neck then use your legs (by digging in your heels or hooking them on the rope loop, and flexing the knees) and torso (by gently arching the Lumbar regions) to pull the rest of the body away from your fixed head and neck. Your intent should be to pull that portion of the body below the area of pain away from the segments of the spine above the area of pain without activating the neck or upper back musculature. In Figure 1, the base of the posterior skull is pinioned against the edge of a couch back so that the weight of the body, flexion of the knees, and the extension of the hips or Lumbar spine will, in concert, pull

282

the inferior aspect of the body away from the neck avoiding the use of muscle groups attached to the problem disc unit.

Activating the muscles of the Upper Thoracic or Cervical regions interferes with the goal of placing TRACTION on and separating the vertebrae of the affected disc unit. The beauty of this technique is that none of the upper body muscles attached to the Cervical spine need be activated to accentuate this form of TRACTION. Only the leg muscles need be activated to pull the body away from the head and neck.

Sometimes simply pulling the body away from the neck is insufficient to generate adequate TRACTION force to successfully open the intervertebral disc space. In that event, one hand can be freed up to supply a resistant force while the other continues to link the head or neck with the platform's surface.

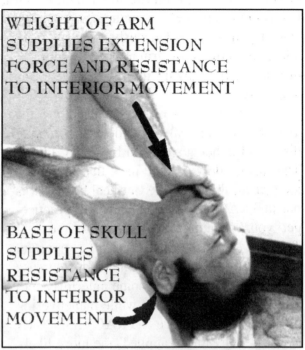

Figure 3 Using the weight of the arm to put a lever action on the jaw to increase TRACTION and EXTENSION for a high midline posterior pain

In Figure 3, the weight of the free hand and arm pushes superiorly on the underside of the jaw. The hand and the back of the skull are positioned such that the edge of the mattress forms an immobile ridge that will not allow the posterior base of the head to move inferiorly. Pushing the chin superiorly with the palm of your free hand (as if you were trying to view something on the top of your head) turns the jaw into a lever which assists in pulling the head off of the neck or neck off of the shoulders.

This magnification of TRACTION without activating the paraspinous, trapezius, or erector spinae muscles (which would, if contracted, defeat the purpose and interfere with the TRACTION), can also be combined with a FLEXION force to increase FLEXION

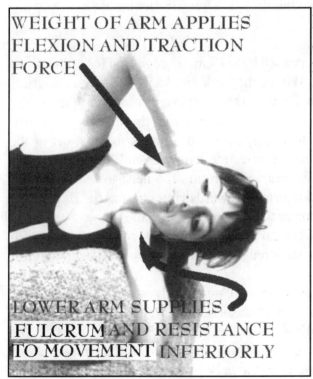

Figure 4 Positioning for increasing FLEXION IN TRACTION for a Middle Cervical disc with pain to the Right

IN TRACTION as in Figure 4.   Here, a mid-level Cervical pain to the right is addressed with both a resistance to inferior movement which facilitates TRACTION, as well as a simultaneous balancing fulcrum-effect on the down-side arm wherein the hand is positioned slightly above the site of pain to simultaneously magnify FLEXION at the problem disc unit.   This positioning allows the down-side arm to act as a source of resistance to prevent the neck above the problem disc unit from moving inferiorly, hence, the TRACTION can separate the painful disc unit's vertebrae..

The position of the hands along the axis of the Cervical spine determines what disc level is being stretched by TRACTION. The further down on the neck that the hands are placed, the lower the Cervical level that is put in TRACTION. You can, with practice, get your fingers almost down to the mid Thoracic level.   This is an important consideration because it is often helpful to use your fingers to push the spine anteriorly into an EXTENSION position while maneuvering because the more TRACTION IN EXTENSION that is applied, the more likely the disc will centralize (See Figure 5) when it is in the Low Cervical or High Thoracic region.

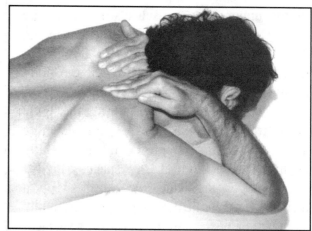

Figure 5 Hand position for a Low Cervical/High Thoracic disc problem

When the problem disc is in the Low Cervical/High Thoracic region, TRACTION can actually be assisted by the fingers pulling on the skin of the neck and back. This has the effect of increasing the ability to put the problem disc in TRACTION. Believe it or not, the fingers can also be used to slightly move the actual vertebral bodies by manipulating the spinous processes.

In contradistinction to the lower neck, when grasping the head/neck to lift it off of the shoulders to effect TRACTION in an Upper Cervical disc, the hands should be held with the palms' side touching the neck skin so that the fingers wrap around the neck to touch or even overlap in the back. The thumbs should be aimed inferiorly towards your chest as the fingers cup and cradle the neck. The lower the pain is in your neck, the lower your hands should be placed upon the neck. Also, as you get lower on the Cervical spine, the neck widens and it makes it more difficult for the hands to grasp the neck with the strength necessary to hold on tight with just the fingers perpendicular.

At any level of the Cervical spine, the fingers alone are not usually strong enough or can't get a significant grip to pull with the force necessary to effect sufficient TRACTION. So, in order to induce TRACTION at the ideal disc site regardless of whether it is low or high in the neck, the inferior medial aspect of the palm's surface that can simply be described as the "karate chop" portion of the hand should be tucked into the muscles of the neck just superior to the site of pain so that the neck is grasped between the two arms pressing together, like a nut cracker. In this manner, additional restraint and gripping function can be brought to bear by the hands, wrists, and forearms as they press against the neck without much strenuous muscular activity that might interfere with the disc unit's separation.

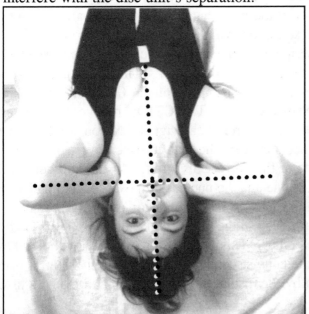

Figure 6 High Cervical disc hand/forearm placement perpendicular to axis of spine.

For all levels of Cervical pain, this technique also includes positioning the karate chop portion of the hand, the wrists, or the forearms (depending on whether your pain is at the High, Middle, or Lower Cervical regions respectively) at the base of the skull so that they abut against the inferior aspect of the mastoid processes (those bony bumps behind the ears). These protrusions of the skull offer a great anatomical anchor point against which the arms can push to create TRACTION.

When the problem disc is high in the Cervical spine, the fingers and forearms are better positioned so that their long axis is on a plane more perpendicular to the spine so as to be able to cup the upper neck (See Figure 6).

The finger's, hand's, and forearm's positions should change if the problem disc is lower on the neck so much that, when dealing with the base of the neck or Upper THORACIC spine, the fingers, hands, and forearms should be aligned almost parallel to the plane of the spine. The more the distal forearms (that part of the forearm farthest from the body) become more parallel to the neck's axis, the greater the amount of contact between them and the greater the friction to generate TRACTION (See Figure 7).

Of note, when the hands move more inferiorly to put TRACTION on Lower Cervical areas some part of the forearm should remain in contact with the mastoid processes so that when the forearms are extended at the elbow, they can assist in continually lifting the head off of the shoulders. The larger the surface area on the neck that interfaces with the arms, hands, or fingers, the more forceful a TRACTION can be generated because friction between the two surfaces is maximized.

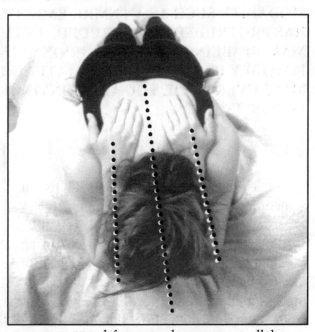

Figure 7 Hand/forearm placement parallel to axis of spine for Low Cervical/High Thoracic pain.

Remember, it is always important to apply TRACTION, FLEXION, or EXTENSION at

285

or slightly above the precise disc level that is producing the pain. You will know you are applying these forces at the right level when the character of the pain changes. When you are stretching the fibers of the affected disc, the stretching sensation will be superimposed upon the pain sensation. Quite often, when the fibers on the periphery of the painful disc segment are stretched, the referred pain will be alleviated during this phase of the maneuver. The pain can suddenly leave the shoulder or other distant part of the area of distribution of the Cervical nerves and become apparent as obviously originating in the spine when the TRACTION relieves pressure on the herniation. As the TRACTION proceeds, this pain's relief can signal that you are doing the maneuver correctly and separating the distance between the two Cervical vertebrae, thus convincing you that you are taking pressure off of the correct disc unit. As the intervertebral distance elongates along the axis of the Cervical spine and the nucleus pulposus, accommodating to the negative pressure created by this separation, sucks the bulging portion of the disc centrally, a squishy crunching (crepitus) often can be heard deep in the neck. This sound is generated by the cartilaginous structures moving against each other. This negative pressure generation takes the outwardly bulging pressure off of the ligamentous structures that surround the central disc material, relieves the pressure placed on them by the displaced disc material and that, in turn, lessens the cause of the referred pain.

IF, DURING ANY OF THESE PROCESSES, YOU INDUCE A SENSATION THAT YOU ARE DIZZY, FEEL LIKE FAINTING, THE PAIN GETS GREATER OR SENDS SHOCK-LIKE IMPULSES DOWN THE ARM OR SHOULDER, OR UP INTO THE HEAD, CAREFULLY STOP THE MANEUVER AND RELY UPON SOME DIAGNOSTIC MODALITY SUCH AS AN NMRI, EMG, OR CT SCAN TO DETERMINE IF THE DISC HAS PROTRUDED OR EXTRUDED. IN THAT CASE, ONE OF THE SPINAL NERVES MAY BE BEING IMPINGED UPON BY A BONY STRUCTURE, SCAR, OR THE POSSIBLY PROTRUDED DISC MATERIAL; AND YOU SHOULD STOP DOING ANY MANEUVER UNTIL YOU ARE CONVINCED NO HARM WILL BE OCCASIONED BY PERSISTING.

Get a Rope

To attain sufficient TRACTION, it sometimes requires that you hang your upper torso well off of the edge of a bed, it will be worth your while at this point to obtain an assistant or, better, a rope tied to the head of the bed before you start. Either one can be used to hold onto your leg(s) to prevent you from sliding off of the bed while undergoing the obligatory hanging components of the neck MANEUVERS (See Figure 8). A rope is best because an assistant usually gets bored or tired and can't hold on as long as it takes sometimes to let the TRACTION take effect. The rope

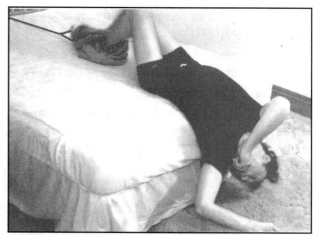

Figure 8 A Rope with loop on heel for neck MANEUVERS. (Towel used to protect skin on leg)

286

should have a smaller loop (about 10 inches in diameter) knotted in it so that the free end of the rope can be fed through the smaller loop making a larger loop, the size of which can be controlled by adjusting the length of the rope's free end. The leg at the knee or, better, one foot can be put through it; and, by hooking the knees or heels on the loop, one can avoid the use of the arms or legs to keep from sliding off of the bed Using one foot is probably the best method because, during the rolling THERAPEUTIC CIRCUMDUCTION component, an extended foot makes the leg easier to complete a roll, and you can use the knee for pulling your torso inferiorly to increase TRACTION. In this manner, all the extraneous sources of muscular contraction are eliminated which improves your chances of adequately relaxing the Cervical spine so as to allow TRACTION to be successful.

These PRINCIPLES will be further discussed later at the specific point in the MANEUVERS when they are particularly relevant; but for now its probably best to just start with the most basic and effective MANEUVER and use the descriptions as a means to elaborate on these and additional points. For a more detailed description of managing the rope, Chapter 4's Section on ROPE-ASSISTED TRACTION provides explicit directions.

THE BED-BASED CERVICAL MANEUVER
or
"THE HEAD-HANG"

In my experience treating neck pain, **the most commonly encountered neck problem is that which is located very low in the neck and lateralized to (or felt mostly on) one side. This also happens to make it the most difficult pain to deal with because the problem disc unit usually is so low in the neck that the pain is felt more in the shoulder or even as low as between the shoulder blades. This is understandable because many of the nerves that supply the muscles of the upper shoulders and back actually exit the spine at the Cervical levels; and** when these nerves are stimulated, they refer the pain to areas that are perceived to be distant to and distinct from the actual neck. Since it is so prevalent, the MANEUVER best suited to remedy this condition seems the most appropriate with which to begin.

This first and easiest MANEUVER to attempt is the **most effective for lateralized pain (pain that feels as though it is coming from the side) at the base of the neck. This type of pain includes pain originating in the disc but presenting as pain radiating to the sides of the neck, shoulders, shoulder blades, and even arms.** Although, with modifications, **it can be used for pain at any level of the Cervical spine**, pain centered in the midline posteriorly, or even pain in the most superior region of the Thoracic vertebrae, **this MANEUVER is the most generally applicable, universally effective, and functional set of movements** to both introduce neck MANEUVERS and put the PRINCIPLES of *The O'Connor Technique (tm)* as they relate to the Cervical spine into practice.

It is most easily accomplished by using a platform such as a bed. Any platform will suffice so long as it holds the body safely off of the ground far enough to hang the head, shoulders, and arms. For the purposes of this depiction, a bed is used and, in general, a bed is the most readily available platform for most people.

The **BED-BASED NECK MANEUVER begins by starting in the FLEXION IN TRACTION position with the area to which the pain radiates (which is also the site of the disc herniation) aimed towards the ceiling.** The site and the position of the herniated disc material can be determined through the DIAGNOSTIC CIRCUMDUCTION process described in the chapter SELF-DIAGNOSING YOUR DISC; however, to simplify matters, one can operate on the assumption that the site toward which the pain lateralizes characterizes the direction and location of the herniation. FLEXION IN TRACTION is particularly pertinent to, and effective in, the Cervical region, more so the lower discs than the upper; but it is relevant to all levels. I begin the MANEUVER with a FLEXION IN TRACTION because it is consistently more effective to start all MANEUVERS that way. Even though it may not be as frequently necessary to utilize as the simpler EXTENSION IN TRACTION MANEUVER, FLEXION IN TRACTION, nevertheless, should be the initiating component in the full MANEUVER sequence required to be practiced if you wish to insure that the most complete effort is made to re-centralize disc material, especially in the presence of longstanding pain. FLEXION IN TRACTION usage also best fulfills the oftentimes required increase in mobility. It must be accepted that this endeavor may be time consuming; and pursuing a continuous, repetitive, effort is not unusual before success is achieved whenever the pain has been longstanding. Towards that end, the described FLEXION IN TRACTION actions can also be combined with the concept of DYNAMIC POSITIONING to merge the successfulness of each.

It may seem obvious, but you start this MANEUVER by sitting on the side of the bed with your hands in a protective cradling of the neck (See Figure 1) and in the configuration most likely to be used later for TRACTION. One should always protect the neck when there is a possibility it may go into an uncontrolled FLEXION while WEIGHT-BEARING. Next you lower yourself down on the surface so that the side of your body to which the pain radiates is aimed towards the ceiling. While lying down, be sure to carry your neck with your hands so that it is not caused to flex while bearing weight. A pillow is optional and can be used to accentuate FLEXION IN TRACTION. When used, it should be placed in advance so that you can lie down upon it as in Figure 1. **Then you slowly let your head hang over the end of the bed, adjusting your legs such that your feet are headed towards the head of the bed where the rope awaits.** (See Figure 2).

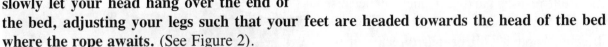

Figure 1 Starting position showing hands cradling neck for Right sided Low Cervical pain

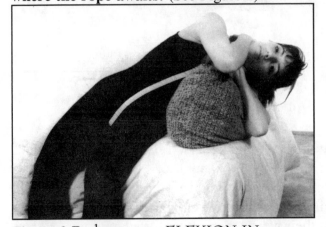

Figure 2 Reclining into FLEXION IN TRACTION position for Right-sided Cervical pain showing pillow in use.

The MANEUVER depicted in Figure 3 assumes positioning to be used for a disc pain that radiates or is felt in the right neck, shoulder, or upper back area. If your pain were to be on the left, then the left side would necessarily be the up-side starting position **Since the reader's pain could be either to the left or the right, I have taken the liberty of showing no preference, and I interspersed pictures depicting positions for both left and right sided pain. Please pay note of this distinction for each picture wherein I annotate whether the position is meant to be used for a left or right sided pain. If your pain is on the opposite side, then you should place yourself in the opposite sided position while performing the MANEUVER.** This saves me from having to separately describe the entire sequence three times. But don't get confused, I only make the distinction pictorially, in the text, I speak of the painful side or the down-side, etc. so that the reader will always know which position is appropriate.

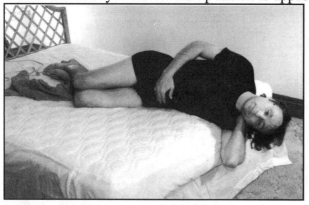

Figure 3 FLEXION IN TRACTION position (without pillow) for Low Cervical pain lateralized to the Right

If the pain is in the midline posterior neck, begin by placing that area up by lying face down with your head hanging over the foot or side of the bed. (See Figure 4).

The lower in the neck the problem disc exists, the more you should hang over the edge. When the problem disc is very low in the neck or between the shoulder blades, it is necessary to hang your arms far over the edge. Hanging the arms is the best way of exerting sufficient TRACTION on those vertebrae that are connected to the shoulder and arm musculature. It is for this reason a bed makes the best platform from which to operate since few other easily acquired platforms are available that will raise you that high off of the floor while reclining.

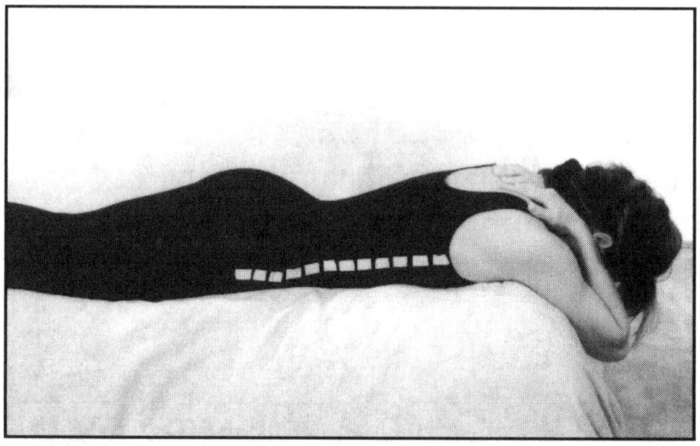

You should be able to tell when you are hanging in the right position because pain from the site of the herniated disc will change character. Usually, it becomes obvious that you are stretching the disc in question because the pain will localize to the site of the stretching and it will be felt directly in the spine instead of being referred to the shoulder or medial shoulder-blade region. This change in pain and stretching sensation signifies that you are putting the ideal disc in FLEXION IN TRACTION. If you do not experience this change in character of the pain, you must continue to re-position yourself superiorly or

Figure 4 FLEXION IN TRACTION position for midline posterior neck pain.

inferiorly (either to hang more over the edge of the bed or pull yourself back onto the bed) until you are certain that you are stretching the ligaments of the problem disc.

Although precipitous hanging is sometimes necessary for low Cervical discs, the basic MANEUVER positioning doesn't always require this level of effort. Instead, a simple placing of the arms resting on the head and neck so that their weight hangs over the edge of the mattress is usually sufficient for uncomplicated disc pain. (See Figure 5).

Now, you must attempt to maximize both the degree of TRACTION and FLEXION. This is done by placing the down-side hand against the neck as close to the painful disc as possible, cupping it with the fingers, while the upper arm is held parallel to the vertical end of the mattress (See Figure 5). The down-side elbow, forearm, and hand becomes a fulcrum upon which the Cervical and Thoracic spine "teeter-totters." If this elbow is fixed against the end of the mattress,

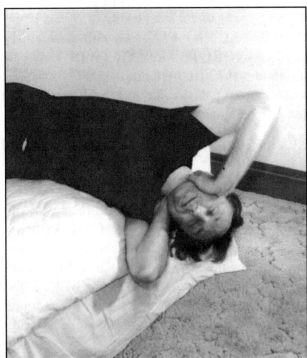

Figure 5 Weighting of head and neck with up-side arm to magnify a hanging FLEXION IN TRACTION for a Low Right-sided Cervical pain

the amount of FLEXION IN TRACTION stress placed upon the disc unit in question can be varied by the degree to which the head, neck, and upper thorax hangs over the end of the bed. By using your feet and legs hooked to or wrapped around by the rope, you can position yourself hanging so far over that the problem disc, no matter how deep in the neck or upper thorax it exists, can be put in the necessary amount of FLEXION IN TRACTION to effect sufficient partial centralization of the disc material.

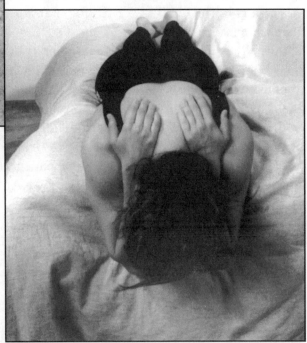

Figure 6 A FLEXION IN TRACTION accentuation with hand positioning shown for Low Cervical disc with midline pain

If the pain is not to one side, but in the midline posterior, a nearly equivalent effort is generated by both elbows doing the same sort of balancing act (See Figure 6). As the forearms are extended at the elbows, the mattress stops the upper arms from moving inferiorly and the head and neck are pulled off of the shoulders. This is an excellent time to use the torso and the legs to pull the body away from the fixed arms thus inducing TRACTION at the putative disc unit.

For an Upper Cervical disc level problem, the hands are cupped on either side of the jaws. For a Lower Cervical/Upper Thoracic disc, the wrists are forced against the both sides of the base of the neck with the fingers running parallel to the plane of the body on the back (See Figure 6). If all are simultaneously combined, the weight of the arms, pulling with the legs, and the act of extending at the elbows will increase the amount of TRACTION IN FLEXION to the maximum allowable by anatomy alone without the aid of complicated and costly apparati.

Next, while the painful site is aimed towards the ceiling (regardless of whether it is your side or your posterior) and while maintaining TRACTION supplied by gravity and the

elbow/arm axis, you do some CIRCUMDUCTIONS by sort of cork-screwing the chest while the head remains fixed with the arms, RELAXATIONAL BREATHING, and consciously work to achieve the highest degree of MOBILITY. CHIROTATIONAL TWISTING can also be tried here to improve the chances of mobilizing the disc material.

Now is an excellent opportunity to gently rock from side to side in a NARROW-ARC ROCKING manner with your painful site continuing to be aimed at the ceiling and the problem disc kept in FLEXION IN TRACTION. This is the NARROW-ARC ROCKING described previously. By "side-to-side," if you are dealing with a lateralized herniation pain and the painful side is aimed upwards, I mean it is as if you were almost trying to roll to your abdomen and, then, alternating by starting to roll onto your back; but the full roll is never completed.

In practice, it is not a good idea to extend the spine using the muscles of the spine associated with the problem disc region while in a FLEXION IN TRACTION during this or any of the MANEUVERS for that matter. The reason being because when you contract the back muscles associated with the disc, it is the physical equivalent to a WEIGHT-BEARING action. Recalling one of the caveats of *The O'Connor Technique (tm),* **if you are in FLEXION, you should not bear weight.** I mention this here because hanging over the edge of a bed, one is tempted to use the back muscles to attempt to move the spine. This should be avoided by using the arms, legs, or torso instead to accomplish the same movement.

You may feel free to periodically relax, take a break of sorts, and let the resting FLEXION IN TRACTION function to bring all the ligamentous and muscular elements to full length. This may take awhile, so be patient, read something (like this book), and be prepared to spend some time in this posture as a DYNAMIC POSITION if your disc is a difficult one to manage.

At this juncture, anatomically, the posterior longitudinal ligament and the peripheral fibro-cartilaginous ligaments that hold the vertebral bodies together are being stretched. When they stretch, they come to their full length. This pushes adjacent disc material centrally. As you rock back and forth, the maximum amount of tension is placed upon successive fibers so that regardless of where the protruded disc material is, it will be contacted and moved centrally. This TRACTION IN EXTENSION effect can also be assisted by RELAXATIONAL BREATHING and exhaling to achieve the maximum amount of relaxation and, hence, TRACTION. Gentle "hula"-like THERAPEUTIC CIRCUMDUCTIONS can be performed here as well. In fact, THERAPEUTIC CIRCUMDUCTIONS can be performed at any juncture to free up the aberrant disc material. Just as in any mechanical part being fitted into another, jiggling it makes it go easier. You are encouraged to wiggle, gyrate, "INCH-WORM," or make "tad-pole"-like movements with the neck so long as, after each, you relax and let TRACTION return before going on to the next step.

When the disc unit is in FLEXION IN TRACTION, as it should be at this point, it is an excellent time to perform an assisted type of CHIROTATIONAL TWIST. For the Cervical spine, especially in the presence of pain that radiates to one side, the wringing action can be accentuated by assistance from the hands. This is done by placing the palm of the up-side hand on the down-side aspect of the jaw and pushing it counterclockwise while at the same time the down-side hand is placed on the up-side aspect of the posterior skull area and pulled so that the head turns counterclockwise, all the while TRACTION is being maintained. This lets you get the disc unit into as much of a CHIROTATIONALLY TWISTED configuration as possible before you actually do the thrusting to perform a forceful CHIROTATIONAL TWIST, but this is not too difficult or dangerous so long as you gradually increase the amount of force as you quickly jerk the head to twist the neck's vertebrae. Refer to the section of this book that discusses CHIROTATIONAL TWISTING for details as to what is happening during this action. If at this point the prospect of twisting your neck is disconcerting, forego this action until you feel comfortable.

To elaborate, for a left sided pain, you would be lying on your right side, the up-side (left) hand's palm would be on the down-side of the jaw pushing it so the head would be rotated as far to the left (counterclockwise) as comfortably possible. The down-side hand would be participating in this twisting of the head by its fingers pulling floor-ward on the back of the head (turning the head counter-clockwise). You would then rapidly, not too forcefully, and carefully twist the head and neck further counterclockwise so that with each thrust you slightly exceed the natural limit of the range of motion. You can gradually increase the force so long as no pain is occasioned until you are getting a good twisting action to maximally tighten the peripheral ligamentous fibers.

The lower in the Cervical spine that the problem disc lies, the lower on the neck you would want to position your hands instead of keeping them on the chin and head, so as to be twisting the superior aspect of the neck on the inferior aspect of the neck (instead of the head on the superior part of the neck as described immediately above). This creates the "wringing" action that often successfully centralizes disc material. If unsuccessful in one direction, you can reverse the position of your hands and rotate your head/neck in the opposite direction while still maintaining FLEXION IN TRACTION, and this time, get it to go counterclockwise. One of these two should get the desired result if the disc is going to centralize with this action. If not, keep on with the MANEUVERING.

You can apply this type of CHIROTATIONAL TWISTING during any neck MANEUVER when your problem disc is in FLEXION IN TRACTION, and you can also use it when the disc is, later, in EXTENSION IN TRACTION.

After you have tried the CHIROTATIONAL TWISTING, rest again in FLEXION IN TRACTION (See Figure 7). Now comes the most critical and unique movement of this particular MANEUVER, the PASSIVE THERAPEUTIC CIRCUMDUCTION IN TRACTION. **In this action, you must roll towards the side of pain until you are 180 degrees rotated from your original position while all the while maintaining TRACTION.** At the end

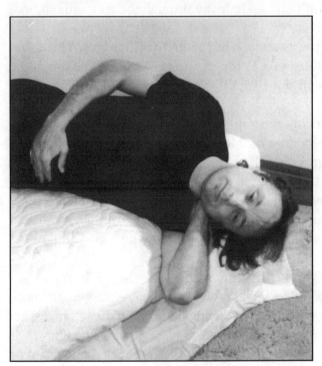

Figure 7 Resting in FLEXION IN TRACTION for a Low Cervical Right-sided pain

293

of the roll, **you want to have the painful site that was originally aimed towards the ceiling, eventually aimed towards the floor.** For example, if your right side was up during FLEXION IN TRACTION, the rolling should leave you with the right side down but still hanging in TRACTION.

In the case of a midline, posterior pain, you would eventually want to end the roll so that the anterior aspect of the body is in the up (supine) position.

In either case, **the affected disc should be caused to go from FLEXION IN TRACTION to EXTENSION IN TRACTION via a PASSIVE THERAPEUTIC CIRCUMDUCTION (rolling).** By passive, I mean that the muscles at the disc unit being manipulated should not be activated. They should stay in the most relaxed and stretched-by-gravity condition. The roll can be accomplished by rolling like a log or be done in place by sequential adjustments in which you roll in place a little, adjust your torso to put the problem disc unit over the same spot that you were in before you rolled, and making sure your are in TRACTION, roll in place a little more, re-adjust, insure TRACTION, and so forth.

By adjusting your position relative to the edge of the surface upon which you are lying, the maximum amount of FLEXION at the onset and EXTENSION at the end of the roll should be kept at the problem disc level where the pain originates. For this reason, anticipating where you eventually want to end up in maximum EXTENSION IN TRACTION should dictate to what degree you are hanging over the edge of the bed or surface upon which you are rolling. Too, if you choose to roll like a log, you don't want to roll off the side of the bed before you complete your roll. So, in this instance, before you roll, position yourself on the bed so that you have a sufficient area on the bed to roll onto so you won't end up halfway through the roll without bed-space upon which you can come to rest.

Insuring that you have enough space to roll when you are actually rolling over like a log, you may find that the rope holding your foot causes you to roll in a "fan"-shape. The top of the "fan" being curved, changes the site upon which the FLEXION and EXTENSION forces are applied by the straight edge of the mattress.

By that I mean, all else being equal, a person starting their roll in the middle of the "fan" and rolling towards the edge will increase the degree of TRACTION because the disc unit is moving inferiorly relative to the end of the mattress which restrains the upper body hanging over it. Similarly, if a person starts at the side of the proposed "fan" and rolls towards its center, TRACTION will be decreased. However, by using the arms in an improvisational manner, these rolls can be used in your favor to generate unique types of TRACTION when artfully coordinated with arm movements.   Rolling-in-place eliminates this problem for those who cannot figure out how to use it to their advantage

It is essential to maintain TRACTION during the entire roll (See Figure 8). To maintain TRACTION on the neck while rolling, the original down-side hand is kept on the neck with the fingers cupping the posterior/lateral aspect of the neck with the palm on the lateral aspect of the neck. Constant efforts should be made to hold onto the neck and extend at the elbows as if you were trying to pull your neck off of your shoulders. A pillow or large rolled towel can be put under the down-side armpit to assist this, but it is not necessary so long as you hang off of the edge sufficiently. In order to give your elbow a place to support the weight it is bearing, at the same time you are extending at the elbow, plant the downside upper arm against the mattress edge and push the elbow into the surface. If your mattress has a box springs, there is a separation between it and the mattress that provides a good surface for the elbow to be planted into so that you can pivot on the down-side arm to work on Middle Cervical region discs. Using your shoulder and your chest wall planted into the surface of the end of the mattress works best for Lower Cervical/Upper Thoracic regions.

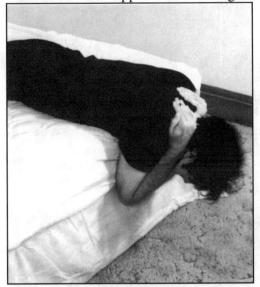

Figure 9 Rolling Counterclockwise towards Right for Right-sided pain while maintaining TRACTION with arms

Ideally, one should roll towards the side of the pain (See Figure 9). For example, if the pain is lateralized to the right, you will be starting with the right side up. As you roll to the same side, clockwise to the right, this will first put you in the face down position. As you continue to roll to the right, or clockwise from your perspective, you eventually bring the affected disc to the EXTENSION IN TRACTION position with the right (painful) side down.

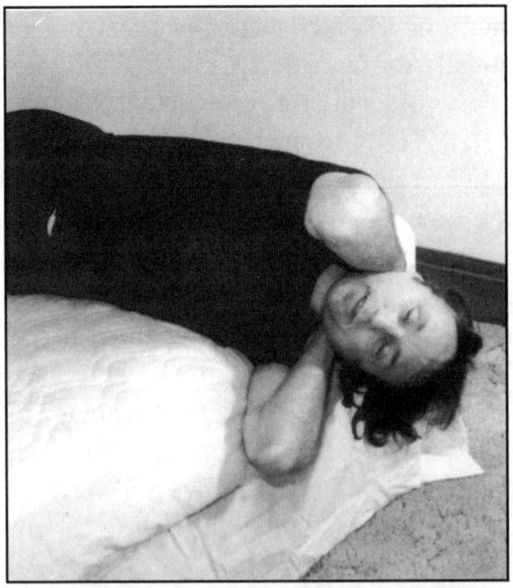

Figure 8 Using both arms to maintain TRACTION while beginning to roll towards the Right (Counter-clockwise) for a Right-sided pain

In order to execute this roll, your feet, legs, and torso should do most of the work while holding onto the rope with the loop in it. Someone can hold onto your feet to keep you from sliding off the bed, but they usually get tired too easily to rely upon. Don't be afraid to use your elbow and neck (for Middle Cervical regions) or your down-side shoulder or chest wall (for Lower Cervical/Upper Thoracic regions) to carry your weight while you pivot on them to bring your hips off of the mattress to adjust your position to effect the roll. This actually is very close to the same action as the "INCH-WORM" technique; and it can be the actual "milking" action that lets the disc material move. While you are in FLEXION IN TRACTION this pivoting on (or sequential planting of the downside to adjust the position of the torso for the next similar movement that in total is equivalent to a roll) actually accentuates the FLEXION, and when your rolling finally gets you around to EXTENSION IN TRACTION, the pivoting accentuates the EXTENSION.

How you roll is almost as important as the necessity to roll. As you execute your roll, what was once the up-side will obviously become the down-side. As this transition is made, the operant TRACTION hand is changed because the hand that is bearing weight is always the down-

295

side one except when you are lying on your face-down position where both arms contribute equally to maintaining TRACTION.

As you roll, you must practice maintaining TRACTION by moving in small increments so that you can be sure that TRACTION persists as much of the time as possible because you never really know when the exact instant the disc material will go in, and you should be in TRACTION when the time comes. The up-side arm can be used to assist this TRACTION by either stretching it over your head to let its weight work for your advantage or you can use it to push down on the up-side of the head or neck to increase the degree of EXTENSION.

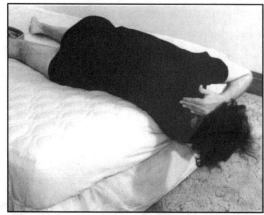

Figure 10 Completed counterclockwise roll towards Right for Right-sided pain ending with disc unit in EXTENSION IN TRACTION

You should adjust your down-side elbow, shoulder or armpit/chest wall relative to the position of your body hanging over the edge of the mattress to keep the disc unit at the fulcrum point of a balancing, "teeter-totter," effect. You should, as much as possible, retain the sensation of stretching at the problem disc site. If this is not done, you are putting the essential forces on the wrong disc and the MANEUVER most probably will be ineffective. For Upper and Middle Cervical regions the forearm is the fulcrum and the "teeter-totter's" "board" is the Cervical spine. For Lower Cervical/Upper Thoracic discs, the down-side shoulder or chest wall should be bearing the weight so as to support the teeter-totter "board" that is the spine. The problem disc unit, while balancing on top of the fulcrum created by the weight-bearing elbow/forearm, shoulder, or chest wall has the maximum EXTENSION forces placed on it in this manner.

When the roll is completed you should be positioned in an EXTENSION IN TRACTION. This should then leave you with the elbow/shoulder of the same side as the pain is lateralized to in the "down" position (See Figure 10) By that, I mean if the pain is to the right side of the neck or shoulder, the right elbow should now be hanging over the mattress end and the pain aimed towards the floor.

When the pain site happens to be in the midline posterior, understandably, you should continue to roll until at the end of the roll you are lying on your back with your head and neck hanging over the end of the mattress as in (Figure 11).

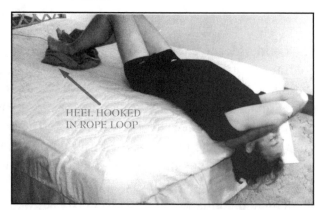

HEEL HOOKED IN ROPE LOOP

Figure 11 Hanging EXTENSION IN TRACTION for midline posterior Cervical pain.

If, as you roll into an EXTENSION IN TRACTION posture, you get an arresting, painful sensation, this can mean that the disc material is not ready to centralize. It may be necessary to again accentuate the degree of TRACTION if the disc has not yet moved. This is done by sliding your trunk superiorly as though you were "pole-vaulting" on your upper arm (humerus) until the shoulder is directly above the elbow (See Figure 12). The head can hang

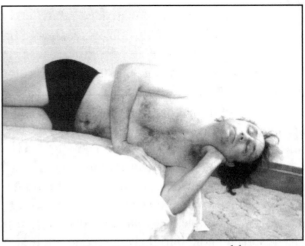

Figure 12 TRACTION accentuated by balancing on down-side arm for a Left-sided pain (this can also be seen as the "neutral position")

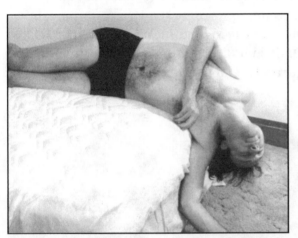

Figure 13 Full PASSIVE EXTENSION IN TRACTION for Left sided Cervical pain.

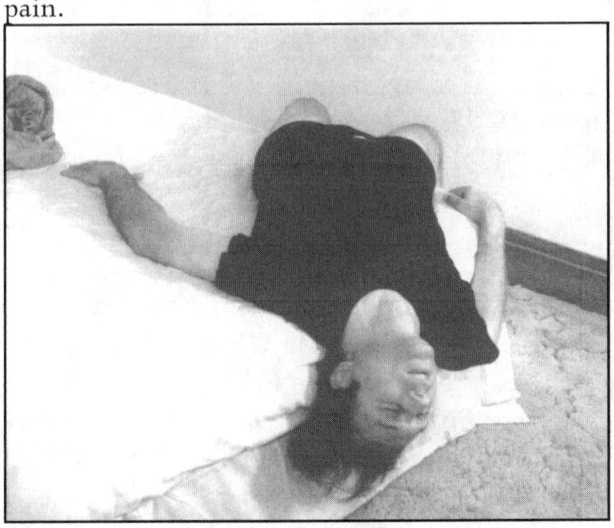

gently above the position of the down-side hand but the hand should attempt to keep that part of the neck superior to the painful disc site straight so as to not apply EXTENSION forces to an unaffected disc. (Notice that at this juncture, you are pushing the head/neck off of the shoulders and keeping it horizontally straight along the axis of the neutral spine. Note that Figure 12 is for a Left-sided pain so that the left side is the down-side in EXTENSION IN TRACTION.)

By continuing to slide the upper chest/trunk superiorly off the edge of the bed, you come to a point where the shoulder is hanging over and subsequently superior to the point on the surface of the bed where the elbow is anchored. Then, when the neck is in full TRACTION in a straight configuration (also known as the neutral position because the cervical spine containing the problem disc is not in EXTENSION or flexion), it is allowed to go into a full PASSIVE EXTENSION (See Figure 13) by removing the support of the down-side hand. When you finally relax, as the upper trunk hangs over the upper arm, simply the weight of the head, neck, and

Figure 14 Initiating CASCADE off of bed keeping neck in EXTENSION towards Right for Right-sided pain

shoulder superior to the down-sided elbow and arm can act with gravity-assisted EXTENSION IN TRACTION on even the lowest reaches of the neck where it merges into the chest if you hang far enough over the edge.

Now, you may not need to go any further, you may end the MANEUVER if you feel that the disc moved centrally enough to eliminate the pain. To determine whether you have done enough to centralize the disc material, you can test whether it is "in" by simply rolling over the problem site with the painful side down. This is a PASSIVE DIAGNOSTIC CIRCUMDUCTION. Since when you are in EXTENSION without TRACTION, cascading off of the edge of the mattress sequentially puts each disc in a semi-weight-bearing state. During this stage, when the problem disc is in a partially loaded condition, you should be able to tell if there is an obstruction to range of motion at the problem disc site. If so, the disc material is not centralized, and you should try the preceding techniques again at least one more time because quite often the first attempt moves the disc material enough to make a second attempt successful..

If there is no restriction of range of motion, you can **return to WEIGHT-BEARING EXTENSION by leaving your head in EXTENSION in a direction towards the site of pain, sliding your legs over the side of the bed (See Figure 14), and letting the neck CASCADE IN EXTENSION over the edge of the mattress.**

As you let your spine bend backwards over the corner of the bed, the feet should be tucked underneath you such that the anterior aspect of the feet (the top part that you see when you ordinarily look down at your feet) is kept level to and touching flat on the floor as much as comfortably possible. This insures that you will stay in the maximum amount of EXTENSION as each individual disc is put into EXTENSION IN TRACTION as it moves over the edge of the mattress. It is sort of like coming to rest seated on your heels, like a traditional Japanese person sits on the floor; only, it is usually necessary to spread the lower legs apart so that you can sit completely on the floor to keep the neck in EXTENSION on an average height bed. In

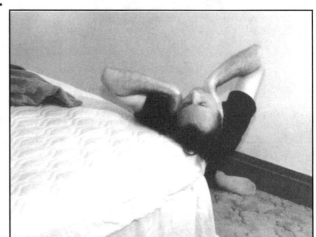

Figure 15 Using hands to increase TRACTION IN EXTENSION (note foot position)

addition, using the hands to keep the head pressed against the surface of the mattress increases friction to enhance the TRACTION aspect of the cascade (See Figure 15). Once you have come to rest, you only need to find the most advantageous means of getting up to a standing position while keeping the neck in EXTENSION towards the site of pain.

After coming to the upright stance, you should execute a final THERAPEUTIC CIRCUMDUCTION.

This must be done without contracting the neck muscles. The object is to get to standing while keeping the neck extended towards the side of pain (directly over the herniation site). This serves to keep the disc material trapped, preventing it from decentralizing.

298

This rather anti-climactic finale is best undertaken once you are standing upright. **You then carefully and repeatedly CIRCUMDUCT the neck IN EXTENSION pivoting at the level of the problem disc unit and especially while EXTENDING directly over the previously painful site of the problem disc (See Figures 16-18) which for all intents and purposes is directly over the herniation.** The disc may not be ready for full WEIGHT-BEARING immediately. If the problem disc is in the High or Middle Cervical region, you can reach up and lift the head off of the neck with an UNWEIGHTING gesture, at first, to make sure that the disc material has a place into which it can move. When it is low in the neck or high in the Thoracic region, you can unweight the disc by pushing down on your hips with your arms to facilitate the final movement of disc material (See Figure 16). You may have to lean quite a great deal as you do it to insure that you are bending the disc unit as much as possible.

For middle to high neck discs, you can reach up with your hands to lift the head off of the neck or the neck off of the shoulders while CIRCUMDUCTING to slightly UNWEIGHT it just in case. **Do not expect the arms and hands to UNWEIGHT a Lower Cervical/Upper Thoracic disc because the shoulder muscles will push the problem disc unit closed when they contract. Be certain when you lift that you can feel the problem disc unit being stretched.**

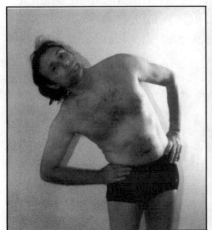 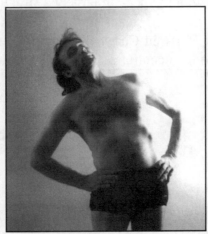 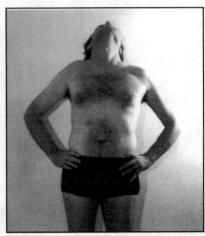

Figure 16 Cervical
THERAPEUTIC
CIRCUMDUCTION

Figure 17 Cervical
THERAPEUTIC
CIRCUMDUCTION

Figure 18 Cervical
THERAPEUTIC
CIRCUMDUCTION

Gradually, in either case, you can release this UNWEIGHTING effect and CIRCUMDUCT while fully WEIGHT-BEARING. If, at this point, you have no arrested motion, the disc material is most probably back in its centralized position and all you need do is MAINTAIN EXTENSION and AVOID WEIGHT-BEARING FLEXION to keep it that way.

However, if you aren't convinced that the disc is "in," you should persist in MANEUVERING until you are reasonably certain that the disc material has moved completely to its central location in the disc. If such is the case and you don't feel any disc movement has occurred, in order to proceed with MANEUVERING, you can repeat the entire above-described MANEUVER or attempt the other types of MANEUVERS that differ slightly from the above and are described later.

Alternatively, you can continue to hang in an EXTENSION IN TRACTION type of DYNAMIC POSITIONING. This is done for Lower Cervical discs by positioning yourself such that rocking forward or backward on the elbow while the upper arm is extended puts TRACTION on the vertebrae at levels of the Low Cervical and Upper Thoracic region (See Figure 12 above). Depending upon how much you hang your head and neck over the elbow's anchor point determines how much TRACTION is applied. The more you move the trunk superiorly the more you are balancing on the upper arm (humerus). This is a beautifully simple position because it requires no muscular activity to maintain a great degree of TRACTION. You effectively are balancing such that the weight of the head and neck supply all the TRACTION force to stretch the vertebrae of the affected disc unit while it remains in EXTENSION.

By using the down-side hand with the elbow planted on the most convenient surface of the bed to support the neck at a site superior to the disc pain area, you can also bring the neck to a straightened configuration while keeping TRACTION applied. Then, you can alternate this straight position with a maximum EXTENSION by removing the down-side arm support which allows the neck to hang in EXTENSION. This should be done such that TRACTION is maintained by the down-side hand and arm until EXTENSION to the maximum is completed. When the TRACTION is applied with the neck in largely a straight, neutral, position or when it is in maximum EXTENSION, you can, again, try a few CHIROTATIONAL TWISTING movements of the head and neck (for mid-Cervical region) or neck and shoulders (for Lower Cervical/Upper Thoracic discs) to help centralize the disc material.

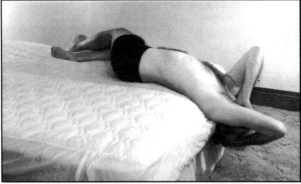 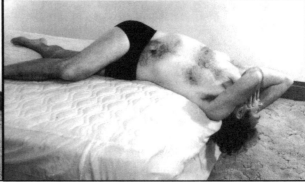

Figure 19 CHIROTATIONAL TWISTING while in EXTENSION IN TRACTION   **Figure 20** CHIROTATIONAL TWISTING while in EXTENSION IN TRACTION

These can be accomplished by either fixing the head and neck and rotating the torso or fixing the torso and moving the head and neck with the arms (See Figures 19-20).
The Cervical spine need not stay in a neutral position for these CHIROTATIONAL attempts, it can be allowed to hang in EXTENSION, but before proceeding with this series of movements, return to the neutral position as in Figure 12, above).

If the (essentially passive) rolling to EXTENSION effect is not successful, there is another little trick that can be brought to bear. It can be looked upon as an ACTIVE THERAPEUTIC CIRCUMDUCTION which is accomplished by progressively changing the point where maximum EXTENSION force (pincer effect by the edges of the vertebral bodies)

is applied to move disc material circumferentially. **This action can be seen as a SEQUENTIAL ARCHING CIRCUMDUCTION. While arching (arching being the act of extending the disc unit by muscular action), first in one direction (from immediately anterior to the painful site through the range of motion of the disc unit to the posterior midline) then, if unsuccessful, in the opposite direction from the posterior midline to anterior to the painful site, disc material that has been trapped in circumferential tears can be moved.** To elaborate on this action, if your pain is more on the left, you should start the arching EXTENSION, laterally as far to the left of the midline as possible (9:30 position), you would then circumduct the upper torso counterclockwise (bending towards the left lateral and moving towards the posterior midline) while maintaining the arch so that each point where the maximum EXTENSION force is applied on the vertebral bodies moves progressively closer to the midline (the 6:00 position).

Basically, what you are doing is figuratively equivalent to drawing a circle on the wall as if a pencil was coming right out of the top of your head, first in one direction and then in the other. The direction in which you would aim your head first would be to the side that the pain was on, then circumduct the head towards the posterior.

In an almost identical fashion, you can employ the SEQUENTIAL ARCHING CIRCUMDUCTION technique, to achieve the same end. In that technique, you arch and relax, arch and relax, along an arc parallel to the posterior rim of the vertebral bodies, each time closer to the midline than the arch before. Each time you use the posterior neck muscles contracting into an arch, you follow by relaxing the arch and restarting the arching again, only the next time closer to the midline by an incrementally small circumductional movement. That is, with each increment you arch, then move the point where the vertebral bodies pinch together a little more along the periphery of the disc, and then arch again. This sequential arching that moves along points of the periphery of the disc can gently force and move the disc material circumferentially between layers of ligamentous tissue as well as centrally along a radial tear. For that reason it should be looked upon as a highly regarded adjunct to disc material mobilization. If doing this in one direction isn't helpful, try arching first laterally on the other side and progressively direct the force towards the midline or start at the midline and progressively direct the arch to one side or the other. If your disc is degenerated significantly, you could be playing the "BB-in-the-maze game" described earlier in the chapter on THERAPEUTIC CIRCUMDUCTION.

This technique is very similar to the PASSIVE THERAPEUTIC CIRCUMDUCTION method that occurs during a roll; but, now, it is combined with arching that allows a certain measure of force to be applied. Yet, it is not really much weight-bearing force. It is only the force that your back muscles can comfortably generate. If any pain were to intervene, you can instantaneously stop the contraction of muscles to unload the vertebrae by returning to TRACTION.

Also, this technique can be combined with an EXTENSION INCH-WORMING in which your pushing the head and neck away from the shoulders restrains them from moving inferiorly as you perform the spinal EXTENSIONS (by contracting the erector spinae muscles at the posterior aspect of the neck and thorax) and you attempt to pull the posterior aspect of your head closer to the posterior aspect of your shoulders (just like a real inch worm only on its back). The problem disc should start in passive EXTENSION in a mild head hang during the TRACTION phase, and this action keeps the disc in maximum TRACTION until the EXTENSION contractions cause the disc unit to close posteriorly first. This ACTIVE HYPEREXTENSION serves to squeeze disc material more anteriorly and centrally.

Combining this type of action with a SEQUENTIAL ARCHING THERAPEUTIC CIRCUMDUCTION described earlier is particularly useful at mobilizing difficult disc problems.

As an aside, this type of movement need not be restricted to a HEAD-HANG, it can be used in a supine position with the Cervical or Upper Thoracic spine supported in EXTENSION with pillows or a towel. It is extremely effective if you repeat it in a rhythmic manner that involves pushing the head with the neck away from the trunk with the arms and pulling with the legs, while exhaling (RELAXATIONAL BREATHING); then, just as the disc unit is in maximum active TRACTION, you contract the erector spinae muscles into an ACTIVE HYPEREXTENSION.

As this series of actions is repeated and combined with CIRCUMDUCTION, you can effectively milk the disc material centrally along circumferential tears like that described in Chapter Four associated with its Figure 42. The beauty of this "sub-MANEUVER" is that it can be done without going through the rigmarole of an entire HEAD-HANGING MANEUVER anytime it has been shown to work successfully. It can be done in bed simply when lying down with a Cervical support as a morning stretching activity to centralize disc material that may have spontaneously migrated during the night's sleep. By sequentially INCHWORMING through all the possible areas where the disc material may be peripheralized you are less likely to miss the precise location that would lead to a movement of disc material centrally back along the radial fissure axis.

After returning to a neutral position with the neck in TRACTION, you can decide if you have successfully induced enough EXTENSION IN TRACTION to move the disc by doing a little bit of DIAGNOSTIC CIRCUMDUCTION to test whether or not the arrested rotation has been eliminated. This can be done by simply rolling through the range of motion in the vicinity of the pain while the disc unit in question is in EXTENSION. The presence of wedge-like arrested circumduction should tell you if you have centralized the disc material. If you did not successfully move the disc material centrally, it is probably because you did not achieve enough TRACTION while rolling into EXTENSION.

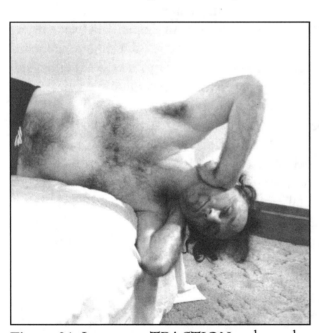

Figure 21 Increasing TRACTION with weight of up-side arm while in EXTENSION IN TRACTION for Left sided Cervical pain.

In order to exert more TRACTION than just simple hanging and gravity will allow, reach up with the up-side hand and push the up-side jaw from its inferior aspect superiorly (See position of right hand in

Figure 21). If you do this while keeping the neck musculature relaxed, you will be able to separate the disc unit in question's vertebral bodies enough to either allow for the suction action to work or give the disc material a sufficient volume of space to occupy when you immediately thereafter go into a hanging EXTENSION.

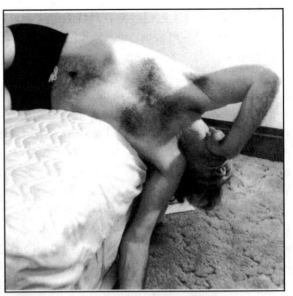

Figure 22 Maximizing EXTENSION IN TRACTION with the arm's weight for Left sided pain low in Cervical region

While accomplishing this method of generating maximum TRACTION and progressing to EXTENSION, the weight of the up-side hand can be pushing the head/neck downwards simultaneously as the down-side arm relaxes its support allowing the neck into an EXTENSION towards the side of the pain (the down-side) without necessitating the use of muscle contraction (See Figure 22). This, then, serves to trap any off-center disc material in a pincer-like movement as the neck assumes maximal EXTENSION IN TRACTION when the head hangs farther over the end of the bed. For Upper and Middle Level Cervical discs, one need not extend very far off the edge of the bed.

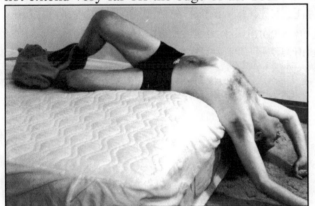

Figure 23 Maximal Hanging EXTENSION IN TRACTION for disc pain Low in Cervical or Upper Thoracic regions

However, **If your pain is in the Low Cervical or Upper Thoracic region, you finish this component of the MANEUVER by going all the way superiorly with the shoulder and upper torso as though the base of your neck was pole-vaulting using the upper arm bone (humerus) as the pole.** As the humerus begins to become parallel to and rest on the surface of the bed, the neck is allowed to assume a maximally extended posture towards the down-side (which also should be the painful side.) As a resting position, you can continue to roll into complete EXTENSION resting on your back in the maximum amount of hanging (See Figure 23) or you can roll from side to side as you hang to allow for a PASSIVE CIRCUMDUCTION IN EXTENSION AND TRACTION.

Finally, to complete the MANEUVER for an Upper or Middle Cervical Level disc, without contracting the muscles, balance your head and neck in a position extended towards the painful site and get to an upright posture by the most advantageous manner you can that insures you do not straighten your neck until you have assumed a fully weight-bearing stance in the upright position (See Figure 24). BY ALL MEANS, DO NOT ATTEMPT TO GET

UPRIGHT BY FLEXION WHILE WEIGHT-BEARING. Such a move could result in the disc going right back "out."

Alternatively, you can always dismount as described previously in this chapter and shown in Figures 14 & 15, above. You simply hang your legs over the side towards which you are facing so that the longitudinal axis of your body cuts across the corner of the bed. Then, you can slide your legs and hips off and swing yourself into a CASCADE or "waterfall"-like-slide to your knees while wiggling and circumducting so that, your painful side is continuously contacting the mattress. Putting your hands on your head or neck, so that the weight of the arms pushes the

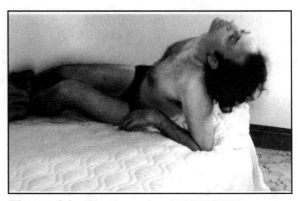

Figure 24 Final maximal WEIGHT-BEARING HYPEREXTENSION angled towards the site of pain for Upper/Middle Level Cervical pain to Left side..

head and neck into the mattress, allows the friction resistance of the surface of the bed to cause your head to be dragged, giving a final bit of EXTENSION IN TRACTION directly over the site of the herniated disc. **Then, while the neck is fixed in the laterally or posteriorly extended position, WEIGHT-BEARING is, again, intentionally allowed. This type of dismount is probably the best for pain located in the Low Cervical or Upper Thoracic region.**

Finally, once standing, a PARTIAL WEIGHT-BEARING THERAPEUTIC CIRCUMDUCTION leading to full WEIGHT-BEARING, similar to that described above and pictured in this section's Figures 16-18, should be accomplished to seat the disc material and/or test whether the disc material has completely centralized.

The above MANEUVER can be effectively used when the pain is located anywhere in the Cervical or Upper Thoracic region; however, a slightly different Cervical MANEUVER is best employed if the pain emanates from just the Upper or Middle Cervical region. This MANEUVER is very similar to the above described MANEUVER, only with this MANEUVER, **the head is positioned initially face down over the edge of the bed's mattress so that it hangs in FLEXION enough to feel the TRACTION on the site of disc pain (See Figure 1).**

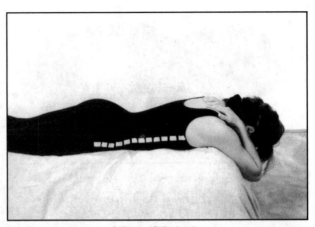

Figure 1 Prone TRACTION at rest.

This is the initial FLEXION IN TRACTION component and this component can be dispensed with if your past successful experience with the use of this MANEUVER demonstrates that it is unnecessary; but I would recommend that you take the time to do it every time you have pain in the Upper or middle neck regions, inclusive of discs C2-3---C4-5.

In this MANEUVER, the upper neck at the base of the head is initially put in simple TRACTION. The neck above the problem disc should be trapped between the "karate-chop" portions of the palms or wrists (with contribution of the forearms) and pushed directly superiorly along the vertical axis of the spine by extending at the elbows so that the forearms push the head straight out along the axis of the spine and away from the torso. The arms should act to **push the head to a position as much in line with the plane of the body and level with the surface of the bed as comfortably possible.** This action provides the TRACTION force. When the problem is lower on the middle of the neck, the fingers can be used to grasp the skin of the neck to improve TRACTION.

Then, the torso, in an "INCH-WORM" IN TRACTION like manner, should be moved inferiorly to separate the head and neck (above the problem disc) away from the rest of the body. The rest of the body in this case constitutes the torso and neck below the problem disc. The body below the affected disc can use the legs and torso to pull itself away from the head. This action accentuates TRACTION at the problem disc site by literally pulling the body apart from both sides of the problem disc. Keeping the arms over the edge of the bed prevents the head and that portion of the neck superior to the hands from moving inferiorly as the legs pull; thus, TRACTION is increased.

After enough TRACTION is applied to feel the problem disc unit's vertebral bodies separate, **a rolling should be accomplished in the opposite direction to the side to which the pain lateralizes such that the painful area of the neck is pointed towards the ceiling while the head and neck stays straight and parallel with the surface of the mattress (See Figure 2). The down-side hand and arms are then allowed to partially relax in such a way so that the**

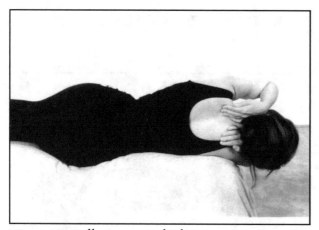

Figure 2 Roll Counter-clockwise to attain a FLEXION IN TRACTION for a Left-sided Upper/Middle Cervical pain

head falls into FLEXION IN TRACTION directly away from the site of pain while active TRACTION is continuously maintained. You will notice that as you complete the roll, the down-side hand begins to bear the weight of the neck. This weight should be borne right at the problem disc level, forcing the maximum FLEXION to be felt as the neck/head falls into FLEXION. If this is not the case, by adjusting the position of the head relative to the body, you can make it so.

While the head/neck is straight or after it goes into FLEXION IN TRACTION, or any position in between, the head can be gently CIRCUMDUCTED or rotated/twisted to its maximum range of motion in both directions, generating a CHIROTATIONAL effect while TRACTION is maintained. These actions mobilize and maximize the stretching of the peripheral ligamentous structures of the disc, giving the highest probability of centralizing peripheralized disc material. Doing this can make the subsequent movements markedly more efficient and productive.

Next, using only the hands and arms to effect movement (do not lift the head with the neck muscles) the head is carefully brought again to the straight line configuration along the vertical axis of the Cervical spine while TRACTION is judiciously maintained with the arms. If TRACTION happens to be interrupted, pause, and re-establish it before continuing your roll. **At this point, complete your roll to the face up position (See Figure 3).** Remember, at any time you feel disc material catching or failing to move, you can do A C T I V E   T H E R A P E U T I C

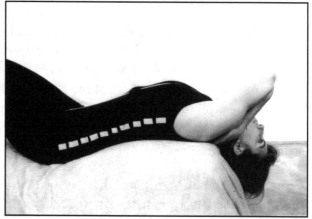

Figure 3 Completion of roll to face up position

CIRCUMDUCTION or INCH-WORM type movements to free-up and centrally mobilize disc material.

Now, you relax, lying on your back in slight EXTENSION IN TRACTION, and gently INCHWORM the neck until it is extended several inches over the edge of the mattress. By relaxing in this configuration, a DYNAMIC POSITION can be capitalized upon. After you have determined that this position has sufficiently served its purpose, then again adopt the straight, in line, neck configuration. In order to do this and still persist in TRACTION, the hands can be placed in tandem on the back of the neck, one superior to the other, such that both hands' palms

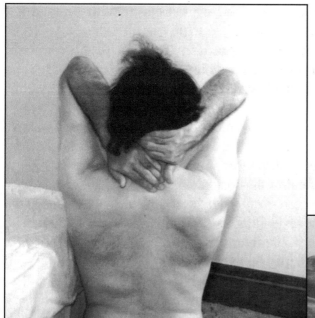

Figure 4 Tandem position of hands to support neck.

and fingers cup the neck. The karate chop portion of the one hand should be tucked into the space below the round bump on the back of the lower part of the skull (the posterior inferior occipital protuberance, (See Figure 4). The other hand's knuckle of the index finger and thumb should be seated against the mattress. This way, the two hands together support the neck and allow the head and neck to extend much farther beyond the edge of the mattress than would otherwise be possible.

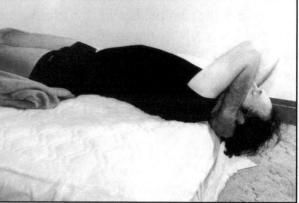

Figure 5 Hands in tandem supporting head far over edge of mattress

By moving the chin towards the chest in a nodding gesture, the space into which the hands will fit can be opened to allow for them to obtain the optimal configuration and space so that when the head is allowed to tilt backwards (towards the floor) when relaxed (as if looking superiorly), the posterior inferior occipital protuberance catches on the karate chop portion of one hand, causing the base of the neck to be put in TRACTION simply by the weight of the head tilting/extending superiorly over the platform created by the hands (See Figure 5).

Once this TRACTION is accomplished, you can maintain the relaxation and effortlessly induce an EXTENSION IN TRACTION by sliding yourself inferiorly (by using the leg attached to the rope to pull you), removing the hands, and hanging the head over the edge of the bed to let the lump at the base of the skull (the posterior inferior occipital protuberance) rest against the end of the mattress so that the problem disc unit is placed in EXTENSION IN TRACTION when the chin is tilted superiorly by the action of gravity. By this method, you let relax the muscles of the Upper thorax and neck while the Cervical vertebrae are experiencing TRACTION without the contraction of any muscles. Again, using the legs to pull while taking deep breaths and letting them out as though you are sighing, as well as making minor "INCH-WORM" adjustments, can help to relax the muscles sufficiently to experience the optimal degree of sustained TRACTION at this juncture.

Now, by letting the head hang with the lump at the base of the skull as the pivot point, you give the relevant section of the spine a chance to stretch and rest in a DYNAMIC POSITIONING mode. This may require a few minutes of relaxed waiting, so have a book (this one would be

307

nice) waiting. The fibers need to be given the time for their natural elasticity to come to full stretched length. Adjust your hands and your position on the bed so that you feel the TRACTION occurring at the very same level from which the pain originates. To increase the weight of TRACTION on the neck you can rest your hands and arms on your cheeks and forehead, causing the chin to tilt more superiorly. This is a sustained TRACTION IN EXTENSION that requires no muscular energy at the neck to maintain.

If you don't feel as though any disc material movement has occurred and you want to increase the level of TRACTION to encourage movement, you can use your arms to push the head away from the body by tucking the medial aspects of the forearms (the part of the forearm near the wrist on the opposite side as the thumb side) against the bony bumps on your skull behind your ears (the mastoid processes). This will push the head away from the body when you extend at the elbows. This is an excellent strategy because extending at the elbows does not require an activation of the neck or shoulder muscles which would interfere with TRACTION. Try to make sure that you don't tighten up your neck or shoulders when you do this. To facilitate this action, take in a deep breath and, as you exhale, extend the elbows to push the head off of the shoulders (see section on RELAXATIONAL BREATHING). You will notice as you do that your neck relaxes and allows for more TRACTION as you do so.

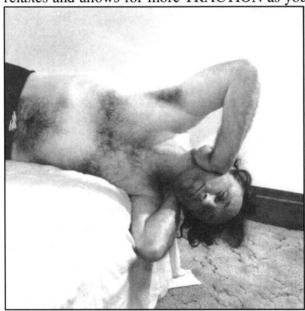

Figure 6 EXTENSION IN TRACTION
directed over site of pain when it is Left-sided
and in Upper/Middle region

Now, we come to another important consideration when putting the neck in EXTENSION IN TRACTION. **The following method of generating EXTENSION IN TRACTION is relevant to all levels of the Cervical spine and even extends to the Upper Thoracic region.** The Middle to Lower part of the neck is especially difficult to get into the necessary amount of TRACTION and sometimes it takes some real intense effort repeatedly attempted until successful.

In order to advance the MANEUVER into a directed EXTENSION IN TRACTION it becomes necessary to get your neck, again, into a position so that the Cervical spine is bent towards the side or site that the pain is greatest.

This brings one to the directed hanging EXTENSION IN TRACTION part of the total MANEUVER. **While supine, move superiorly and again support your neck with your hands in a tandem fashion so that the hand closest to the head is the hand on the same side as the pain. Then, while keeping the head and neck supported with the hand closest to the head and pulled away (superiorly) from the body, roll your whole body towards the area where the pain is greatest so that the painful site is aimed towards the floor (See Figure 6). Then slowly and carefully remove the down-side hand and let the head fall gently into a hanging EXTENSION posture directly over the**

painful site (See Figure 7). This turns the EXTENSION IN TRACTION into a HYPEREXTENSION IN TRACTION.

At the same time, like one trying to pull one's head out of a small hole (which can be seen as the "hole" that was formed by one's forearms) use the abdominal muscles and the legs to drag your body inferiorly (back towards the bed) away from the point of pain in the neck. As you do this, let the head fall further into EXTENSION over the edge of the mattress. Again, by using the torso musculature to pull the body away from a fixed head/neck (the head is stopped in its inferior movement by the edge of the mattress), no muscles need to be contracted in the neck region.

The point of pain should have been near the edge of the mattress so that as you pulled your body more back onto the bed the neck courses over the more sturdy edge portion of the mattress and the affected vertebrae are mildly forced upwards (into accentuated HYPEREXTENSION IN TRACTION) while going over that "hump."

Once you have achieved HYPEREXTENSION IN TRACTION in this manner, work with it and do some INCH-WORM movements, A C T I V E   T H E R A P E U T I C CIRCUMDUCTIONS, RELAXATIONAL BREATHING and general mobilizing actions to free up any disc material. By maintaining EXTENSION IN TRACTION while you work with the disc, you can be reasonably certain that any movement will result in centralization of the disc material so long as you do not try to lift your head up into WEIGHT-BEARING FLEXION. Feel free at any time to re-support your neck with your hands, re-straighten it, and repeat this process of stretching the neck while it is straight and then letting it go into maximal EXTENSION IN TRACTION.

Also, if the pain is very low in the neck, you move superiorly so far that your head is hanging almost to the point where it touches the ground. This is sometimes necessary for disc problems in the Lower

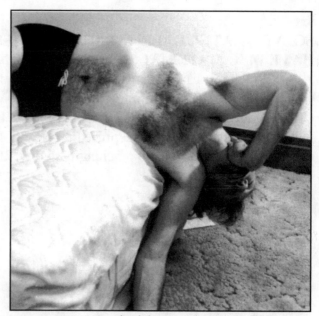

Figure 7 Removal of down-side hand allowing neck to go into HYPEREXTENSION IN TRACTION for Left sided pain

Cervical/Upper Thoracic region. **Although this MANEUVER is best for the Upper/Middle region, it can also be used for the Lower Cervical spine, but you have to hang very far over the edge as in Figure 8.** Understandably, hanging this far over necessitates the use of the rope loop and the leg to prevent your sliding to the floor.

Once you have become successful at relieving your pain, you will have learned exactly what movements to make to get your disc "in" and you can repeat them. So, keep mental notes on what movements you actually made and document them later.

309

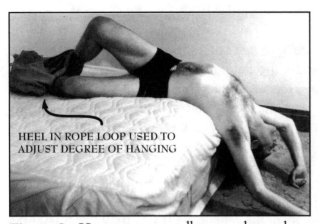

HEEL IN ROPE LOOP USED TO ADJUST DEGREE OF HANGING

Figure 8 Hanging maximally over edge with use of rope loop and legs for Low Cervical/Upper Thoracic disc

ABOVE ALL, IF AT ANY TIME YOU FEEL DIZZINESS, PROFOUND MUSCLE WEAKNESS, INCREASED PAIN, or AN ELECTRIC-LIKE SHOCK GOING DOWN YOUR ARM, STOP MOVING AND GET YOURSELF BACK INTO A NEUTRAL POSITION ON THE BED AND REST FOR A FEW MINUTES. THEN, WHILE SUPPORTING YOUR HEAD IN A NEUTRAL, PAINLESS, CONFIGURATION GET UP BY THE MOST CONVENIENT MEANS; AND REFER TO THE CHAPTER ON DIAGNOSTIC METHODS. YOU MAY NEED AN NMRI or SURGERY TO SOLVE THAT PROBLEM, BECAUSE THESE SIGNS INDICATE THAT YOU MAY HAVE DISC MATERIAL IMPINGING UPON A NERVE ROOT.

When you have satisfied yourself that you have done enough, then dismount from the bed with a CASCADE and terminate the MANEUVER with a PARTIAL WEIGHT-BEARING CIRCUMDUCTION advancing carefully to a FULL WEIGHT-BEARING CIRCUMDUCTION in a manner as described in the preceding HEAD-HANG Section and portrayed in Figures 14-18 of that section so long as no pinching pain or ARRESTED CIRCUMDUCTION persists.

PILLOW-ASSISTED CERVICAL (NECK) MANEUVERS

Large pillows can be used to help perform Cervical MANEUVERS if a bed is not available (or in combination with a bed to realize greater FLEXION and comfort). Couch cushions provide some of the best pillows, but any large soft structure that can be formed into a mound will suffice. When using a pillow to assist you, the basic principles are the same as in any MANEUVER; but, because the pillows raise you off the surface and you are not really hanging from a surface, there are slight differences in technique worthy of warranting a separate description. The following instructions provide a means to that end before discussing the actual MANEUVER.

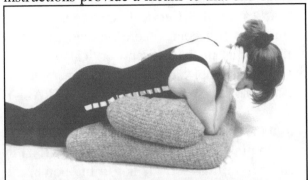

Figure 1 Using couch cushions to induce FLEXION IN TRACTION for a midline Cervical pain

When performing a Cervical MANEUVER for midline posterior pain at just about any level of the Cervical or High Thoracic spine, **you start by positioning the pillows on the floor in a pile and simply lying face down on top of them.** They should be centered under the chest so that your arms and head hang over one edge of the pillows while your torso and abdomen are draped over the other side of the pillow pile. If pain is referred to the center of the back, or posterior midline, then the center of the posterior midline should be aimed towards the ceiling just like in any other MANEUVER where the painful area is facing towards the ceiling. You then hang your head from your neck while supporting the neck with your hands. The weight of all this should be on your elbows (See Figure 1). This is almost the natural position that a person adopts when lying on the floor and supporting the head with the hands while watching TV, except that the face is aimed at the floor.

In this series of movements, pillows are used to sequentially induce a FLEXION IN TRACTION with the painful site aimed towards the ceiling, followed by a rolling CIRCUMDUCTION while MAINTAINING TRACTION with the arms (See Figure 2), and leaves one in an EXTENSION IN TRACTION (See Figure 3) with the painful area aimed towards the floor. This basic series constitutes the bare essentials of all the Cervical MANEUVERS and the PILLOW-ASSISTED ones are no different. Too, when it comes to employing the various MOBILIZATION techniques such as NARROW-ARC ROCKING while in FLEXION IN TRACTION, THERAPEUTIC CIRCUMDUCTIONS, CHIROTATIONAL

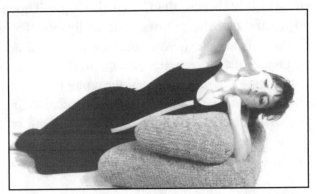

Figure 2 Rolling Clockwise while maintaining TRACTION

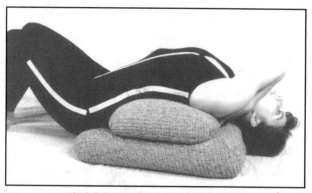

Figure 3 EXTENSION IN TRACTION for a midline Cervical pain

TWISTING, RELAXATIONAL BREATHING, INCH-WORMING, and even CASCADING (to a small degree) the same principles pertain. **This particular series of photos (Figures 1-3) depict a very simple but effective MANEUVER that is best intended for Upper/Middle Cervical disc pain, especially if it is centered in the midline posterior.** It is fairly straight-forward and easy when the pain is in the upper reaches of the Cervical spine and in the midline. It becomes more problematic when the disc is in the Lower Cervical or Upper Thorax region and the pain radiates to the side. So, a more complex description is generated for that more common condition and is described separately in the following Section dedicated to LATERALLY HERNIATED DISCS.

The use of pillows, in addition to sufficing as a means to execute spine MANEUVERS at any level, provides one of the most convenient ways to practice DYNAMIC POSITIONING in the home so as to move disc material in a slow and careful manner. If not in the home, the pillows can realistically be replaced by any similarly-shaped object such as a barrel, bale of hay, or the bulk of anything that allows you to hang over it. Of course, the DYNAMIC POSITION you use is dependant upon the goal of your effort. For instance, Figure 2 can serve as a FLEXION IN TRACTION for a pain on the Right Middle Cervical region as well as an EXTENSION IN TRACTION for a left-sided pain. If this is unclear, refer to the Chapter Four's Section on SELECTING THE IDEAL DYNAMIC POSITION for the principles governing this positioning and then apply them to the neck.

Before beginning the next full MANEUVER described in the next Section, it is advantageous to understand how the elbows can be used to generate the TRACTION forces in most of these MANEUVERS. **It is a good idea to take a minute to practice this action separately, in advance, in order to become familiar with its capability and use because the basic technique, although essential for pillow-assisted neck work, can be applied to many situations involving the Cervical, Upper Thoracic as well as the Lumbar spine with only an adjustment of the pillows.** Basically, this technique allows you to turn your own arms into a platform from which you can hang your head and torso so that TRACTION of any disc inferior to the shoulders can be generated. By using the forearms, elbows, and body in a unique configuration with the area of the spine in which the damaged disc resides, a TRACTION can be effected that does not require the use of muscle contraction to maintain.

In essence, the elbows are placed with reference to the pillow and spine in such a manner that they become the point of an inverted triangle upon which the spine is balanced. As the spine "teeters" over and back on this triangle, the weights of the body parts on either side act as the tractive force mechanism.

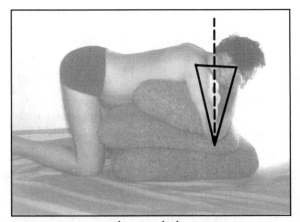

Figure 4 Cervical spine balancing on triangle formed by arms.

To physically perform this action, the upper arms are tucked closely together in front of the chest while the hands cup the neck. The elbows press into the pillow with the weight of the body and are positioned underneath the chest (See Figure 4). This position gives the neck the opportunity to be stretched away from the shoulders as the torso is adjusted superiorly to hang more over the pillows (See Figure 5). As the head and neck is balanced forward and the torso hangs behind the pillow pile, the Cervical discs will experience a stretching effect as the area around the shoulders balances on the forearms and shoulders. Once you have adopted this position, you should be able to experience the effectiveness of the stretching. At this point, you are capable of beginning a MANEUVER because you are essentially in FLEXION IN TRACTION; however, it is probably better to relax for a time in this position and apply the concept of DYNAMIC POSITIONING or any of the other MOBILIZING techniques that are appropriate for this position to loosen up the problem disc.

Depending upon where the hands are positioned relative to the Cervical spine, at what position the shoulders are kept and how far you angle forward determines which disc unit is put in TRACTION. How much you pull your lower torso away from your arms and how far the head hangs superior to the balance point determines the degree of FLEXION (or EXTENSION, for that matter). Once you become competent at this balancing process, you can accomplish the same effect with only one arm acting as the balance point; and, by turning onto one side or the other you can preferentially place your neck in the ideal position for lateral FLEXION or

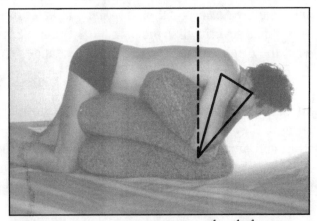

Figure 5 Exerting TRACTION by shifting weight superiorly

EXTENSION if the pain is located more to the side than the midline.

Although premature in this discussion, you may also note that **rocking inferiorly in this configuration puts the neck in an EXTENSION IN TRACTION and on into a WEIGHT-BEARING EXTENSION, if desired, depending upon whether your arms are employed in concert with the pillows to restrain your head's movement in an inferior direction** (See Figure 6). This ability to go from FLEXION IN TRACTION to EXTENSION IN TRACTION can be a very valuable skill because once you have mastered this technique you will have the skill to put the neck into just about any position, anywhere, anytime you need to get out of neck pain. With or without the pillows, your shoulders and elbows can then provide the device you need to put any

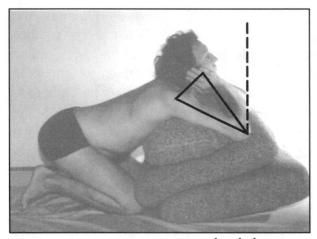

Figure 6 Exerting TRACTION by shifting weight inferiorly

part of your neck in any configuration necessary to MOBILIZE disc material.

This next-to-be-described PILLOW-ASSISTED CERVICAL MANEUVER consists, basically like all maneuvers, of applying TRACTION on the problem disc while it is hanging in flexion (FLEXION IN TRACTION) until the body is rolled (PASSIVELY CIRCUMDUCTED) while maintaining TRACTION into full EXTENSION IN TRACTION. The TRACTION is maintained by both the INCH-WORM-type pulling motion of the torso acting with the weight of the torso hanging inferiorly from the arms as well as by the legs and hips being used to pull the torso away from the point on the neck that is held by the hands as they are balancing on the forearms and elbows. Actually, the point that is the balancing point in the "teeter-totter" that is created should be positioned at or slightly above the area of spinal pain. When that point is stretched by the TRACTION, it should be felt as an alteration in the pain from the same area of original pain. The character of the pain should change. It should, overall, be of lessened severity than the pain felt originally. It should be able to be differentiated qualitatively from the original; but, by virtue of its change, you should be able to tell that you are stretching the proper disc unit.

When the painful disc is extremely low in the Cervical region or High Thorax, it is difficult to find a means of using just the arms to pull the head and neck off of the shoulders because they are connected to the shoulders. The arms must necessarily have a place to originate from and attach to the body. Inconveniently, the muscles of the shoulders (trapezius and the rhomboids) span the area of the Lower Cervical and Upper Thoracic vertebrae, areas that seem to give people the most problems. One cannot expect a simple pushing of the head away from the body with the arms to succeed, because so doing causes the muscles to contract in the area superior to the spinal segment that needs to be placed in TRACTION in order for the vertebrae to separate. The contraction of those muscle groups works against TRACTION by pulling those particular vertebral segments together when they need to be relaxed so as to be allowed to separate.

This dilemma can be solved with rather difficult to accomplish but reasonably successful DYNAMIC POSITIONING so that the shoulder muscles, neck, and head superior to the problem disc all hang in FLEXION IN TRACTION. When the superior aspect of the shoulders are hanging in TRACTION IN FLEXION with the added weight of the arms on the neck, the muscles that otherwise would cause the vertebrae to be compressed are caused to be stretched by the weight of the hanging upper body parts. It is often helpful to have someone hold your head or arms and pull them to assist TRACTION on the Lower Cervical or Upper Thoracic region where natural mobility is reduced and you need all the help you can get to separate the disc spaces. I know it sounds complicated and difficult, but the mastery of this technique can often afford instantaneous relief when no other therapy is successful.

The choice of which way to start the PILLOW-ASSISTED CERVICAL MANEUVERS depends largely upon whether the pain and ARRESTED CIRCUMDUCTION is more towards the sides or midline posterior. The position for a midline posterior pain has been shown above in Figure 1. If the pain is referred more to one side or the other such that the pain is referred to the shoulder blade area or to the side of the base of the neck (as is more often the case), you should try the elbow-assisted TRACTION method first with the painful side up as described in the next section.

PILLOW-ASSISTED MANEUVER FOR LATERAL CERVICAL PAIN

This PILLOW-ASSISTED CERVICAL MANEUVER is dedicated to those painful discs whose herniations are much more laterally-herniated. In these cases, the pain appears to emanate from the side more than the midline of the neck or upper back. The pain, more often than not, appears to originate in the shoulder blade area or upper arm at the shoulder. In these lesions, the disc material has opened a laterally-directed fissure resulting in a more lateral disc herniation; and, DIAGNOSTIC CIRCUMDUCTION usually makes this reality obvious by the arrested motion being experienced near the 3:00 or 9:00 areas to the left or right side of the body respectively. Conceptually, the following MANEUVERS are identical to the posteriorly-directed TRACTION/EXTENSION MANEUVERS only, since the mobile disc material has migrated more to one side than the posterior, these MANEUVERS are designed to cause the disc material to move more medially rather than just straight anteriorly. If the previously described MANEUVERS for a midline lesions are unsuccessful, then probably it means that the disc material is protruding more laterally and has moved through a radial tear that is aimed more towards the sides than the posterior. In this event, a somewhat more complicated strategy is necessary. It relies upon the same principle as immediately described above, only the MANEUVER requires more laterally focused effort.

This maneuver starts by putting your neck in a TRACTION IN FLEXION posture as described above in the PILLOW-ASSISTED NECK MANEUVERS section above in the balancing position shown in that Section's Figure 4. This position should be sustained long enough for you to relax in the TRACTION and become comfortable while stretching the affected disc. This "teetering" balancing action starts the MANEUVER by applying the maximum amount of TRACTION on the affected disc that can reasonably be expected in the pillow-assisted mode.

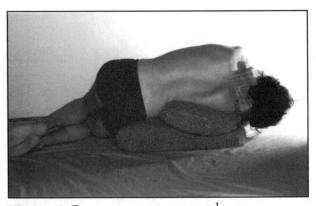

Figure 1 Coming to rest in straight TRACTION for a Left-sided Cervical pain

Then, while maintaining the TRACTION as best as possible, you lie down in a specific manner placing the painful site up, or aimed at the ceiling. The way you lie down insures that the TRACTION is sustained. You do this by putting most of the weight on what will be the down-side elbow and turning as you are doing this to put the painful area up. The inverted triangle support then becomes provided by only the down-side arm while you roll to your side. Once you have all the weight on the down-side elbow, you simply let your upper body gently collapse towards the posterior, leaving just the weight-bearing elbow in place, causing you to come to rest on your side with your arms basically in the same position relative to the spine as they were in Figure 4 in the previous Section, only now you are lying on your side. If you find that you don't have enough room to land on the pillow, just repeat the action starting at one end of a pillow so you have the other end to land on.

The TRACTION is maintained by continually "teetering" your weight on the elbow until you come to rest draped over the pillow, whereupon the weight of your head and neck hanging comes to effortlessly provide TRACTION. When you are draped over the pillow on your side as in Figure 1 (this section), the weight of the head and neck provide a continuous TRACTION force as you rest on your shoulder or chest depending upon where the best position of rest results in keeping TRACTION applied at the disc unit in pain.

The arms can assist in maintaining this TRACTION not only by their simple "teetering" but by extending at the elbows (as though you were lifting your head off of your shoulders) and by using the fingers to push into the skin while flexing the wrists. By placing the tips of the fingers inferior to the painful disc level and flexing them while at the same time pushing superiorly with the "karate-chop" area of the palm while the wrist is flexed, you can push your head away from your body. These techniques for accentuating TRACTION were described previously in the beginning of the CERVICAL MANEUVERS

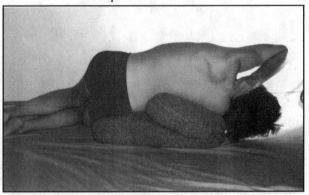

Figure 2 Using weight of up-side arm to increase FLEXION IN TRACTION for Left sided pain low in neck

Section associated with Figures 1, 2, & 5 of that Section. The TRACTION can be increased by also using your legs to pull your torso away from your neck. **This TRACTION should be maintained as much parallel to the axis of the spine as if you were trying to pull your head and neck straight out and away from your shoulders (as seen in Figure 7 of the same above Section).**

The head is then allowed to hang in TRACTION IN FLEXION by relaxing the down-side arm's TRACTION force. When your head begins to fall into the flexed position away from the area of pain, the TRACTION generated by the weight of the up-side arm should be continued until the affected disc unit is in the fully resting flexed position before the TRACTION is relaxed. You should rest in this position for a time with your neck in FLEXION with the painful site up and the TRACTION being passively maintained by the weight of the head and the neck above the point of pain hanging over the pillow. Adjusting your position on the pillows should be done to make certain that you get the most TRACTION directed at the problem disc unit as you lie on your shoulder or chest draped over the pillows. If you feel that not enough TRACTION is being generated passively and want to increase this FLEXION IN TRACTION, you can get more pillows. This is a good position for FLEXION IN TRACTION type of DYNAMIC POSITIONING so long as TRACTION and FLEXION are applied at the site of the disc problem. Refer to those sections of the book if you are unclear as to what is intended and what is mechanically occurring in this position.

Here is an excellent opportunity to do some NARROW-ARC ROCKING, INCH-WORMING, THERAPEUTIC CIRCUMDUCTIONS, and even CHIROTATIONAL TWISTING, probably all of which can be combined with TRACTION to improve their effectiveness so long as the flexion component is not sacrificed. The FLEXION IN TRACTION can be accentuated by using the weight of the up-side arm resting on the head and pushing superiorly (See Figure 2).

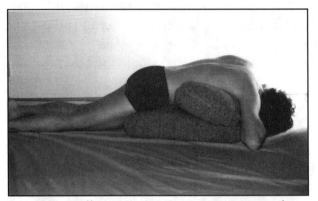

Figure 3 Rolling CIRCUMDUCTION at the face-down position (while allowing the neck to bend anteriorly)

The next move requires that you bring the neck back to a neutral, straight, configuration and then roll clockwise to the face down position while maintaining TRACTION (See Figure 3). Before rolling to come to rest on the same side as the pain to effect this MANEUVER, you must **try to maintain the TRACTION at all times in a straight neck, in-line, configuration before the actual bending is accomplished.** You may find that this is difficult. If your movements or adjustments of posture while you are getting into position result in the TRACTION being lost, stop and relax, keep the superiorly directed force that is putting TRACTION on the neck applied, take a few deep breaths and exhalations, and allow the relaxation of the para-spinous muscles. This RELAXATIONAL BREATHING will assist effective TRACTION during the exhalation phase. The manner in which you apply TRACTION should keep your head and neck aligned in a straight configuration until you are ready to let it bend.

While keeping TRACTION on the painful disc, your rolling CIRCUMDUCTION on the pillow often allows it to fall into a bend towards the side of pain. That is not a big problem, it can hang in a laterally or anteriorly bent configuration. Once it is bent, can you even release the TRACTION so that the pressure will be applied to the disc material to move it medially or centrally. While during the roll, when the neck is in some form of EXTENSION, this allowance is very much like the SEQUENTIAL ARCHING THERAPEUTIC CIRCUMDUCTION. Actually, you can even do it intentionally to try to mobilize difficult disc material; but before you continue the roll, try to straighten out the neck in TRACTION.

If you are able to maintain TRACTION, the effect of eventually bending your neck towards the side of the pain will be nearly identical to an EXTENSION MANEUVER only it will be directed towards the side of the pain rather than posteriorly. By so doing, laterally protruded disc material can be moved more towards the midline and reposition itself centrally.

This rolling can be combined with any number of MOBILIZING moves as you see fit, however, the intention is to maintain TRACTION until you have rolled completely 180 degrees so that you are, at the completion of the roll, still in TRACTION and the painful side is now facing towards the floor (See Figure 4).

Once you have arrived at the painful site down position, you maintain the TRACTION as you let the head hang towards the floor by removing the support of the down-side hand. This is the EXTENSION IN TRACTION component of the MANEUVER. You see, when the disc has herniated laterally, you must bend the neck towards the same side as the pain if you want to trap the disc material and move it centrally. It is most effective if you bend the neck towards the side of the pain without using or contracting the actual muscles of the n e c k or shoulders; but, rather, do so by a form of DYNAMIC POSITIONING.

Simply extending or hyper-extending directly to the posterior is insufficient when the disc has protruded mostly laterally because the force moving the disc back to the center must direct it more towards the midline rather than anteriorly. If a piece of disc material is resting somewhere along a radial tear and you inappropriately attempt a MANEUVER that is designed to move it strictly anteriorly, it will run into more of the annulus fibrosus portion of the disc rather

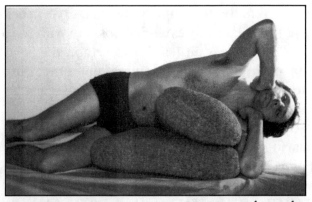

Figure 4 Maintaining TRACTION at the end of CIRCUMDUCTION in preparation for an EXTENSION IN TRACTION when the pain is Left-sided

than the vacant nucleus pulposus region where it belongs. To get it back to the center (the nucleus pulposus region) requires that it be moved medially (towards the center of the body) from the side to which it had herniated. The following directions teach you a method to do just that; however, at this point, MOBILIZATION techniques can be used to free-up stuck disc material..

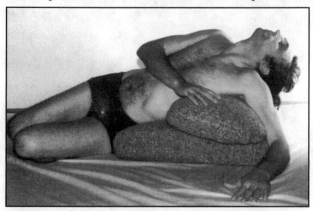

Figure 5 Fixing neck in Left lateral EXTENSION directly over the painful Left-sided herniation to get to weight-bearing, upright posture.

Also, turning just your torso to aim the anterior chest more towards the up position and then alternatively re-rotating to the more anterior-chest-down position while keeping the head's position fixed with the hands and arms can encourage the disc to move by inducing a CHIROTATIONAL action on the most peripherally located capsular ligaments which can often "wring" the malpositioned disc material centrally. **While your neck is in a maximally EXTENDED position and hanging in TRACTION, use the up-side hand to carefully twist your head anteriorly to its maximal range of motion. Then roll it back posteriorly to its maximum range while keeping the torso's position fixed while the head is kept in TRACTION with the hand by which it is being supported.** This also twists the peripheral ligaments in a wringing fashion very similar to what a chiropractor does, only this technique is much less violent or forceful because you can do it gently and, if pain is generated, you rapidly can determine when to stop.

Finally, to complete the maneuver, position yourself so that your head and neck are kept in the laterally extended position with the neck bent towards the site of pain (See Figure 5). If that site is difficult to ascertain, the head can be bent as much as possible towards the 3:00 or 9:00 position depending upon the side of the pain) and get to an upright posture by the most advantageous manner you can that insures you do not straighten your neck until you have assumed a fully weight-bearing stance in the upright position (See Figure 6). Lastly, you would do well to seat the disc material by CIRCUMDUCTING IN PARTIAL WEIGHT-BEARING EXTENSION This is done by lifting the head off of the neck for High Cervical discs, the neck off of the shoulders for Middle Cervical (See Figure 7), or the shoulders off of the Thorax by supporting and suspending the Lower Cervical and Upper Thoracic region by the outstretched the arms on the hips or floor. That way you can roll the disc unit through its posterior range of motion before fully RE-WEIGHT-BEARING and CIRCUMDUCTING.

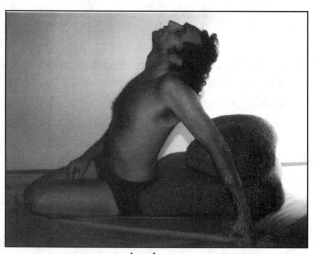

Figure 6 Bringing the disc to WEIGHT-BEARING IN EXTENSION aimed towards site of pain

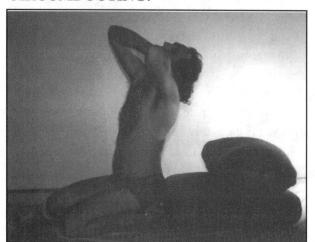

Figure 7 CIRCUMDUCTING in partial WEIGHT-BEARING EXTENSION

An Alternative Lateral Cervical Pain Maneuver Strategy

There is another variation on the PILLOW- ASSISTED CERVICAL MANEUVERS which can be employed when on a bed or on the floor with pillows. It also doubles as an especially helpful DYNAMIC POSITIONING technique whenever the disc seems to be only partially seated centrally or repeatedly keeps going "out" after you are convinced that it was "in" after doing the other MANEUVERS. If your disc has not become pain-free as a result of the above MANEUVERS; hopefully, the preceding MANEUVERS have at least pushed peripheralized disc material centrally enough to allow this next EXTENSION-type movement to be successful.

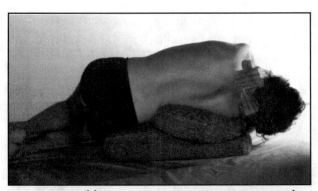

Figure 8 Mild FLEXION IN TRACTION for Left-sided Low Cervical pain

This MANEUVER begins by lying on your back and exerting TRACTION with the hands as described above in PILLOW-ASSISTED NECK MANEUVERS and shown above in that Section's Figure 3. When you successfully feel that the affected disc is in sustainable, comfortable, TRACTION, you **support your head's weight with your hands so that the neck is kept relatively straight, and you roll away from the side of the pain.** That is, if the pain is radiating to the left neck or left shoulder blade area, you will roll from lying on your back to lying on your right side with the left side up. **After you have rolled away from the side of the pain and the painful side is in the up position, you should be draped over the pillow (or the edge of the bed) in a lateral, mild, FLEXION IN TRACTION.** This will put you in a sort of fetal position not highly unlike the natural position a person lying on the ground spontaneously takes when having their face kicked at in a fight. (See Figure 8). Your hands should be used as described in the previous maneuver as if you were pulling the neck off the shoulders. Your position should be adjusted relative to the pillow so that the problem disc is felt to be stretching to the side in FLEXION IN TRACTION away from the side of the pain.

The next goal is to maintain TRACTION while raising the head and neck superior to the painful disc into an EXTENSION IN TRACTION that smoothly flows into a WEIGHT-BEARING EXTENSION by bending the neck in the direction of the site of pain. The bending has to be centered right at the level of the bad disc while it is simultaneously relaxed in TRACTION.

The idea in this move is, again (similar to hanging EXTENSION MANEUVERS), to trap the aberrant disc material between the peripheral surfaces of two vertebral bodies' edges and, in a pincer effect, squeeze the disc material centrally while maintaining a TRACTION-induced separation of the vertebral bodies allowing a space for the disc material to move into. You should be able to maintain the TRACTION until you are up in EXTENSION by using your torso and legs to continue applying a pulling force while the head and neck are prevented from moving inferiorly due to the interference created between the arms and whatever surface you are using, in this case, pillows.

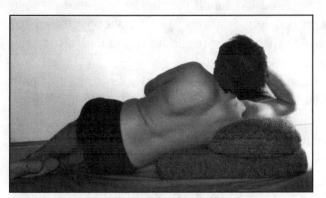

Figure 9 WEIGHT-BEARING EXTENSION for Left sided Low Cervical pain

This is accomplished by first disengaging the up-side hand. This free hand then comes up to push the chin superiorly by pushing the lateral aspect of the jaw from below with the palm, using the other side of the jaw (the side interfacing with the edge of the mattress or pillow or the floor) in concert with the down-side hand, arm, and shoulder as the fulcrum upon which the pertinent disc is bent (See Figure 9).

Now, while the particular segment is maintained all-the-while in maximum TRACTION you plant your down-sided elbow into the surface of whatever you are lying on and elevate your neck and head by pushing the down-side elbow into the surface and raising that part of the head and neck above the problem disc level. Simultaneously, your legs pull your torso inferiorly over the mound of the pillow. As the edge of the pillow or bed contacts the upper arm, TRACTION is maintained. This should be done in a smooth movement so that FLEXION IN TRACTION converts into EXTENSION IN TRACTION. The head

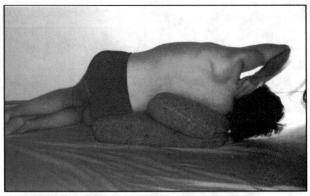

Figure 10 Using up-side arm and hand to accentuate FLEXION IN TRACTION for Left-sided Low Cervical pain

should finally come to rest upon the hand, arm, and elbow as if you were resting your head on your hand, watching TV (See Figure 10). This leaves you in WEIGHT-BEARING EXTENSION.

In order to bring your neck into the bent-towards-the-same-side-as-the-pain-position, you must elevate the head relatively high. This results in a very acute angle of laterally-directed EXTENSION at the neck. If you find this uncomfortable for the presumably normal upper level discs, it may be better to position your down-side hand at a place on your neck immediately superior to the painful disc rather than using the head (unless the affected disc is very high in the neck and this cannot be avoided.) I say this because the non-painful side of your head/neck junction may be put, otherwise, into a very acute angle equivalent to a WEIGHT-BEARING LATERAL FLEXION--which is taboo. This might be too much for the discs at that level to tolerate if they have unappreciated damage from previous trauma. The Cervical spine in the inferior regions has less flexibility from side-to-side than closer to the head and doesn't tend to allow you to bend it excessively; so it is less of a problem.

The purpose of this positioning is to cause your neck to be bent towards the side of pain at the level of the painful disc while TRACTION allows the disc material a place to move into. It accomplishes the same physical forces as a Yoga-type EXTENSION exercise for the Lumbar spine pictured in the beginning of the book only it is directed laterally and at the Cervical spine. In this MANEUVER/DYNAMIC POSITIONING, you are producing an EXTENSION force; but you are not hanging your head in TRACTION; rather, you are making the problem disc unit be bent (laterally extended) by your causing the head and neck (above the problem disc) to rise higher than the torso, as the chest and arm ride over the pillow mound and the arm causes the head and neck to elevate. Since TRACTION is maintained until the last point when the vertebral bones' peripheral rims come together on the same side as the herniation, there is still a space available for the disc material to enter as the EXTENSION squeezes the material centrally.

This position can be adjusted and played with by moving inferiorly and rolling your shoulder and chest across the pillow (if used) as shown above to accentuate the bending towards the painful site. By resting in this position, you convert the action into a DYNAMIC POSITIONING that applies steady pressure on a pincer-captured piece of disc material insisting that it move centrally.

If, at any point in the EXTENSION process, a pinching increase in pain occurs, then you are probably trapping and squeezing a piece of protruded disc material. In that event, by dropping the down-side arm and allowing your neck to fall slowly and gently to the neutral position you can bend the neck away from the side of pain. This should immediately relieve the pressure. Then, again, if you move superiorly on the bed or pillow, you can return to the starting position (See the above PILLOW-ASSISTED NECK MANEUVERS section and the position shown in that section's Figure 4), only this time letting the head hang into an increased bend to the side away from the pain.

This is equivalent to the recruiting of the lateral interspinous ligaments with FLEXION IN TRACTION (described earlier in the so named section) in order to push protruded disc material within the periphery of the vertebral body's outside borders so that a later extension MANEUVER can be more successful. Then, following immediately with repeated straightening in TRACTION by pulling with the feet and torso and a "milking" manipulation (described in the "INCH-WORM" technique) is helpful before proceeding. Applicable here as in any other situation wherein the discs need to be mobilized, CHIROTATIONAL TWISTING, NARROW-ARC ROCKING, and THERAPEUTIC CIRCUMDUCTIONS can be utilized. Above all, don't feel that you need to force any component of this MANEUVER, if it hurts don't do it.

By wriggling, making snake-like movements with your neck and repeating the in-line straight-neck TRACTION process alternating with the FLEXION IN TRACTION bent away from the side of pain, chances are you will be able to free it up, and you can continue with the EXTENSION process until successful. This is such an easy means of converting FLEXION IN TRACTION to WEIGHT-BEARING EXTENSION, that it can be repeated many times in succession until the disc material moves.

Finally, all that is necessary is to get up to standing while keeping the neck in EXTENSION towards the side of the pain as in the other MANEUVERS. This can be accomplished simply by rolling over onto your opposite side so that your head's weight can maintain EXTENSION towards the side of pain, and coming to standing as was done in the PILLOW-ASSISTED NECK MANEUVER FOR LATERALLY HERNIATED DISCS' MANEUVER instructions immediately above in Figures 5,6, & 7 and can be followed by the terminal CIRCUMDUCTIONS described in the HEAD-HANG Section Figures 16-18.

The following abbreviated series demonstrates how the back of a couch can be used to effect the FLEXION IN TRACTION and rolling to EXTENSION IN TRACTION for the Cervical region. There is little reason to repeat all the previously elaborated details because this presumes that the reader has studied the previous neck MANEUVERS to the extent that a familiarization with the concepts has occurred. This one is extremely convenient because using the back of a couch has the added advantage of your not needing to use a rope to hold your body from sliding off the edge of a bed. The weight of the legs alone on the front side of the couch is sufficient to hold you in place. Also, coming to an upright position is simplified because you only need to CASCADE over the front side of the couch. **BE CERTAIN THAT YOUR COUCH WILL SUPPORT YOUR WEIGHT WITHOUT TIPPING OVER. IF YOU ARE UNCERTAIN ABOUT THIS OR YOUR CAPACITY TO ACCOMPLISH IT SAFELY, IT IS WISE TO BE ASSISTED BY SOMEONE STRONG ENOUGH TO HELP YOU IF YOU GET INTO TROUBLE.**

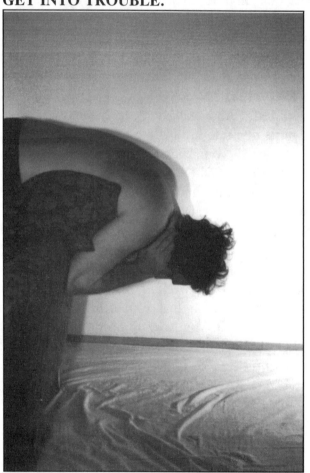

Figure 1 Initial position for couch-assisted FLEXION IN TRACTION for Low Cervical pain in midline

To prepare for this MANEUVER, it is necessary to pull the couch away from the wall if it is situated against one so that the back side has sufficient room to hang your upper torso over the edge. The couch's back's edge is usually sharp and hard so you should also be prepared to stack a couple of pillows on it for comfort.

The starting position for a pain in the midline is face down (See Figure 1) and for a pain that radiates to the side, the painful side should be the up-side aimed towards the ceiling (See Figure 2). The FLEXION IN TRACTION should be focused upon the problem disc by hanging over the edge until the problem segment of the spine's discomfort changes. The lower in the neck that the pain originates, the more you need to hang over the edge. The location of problem disc can be identified characteristically by a stretching sensation deep in the spine that can usually be easily equated with the origination of the pain. I usually ask my patients to tell me when they feel that the problem disc is being stretched; and they always seem to be able to recognize it. This position can be transformed into a DYNAMIC POSITIONING by simply resting in the most

324

appropriate FLEXION IN TRACTION configuration.

The same principle considerations hold for this MANEUVER as all the others. **A rolling PASSIVE CIRCUMDUCTION is accomplished in the direction of the pain while traction is maintained.** For a Left-sided lesion, you would roll to a face-down position and continue rolling clockwise until coming to the point where the painful side is now facing the floor. It is in this manner that the FLEXION IN TRACTION is converted to an EXTENSION IN TRACTION. Anytime before, during, or after the roll, you can use the MOBILIZING techniques such as INCHWORMING, CHIROTATIONAL TWISTING, NARROW ARC ROCKING, and THERAPEUTIC CIRCUMDUCTIONS; however, the SEQUENTIAL ARCHING IN EXTENSION is, by definition, reserved for those postures in which you are in EXTENSION.

In practice, it is not a good idea to try to extend the spine using the muscles of the spine associated with the problem disc region while in a FLEXION IN TRACTION during this or any of the MANEUVERS for that matter. The reason being that **when you contract the back musculature associated with the disc, it is the physical equivalent to a WEIGHT-BEARING action.** Recalling one of the caveats of *The O'Connor Technique (tm)*, **if you are in FLEXION, you should not BEAR WEIGHT.** I mention this here because hanging over the edge of a couch, one is tempted to use the back muscles to attempt to move the spine. This should be avoided by, instead, using the arms, legs, or torso whenever possible to accomplish the same movement.

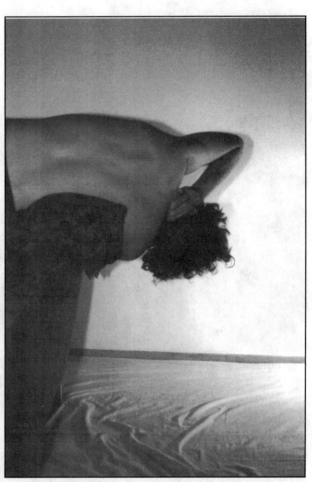

Figure 2 Initial position for couch-assisted FLEXION IN TRACTION for Low Cervical Left-sided pain

Once you have arrived at the EXTENSION IN TRACTION component (See Figure 3 for a midline pain or Figure 4 for a left lateral pain), you can really exaggerate its degree by hanging way off of the edge of the couch without fear of sliding off the edge because the rest of the body below the cervical region is hanging over the front of the couch preventing it.

When in EXTENSION IN TRACTION, the same MOBILIZATION techniques described in the previous MANEUVERS can be employed and the posture can be used as a DYNAMIC POSITION by simply resting in that position for a prolonged time, so long as it does not become uncomfortable.

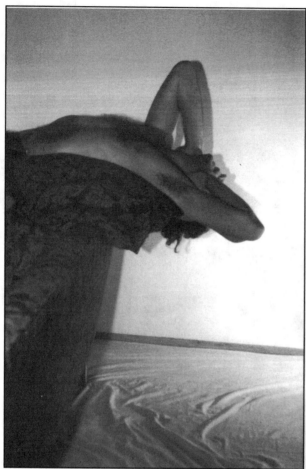

Figure 3 EXTENSION IN TRACTION for a Midline Posterior Low Cervical pain.

After satisfying yourself that you have done everything possible to centralize the disc material, you can test whether it is "in" by simply rolling over the problem site with the painful side down to determine if an arresting type of pain results. This is a PASSIVE DIAGNOSTIC CIRCUMDUCTION. You can add some WEIGHT-BEARING to this CIRCUMDUCTION by sliding your torso

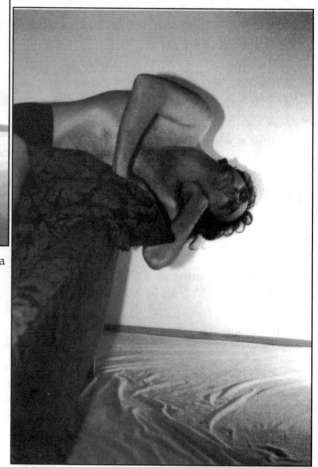

Figure 4 EXTENSION IN TRACTION for a Left-sided pain Low in the Cervical spine.

towards the front of the couch. This removes some of the TRACTION, replacing it with WEIGHT-BEARING. Since when you are in EXTENSION without TRACTION, sliding off of the front of the couch sequentially puts each disc in a semi-weight-bearing state. During this stage, when the problem disc is in a partially-loaded condition, you should be able to tell if there is an obstruction to range of motion at the problem disc site. If so, the disc material is not centralized, and you should try the preceding techniques again at least one more time because, quite often, the first attempt moves the disc material only enough to make a second attempt successful.

If you choose to complete the MANEUVER at this point, you only need to CASCADE off of the front of the couch until you again assume the WEIGHT-BEARING IN EXTENSION component. INCH-WORMING is especially effective during this last phase of the maneuver. As you are CASCADING off of the couch front, you can hook the back of the base of your skull on the top part of the back of the couch. This anchors the head to the couch as the weight of the body provides excellent TRACTION force without any muscular activity associated with the spine, particularly if you use the weight of your arms to pinion the head or neck to the couch. You can even use some of your fingers to hold onto the couch and others to grip the neck or skull to better fix the head to the couch.

As you are finally sliding to the ground, you can end with your feet tucked underneath you or you can go so far as to let yourself slide across the edge of the seat of the couch until you are lying on the ground. Either way, make sure that, if the pain is to the side, you angle your CASCADE so that the painful site is aimed towards the floor to insure that it is put in the maximum amount of EXTENSION IN TRACTION during the CASCADE and keep it EXTENDED in that configuration until you stand up or are fully weight-bearing again.

CERVICAL DYNAMIC POSITIONING

DYNAMIC POSITIONING for the Cervical region of the spine can be as simple or as complex as the degree of complexity of the disc problem. So as to reduce the herein given advice to an understandable order of complexity and to avoid confusion, I am going to fall back upon the most uniformly successful positioning strategy and give that as my foremost recommendation. That is to **keep the affected disc in slight EXTENSION IN TRACTION with the painful site (the herniation) aimed towards the floor for as much of the time as possible.** This is a pretty good rule of thumb notwithstanding all the particulars delineated in the chapter dedicated to the PRINCIPLES of DYNAMIC POSITIONING. As one becomes more adept at self-manipulation and competent in the understanding of vertebral mechanics in general and especially in the context of one's own particular problem, one can advance into more complex positioning strategies.

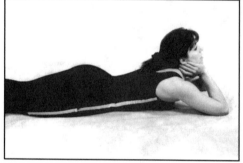

Figure 1 EXTENSION IN TRACTION DYNAMIC POSITIONING for midline Cervical disc herniation.

Even the simple act of watching television with one's head and neck placed in a disadvantageous configuration can result in pain in the presence of disc disease. Conversely, employing the PRINCIPLES OF DYNAMIC POSITIONING can make TV watching an effortless means to centralize displaced disc material. Competently arranging your body position relative to your TV can prevent as well as alleviate pain. Consider how lying for hours with your head cocked to one side resting on your hand or a pillow can induce FLEXION with the weight of the head supplying the force of the "avoid at all costs" WEIGHT-BEARING FLEXION. Then consider how easy it is to simply change your position so that your neck is kept in EXTENSION and UNWEIGHTED such that the involved disc will migrate in the direction necessary to allow for its centralization. If this is done before pain ensues, you reduce the probability of disc material migration and can actually prevent it.

For instance, assume that your neck has a disc that migrates such that it bulges to the right posterior at the C4-5 region. The worst position for this disc and sure to result in pain would be one in which you are resting while WEIGHT-BEARING with the head flexed to the left and anteriorly. The best DYNAMIC

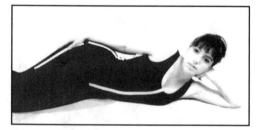

Figure 2 EXTENSION IN TRACTION for Right-sided Cervical disc herniation

POSITION would be to lie on your left side with your neck supported (draped over a pillow or resting on your hand) in EXTENSION to the right (See Figure 2).

Another position could be to support your head (with your hand on your left cheek or lying on a pillow) on its left side resting so that the neck is caused to be extended to the right posterior; however, this position can allow the disc to BEAR WEIGHT IN EXTENSION and should only be used if you are certain that the disc is "in" by virtue of the absence of pinching discomfort when it or CIRCUMDUCTION is attempted. Either way, the disc unit is maintained in EXTENSION so that the posterior intervertebral space is closed to prevent disc material from moving posteriorly.

For now, **you can act upon the assumption that the best time to practice DYNAMIC POSITIONING is when sleeping**. One should sleep in the most favorable position to give the disc a chance to migrate centrally during the minor position changes occasioned during a night's sleep. Again, the area of the neck affected determines, in large part, the appropriate position of sleep.

As a means to apply the DYNAMIC POSITIONING and MAINTENANCE OF EXTENSION principles to the Cervical and Upper Thoracic spine, one must realize that in order to MAINTAIN EXTENSION, support must be provided or else it would require constant muscular energy. Support structures, regardless of the type, must be comfortable and able to be slept in so as to keep the segment of the spine in EXTENSION for a prolonged period. Whatever area they are applied to, they should be placed directly beneath the painful site in question so as to maintain extension effortlessly at the painful disc unit.

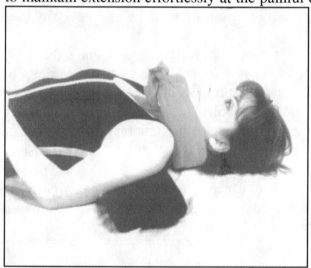

Figure 3 Sleeping position with both High Thoracic and Cervical supports in place

For the Cervical spine, these classically and routinely have been largely limited to the soft or hard collars seen on people walking around who have had "whip-lash" injuries. However, more effective devices exist that are simple to make and use. The simplest is a collar made from a soft towel rolled to the ideal size to fit the hollow of the neck and used especially while sleeping. The height it takes the effected disc unit off of the sleeping surface should be only so much as to maintain slight elevated support. It should not be uncomfortable. It can be secured in front with a shoe lace or large rubber band. A better device can be fashioned out of foam rubber by cutting the edges off of a long rectangular cube-like piece that is as long as necessary to wrap around your neck so that the ends touch in the front. Its height and width should be such that when compressed by the weight of the neck, it completely and comfortably fills the natural concavity or keeps it in slight EXTENSION. Covering it with soft, comfortable cloth can make it pleasant to touch the skin (See Figure 3). This Figure shows both the High Thoracic and Cervical supports in place. The purely Cervical support is best used alone for High to Mid-Cervical lesions. The High Thoracic can be used alone or in combination with the Cervical collar depending upon whether the pain is more towards the Cervical region than the Thoracic. For pain in the high Thoracic region or at the junction of the Thoracic and Cervical regions, the placement of the support directly under the site of pain without the use of the Cervical collar is probably the most effective because the Cervical support can defeat the EXTENSION effect by raising the Cervical spine too high.

One of the most effective and easily-acquired long-term support devices for the back pain sufferer is the feather pillow. The foam rubber devices, although fashioned in what appear to be scientific designs, in practice, cannot accommodate the myriad of anatomical permutations in the real world of back pain. Therefore, by experience using any number of them, I have arrived at the understanding that the best device available is the lowly feather pillow. It should be only about one-half to two-thirds full of feathers. If too full, it loses the ability to be shaped to fit the individual and becomes no better than its inadequate and ultimately painful foam rubber, pieced foam, or polyester batting counterparts. If too empty, it doesn't serve any purpose; so, let your own needs dictate the exact size.

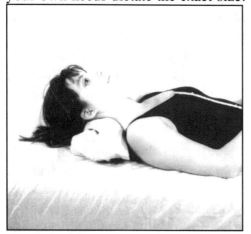

Figure 4 Ideal pillow support for Cervical region

The ideal attribute of the feather pillow is that the exact anatomical contours can be approximated and supported by positioning yourself in the most advantageous posture and pushing or crowding the pillow into filling the space between the mattress and your body. Or, it can be fashioned into a shape and height that is precisely suited for your individual necessity (See Figure 4).

For Upper Cervical disc problems, the head should be effectively immobilized so that regardless of how you may want to move during the night, the neck will be required to remain in slight extension (depending upon your disc fragment's location relative to the center as described immediately above) and mild, passive, gravitational TRACTION. One of the easiest and readily available means I have found to accomplish this end is to use a rolled towel wrapped around the neck and secured loosely in the front. The towel should be a soft, fluffy, one rolled lengthwise to a thickness that, as closely as possible, fills the space formed by the natural Cervical curvature. It should be rolled no greater than that which slightly puts a comfortable EXTENSION pressure on the neck while reclining. Any greater and the HYPEREXTENSION created can be painful in and of itself.

One must be careful to insure that the towel is not so tight around the neck that it impairs the circulation and not so well secured in the front that it could accidently choke one at night during the predictable tossing and turning.

Once the towel is in place, lying flat on a firm mattress without a pillow (or with only a small feather pillow slightly providing a slight amount of support for the head) finds the Cervical curvature supported and maintained in slight EXTENSION IN TRACTION

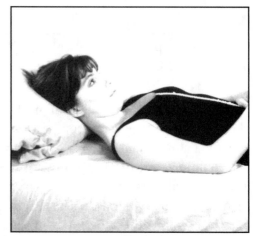

Figure 5 Large pillow placing Cervical spine in WEIGHT-BEARING FLEXION

throughout the night. Without the towel, the Cervical spine is allowed to persist in FLEXION induced by gravity because the back of the head and the shoulders are the main supports and the neck between them is allowed to sink down until it touches the mattress surface without any support to oppose it. This, especially if the head is raised by a pillow, constitutes WEIGHT-BEARING FLEXION--the enemy (See Figure 5). In fact, often sleeping with a pillow that is too large or too firm can cause neck pain in and of itself. Think about it, if one were to remain with the head equivalently flexed while standing for eight hours, the actual degree of FLEXION imposed upon the neck would be almost the same as if you were to walk around all day with your chin touching your chest. Try this for a few minutes and see if the pain makes you glad that you can balance your head directly on top of your neck.

The benefit a towel has over a small pillow is that should you turn on your side during the night, the towel fills the spaces on the side of the neck too, and maintains the neck in a neutral position even if you roll on to your side unconsciously. To insure that the neck is supported on all sides is the best means of stabilizing the neck during the night, especially during episodes of acute pain. Realistically, however, it is unreasonable to expect a person to wear a towel every night and, in practice, it is not necessary. A feather pillow can accomplish the night-to-night MAINTENANCE OF EXTENSION just as well if you can stay cognizant of the necessity to try as best as you can to retain this positioning throughout the night.

One of the easiest positions for sleep with midline neck pain of vertebral disc origin is to remain flat on your back with the towel support in place or the pillow with enough of its bulk tucked into the hollow of neck to MAINTAIN MILD EXTENSION; however this may be easy on paper to say, yet, in reality, that, or any one position, may become too uncomfortable to maintain without occasional turns on the side. If you do turn on your side, make sure you have a proper pillow to support both the weight of your head and fill the space between your neck and the mattress when the shoulders are raising the base of the neck high off of the bed. The best pillow to meet that need is a feather pillow that is only about half full of feathers. It is ideal to have two such pillows if you want to use a pillow to support the neck instead of the towel roll. A pillow is actually more comfortable; but rolling around at night offers little guarantee that it will remain positioned ideally when you need it. When used , it should be crowded under the head to the exact individual height necessary to just maintain a position of comfortable EXTENSION without letting the neck ever enter into WEIGHT-BEARING FLEXION. Those foam rubber shaped pillows sold for neck pain may help if your neck is the exact size and shape to fit the size sold; however, I have tried them and found them actually uncomfortable. I wasn't impressed. If I hadn't received it as a gift, I would have gotten my money back. I don't know who it was made to fit, but I consider myself an average kind of guy; and it didn't fit me.

If the pain is more to one side than straight in the midline of the posterior neck, then one must sleep turned to one side so that the painful site is aimed down, closest to the mattress surface. The highest point of the pillow or the support should be positioned such that it is directly beneath the site of pain. That insures that the problem disc is put in the relatively greatest degree of EXTENSION.

As elaborated in the DYNAMIC POSITIONING Section of Chapter Four, a decision often needs to be made whether to use FLEXION IN TRACTION or EXTENSION IN TRACTION to best allow for the spontaneous centralization of disc material. A degree of increased difficultly is imposed upon the concept of DYNAMIC POSITIONING when the herniated disc material is peripherally displaced so much that EXTENSION is uncomfortable or pinchingly painful. In that event, you must decide whether to sleep in FLEXION away from the painful site by aiming it towards the ceiling. This choice would be appropriate if the disc material needs the stretching of the peripheral ligaments to push it centrally beyond the lips of the vertebral bodies. So, in this instance, the neck would be positioned in FLEXION IN TRACTION with the painful side up until such time as the disc is moved centrally enough to allow for a non-painful EXTENSION position. This may take minutes or numbers of nights. As soon as it moves centrally (and you may become astute enough to feel the actual movement by recognizing the little crunch that immediately precedes painlessness), you can then roll over and make an attempt to sleep more on the other side such that the painful area is aimed towards the surface of the mattress. This would be putting the same disc unit in EXTENSION IN TRACTION; and, therefore, it would feel the greatest degree of support and EXTENSION from the pillow or the towel roll. **If the pain is very far to the side, it may be necessary to sleep fully resting on the same side as the pain with the head supported sufficiently by a pillow so that it is still in mild EXTENSION relative to the source of the pain; yet it remains comfortable enough to allow for sleep.** In this position, the neck or painful site is draped over the pillow or the towel. In the case of using a towel, only a portion of the pillow is used under the head just enough to keep the slight amount of TRACTION comfortable. If you are not using a towel, the larger part of the pillow or an other pillow can be crowded under the neck at the painful site to support the head.

Now, once you have reclined in this position with the towel and pillow and you are ready for sleep, you must put yourself in the optimal degree of gentle traction. First, position yourself so that the towel is supporting the area as best as you can adjacent to the painful area. Relax the neck and reach up holding the head with your hands. Push the head and the part of the neck above the pain off of the shoulders. Using the towel to interfere with the movement of the head, pull your body away from your head by using your hips and legs to pull the lower part of your neck and body below the point of pain away from the head. Then position your body and neck such that the towel is directly beneath the point of vertebral pain as though your neck was the board of a "teeter-totter" board and the towel was the central support bar.

Think about what is happening here. You are placing the involved segment in gentle TRACTION and EXTENSION, giving the structures of the neck an advantageous mechanical position to favor the movement of misplaced disc material anteriorly and centrally. Once you have induced some traction, you can remove your hands and put them comfortably at your sides as you try not to tighten up the muscles that you have just pulled to full length. With some effort, you can maintain this position throughout the night so that when you experience the full effect of sleep's relaxation, your neck is set for re-positioning of the disc material that been displaced.

This is for a pain that originates in the superior portion of the neck. If the pain is lower into the shoulder blades or at the very top of the back where the neck joins the thorax, a different strategy must be employed either in concert with the neck roll or independently. The more likely that the following will be successful by itself depends upon how far down the back the pain originates. The further down, the less likely it will be necessary to employ the towel.

For midline posterior pain, putting the support pillow in the midline directly under the painful site is sufficient and it need not get more complicated than that; however, most of the time the pain is to one side or the other.

For pain deep in the neck at or near the Thoracic level that radiates more to the side than the midline posterior, it may be necessary to place a larger pillow under your armpit and tuck the other pillows under your head and neck. The problem with pain in this area is that the shoulder gets in the way and tends to force the High Thoracic and Low Cervical region into an unwanted WEIGHT-BEARING FLEXION while lying on your side. So, the pillows are necessary to raise the entire upper torso off the mattress so that the shoulder is not interfering with the needed EXTENSION at the painful level.

Neck pain is particularly amenable to DYNAMIC POSITIONING once the pillows are properly positioned because the shoulder and upper arm act as an excellent device to drape the spine over to achieve a DYNAMIC POSITIONING IN TRACTION effect.

DYNAMIC POSITIONING with TRACTION IN EXTENSION is accomplished much more effectively when the process is initiated with an actively induced TRACTION at the onset. Then, after the TRACTION is applied, you relax into a passive position that maintains this TRACTION so long as you don't move or contract the muscles acting upon the disc you previously put into TRACTION. When applying this method to the Cervical spine, the object is to position the head with the hands such that gravity is eventually capitalized upon to pull, in combination with lever actions of the abducted (moved away from the body) upper arm and shoulder, putting continuous, easily maintained, TRACTION on that portion of the head and neck in directions away from site of vertebral pain.

The process is accomplished like this for pain originating in the Cervical region:

1) Lie down on a bed or couch such that the body is slightly diagonally positioned near one side of the bed or the end of the couch. If the pain is midline and posterior the face should be up. If the pain radiates to one side, the side to which the pain radiates should be down. The neck can also be placed directly over a couch pillow or the corner of the bed, just so long as the head is placed so that as it hangs over the edge of the bed or the pillow so that the weight of the head extending passively due to gravity can produce a lever action causing the vertebral column to be stretched.

(2) The body is then moved slightly towards or away from the head, or the head is allowed to hang more or less so that the stretching sensation is felt right at the site where the pain originates. Quite often a crunching sound is heard as the vertebral bodies are moved apart and the disc material is centralized simply from the suction effect. This position should not be painful. If it is, you are applying too much tension too fast or at the wrong site. If a pinching sensation occurs, this means that the disc is extruded beyond the periphery of the vertebral bodies and some patient traction or some FLEXION IN TRACTION might be necessary before EXTENSION is allowed to proceed again.

3) The hands and arms are then recruited to assist in this MANEUVER (See Figure 4 in Section named CERVICAL (NECK) PAIN MANEUVERS). One hand is placed so that its palmar surface abuts on one of the notches at the bottom of the posterior skull (the posterior inferior occipital protuberance or the mastoid

processes). That same hand's arm (the one on the same side as the side that the pain radiates to) is used as a pivot point upon which the neck is draped with the elbow serving as the anchor point. The pillow can be placed superior to the arm or inferior to it (in the arm pit) depending upon how far out over the edge it is necessary to hang. The more inferior Cervical vertebrae that the pain originates from, the farther one must position one's self out over the edge. The other hand (the one on the upward side or on the opposite side of the side of the pain) can gently be used to push the head away from the neck by pushing superiorly on the jaw to cause the head to tilt backwards or extend towards the side of the pain into a more bent position. The other arm that is on the down-side can be hanging over the edge of the bed or be placed so that the elbow is on the edge of the bed so that the shoulder becomes the actual point upon which the neck pivots if the pain is particularly low in the neck or at the junction of the Thoracic and Cervical vertebrae. The hand of the down-side arm should be placed under the neck so that the palm is touching the skin of the neck and the karate chop surface of the palm abuts against the base of the skull adjacent to one of the notches. As the neck is gently allowed to extend by the action of its own weight, the hand and arm act as a fulcrum to give leverage to the head's pulling the neck away from the torso as gravity acts to pull the head earthward.

While the head/neck is first hooked on the hand and while the neck is being stretched, it sometimes helps to gently activate the neck muscles to alternately flex and extend the head and neck rhythmically and with very little actual movement as though one were moving the head almost imperceptibly to silently say "yes" or as if one were trying to touch their ear to their shoulder. Each time the neck extends, the base of the skull should use the hand to pivot on and ever so gently "drag" the neck and body below the point of pain away from that portion of the head and neck above the painful area. All the while, the body can be moved like a porpoise and a snake to maximally mobilize all the vertebral elements.

(4)   Once the ideal stretching occurs and the site of pain is identified by the change in the character of the pain, this site's muscles and ligaments are preferentially given the opportunity to come to their maximum length by simply resting in the exact position that allows the stretching to be maintained. The head should be left in the exact position that allows for its resting and relaxed weight to exert constant tension simply by gravity's action. The head, by hanging over the side of the bed while the neck is supported by the hand and the bed underneath, naturally will extend the neck by the weight of the head. The weight of the head acts as the traction weight now and the traction can be sustained simply by the weight of the head. Therefore, the body can completely relax and let the disc space separate. The angulation of the planes of the vertebral bodies should be such that EXTENSION causes the disc material to move only centrally. This can last as long as you want it to, so long as the TRACTION is passively maintained and the body is positioned relative to the head and neck. So long as the position is comfortable, this should not be a problem.

Now, if you think about it, there are two ways in which a piece of disc material can be moved centrally with EXTENSIONS. You can keep the disc space open with TRACTION and MAINTAIN EXTENSION, as above, letting the displaced material migrate passively centrally; or, alternatively, you can position the disc in EXTENSION and allow WEIGHT-BEARING to squeeze the disc material centrally.

In order to effect the alternative DYNAMIC POSITIONING to use WEIGHT-BEARING EXTENSION, you must position yourself such that the side to which the pain radiates is upwards, very similar pre-positioning TRACTION is applied in a nearly identical manner. Only this time, the opposite hand/arm/shoulder becomes the down-side support. TRACTION is effected with the head/neck held straight in line with the axis of the spine and the head does not use its weight to pull on the neck. Rather, the head is fixed by placing the palm of the hand on the neck. The part of the neck where it is placed depends upon where the pain is located. If the pain is in the superior Cervical region, the hand karate chop portion of the hand can abut up against the mastoid process on the down-side. If the pain is in the Lower Cervical region of the neck or Upper Thoracic region, the hand needs to get as low on the neck as possible using the friction of the hand and the skin of the neck as the anchoring means. The top side hand/arm can be again allowed to rest its weight on the up-side neck or even push superiorly on the jaw.

Now, in order to achieve the EXTENSION while remaining in relaxation, the legs and lower torso are used to pull the body away from the neck which is fixed by the down-side arm and hand against the edge of the bed or the pillow. As the formerly straight neck is being pulled by the body and torso, it is allowed to passively assume an extended position. With that action, the upper sides of the vertebral body's periphery close, hopefully trapping the disc material and causing it to move centrally or downwards. The weight of the body pressing down on either side of the disc supplies the force to move the disc material. The same gentle gyrations of the neck and head can be done during this positioning as described above. This should take the head to the pillow or bring it to rest upon an upright forearm with the elbow supporting the weight. There it can remain in PASSIVE EXTENSION, DYNAMICALLY POSITIONED until the disc takes its time to re-centralize.

It is important to relax in these positions. Simply let the body relax for a good length of time. As the relaxation progresses, the crunchy, squishy sound can occur and quite often when the offending disc does move enough to take pressure off of the outer ligamentous annulus, a warm sensation and localized tingling can be felt where the pain used to be. This is normal and good. If any increased pain is experienced, this implies something is wrong and one should carefully re-position one's self so that the pain is stopped. **ANY TIME THAT ANY MOTION CAUSES DIZZINESS OR INCREASED PAIN TO SHOOT DOWN THE ARM OR RADIATE TO SOME OTHER SITE OF THE BODY OTHER THAN THE VERTEBRAL COLUMN, THIS COULD MEAN THAT A DORSAL NERVE ROOT IS BEING IRRITATED AND THE BEST THING TO DO IS STOP THE WHOLE AFFAIR, AND CAREFULLY REPOSITION ONE'S SELF SO THAT THE PAIN STOPS AND DO NOTHING FURTHER THAT WOULD BRING ON THIS PARTICULAR TYPE OF PAIN. THIS PAIN INDICATES THE NECESSITY TO SEE A NEUROSURGEON SO THAT A CT SCAN OR NMRI CAN BE OBTAINED TO INSURE THAT DISC MATERIAL IS NOT IMPINGING UPON A NERVE.**

Oddly enough, gently and increasingly strong coughing during this MANEUVER while the offending disc space is being stretched creates a favorable set of muscular relaxations and contractions that predispose the neck to allow the disc to centralize.

As a few closing thoughts on preventing neck pain, be ever-cognizant as to what clothing you are wearing and in what positions your neck rests while working. Anything that you wear that puts weight on your neck, can add to your discomfort by putting weight on a particular point of the neck. This constant pressure is like that generated by wearing a heavy coat or jacket with weight in the pockets. It is the equivalent to wearing a rope around your neck with heavy weights. The same effect can be created by a camera bag, strapped valise, or even an arm sling. Any object that keeps steady weighted pressure on a spinal segment detrimentally assists the disc material to migrate if the neck is placed in FLEXION for any reason. So, be aware of this phenomenon and guard against it.

At work, many people are so absorbed in what they are doing, that they neglect to notice that their Cervical and Upper Thoracic regions are in WEIGHT-BEARING FLEXION. Simply looking down on paperwork at a desk or a computer can keep the neck in this disadvantageous posture for nearly eight hours a day. See Chapter Four's Section on AVOIDING WEIGHT-BEARING FLEXION for a more in-depth treatment of this subject and some solutions.

Believe it or not, how you take a shower and the position of your head relative to the shower head can determine whether or not you have neck pain for the rest of the day. Degenerating disc material can be displaced by an action so simple as having to bend your head forward to get it into the shower stream. Add to that the pressure placed on the head and neck by the hands washing the hair or neck is sufficient to induce disc migration pain.

Think about it. When you shower in the morning, your neck muscles are literally still asleep. The protective muscle tone mechanism is not yet fully functioning, the muscles are still lax and have not acquired the tone in the posterior neck to keep the neck in its neutral, extended position that serves to naturally centralize the discs through posture. All of that is disarmed as you dig your fingers into your hair with the weight of your hands and sleepily bend the neck forward into extreme FLEXION in order to allow the water stream to strike it while you scrub. This is especially true for tall persons. The solution is to buy an s-extender for your shower head so that you do not have to flex the neck to take a shower.

The reader is encouraged to examine nearly every aspect of their activities of daily living to detect WEIGHT-BEARING FLEXION postures that contribute to neck and upper back pain; and seek solutions by designing physical positions, conditions or the environment to favor EXTENSION, UNWEIGHTED EXTENSION, or EXTENSION IN TRACTION when and wherever feasible.

THORACIC (CHEST) PAIN MANEUVERS

The basic PRINCIPLES that apply for all MANEUVERS of *The O'Connor Technique (tm)* can be applied when pain originates in the Thoracic region; however, the Thoracic spine is functionally and structurally different from the Cervical and Lumbar regions in that it is more rigid and less likely to rotate. This has the advantage that it is less likely to suffer discogenic pain, but the disadvantage of its immobility is that when discogenic pain occurs, it is usually more difficult to centralize disc material, especially in the Upper Thorax where the shoulder musculature attaches. However, the Thorax also has at least one advantage when it comes to MANEUVERS, there are two body segments of substantial weight on either side of any given disc that can be used to exert significant nearly effortless TRACTION, making the generation of sufficient TRACTION less difficult.

Since the Thorax is in about the gravitational center of the body, either the upper body or the lower body can be used to generate the TRACTION. For this reason, I divide the Thorax into an Upper and a Lower section. **In the situations where the pain is located in the Upper Thoracic region, one should choose the method in which the hanging head and shoulders supply TRACTION forces. Most of the methods that are successful for the Uppermost Thoracic discs are covered in the CERVICAL (NECK) PAIN MANEUVERS section; so, if your pain is located very high in the Thorax, at the level of the shoulder blades, you should go to the Section of the book that describes CERVICAL (NECK) PAIN MANEUVERS and apply them.** Those MANEUVERS that describe how to manage Low Cervical disc problems can give you a great deal of insight into your solution to pain. **Similarly, if pain is located in the Lower Thoracic region, selecting a MANEUVER that uses the weight of the legs and hips to produce the TRACTION force seems to work best. These MANEUVERS can be looked upon as modifications of the Lumbar region's and are, likewise, previously covered in the LUMBAR (LOW BACK) PAIN MANEUVERS Sections.** Depending upon whether your pain is in the High Thoracic or Low Thoracic region, I would encourage the reader to go to those respective Sections and read the MANEUVERS' directions and explanations if a more extensive or in-depth understanding is desired due to a difficult to centralize disc.

Like the other MANEUVERS, a platform-based MANEUVER seems to be the easiest and most effective; and, of course, a bed makes about the most comfortable platform available to most people. However, a difficulty comes in getting your Thorax high enough so that the weight of your legs and lower torso can still produce TRACTION without hitting the floor first. Large, couch cushions can be stacked up on a bed to assist in this endeavor; however, the higher the pile, the more unstable it becomes. You can't easily roll because the cushions fall to one side or the other when you attempt to roll or you fall off the edge of the cushion unless you constantly re-adjust your position. This re-adjusting involves contracting musculature that should be remaining in the most relaxed state it can during the MANEUVER and oftentimes, the purpose is defeated.

With this consideration in mind, one needs to be prepared to practice rolling CIRCUMDUCTION in place and making sure that, with each sequential adjustment, adequate time is allotted to allow TRACTION to sufficiently separate the vertebral bones before continuing the THERAPEUTIC CIRCUMDUCTION component..

UPPER/MIDDLE THORACIC SPINE MANEUVER

For Upper and Middle levels of Thoracic vertebral disc disease, the basic PRINCIPLE of FLEXION IN TRACTION followed by a rolling PASSIVE THERAPEUTIC CIRCUMDUCTION into TRACTION IN EXTENSION then terminating in WEIGHT-BEARING EXTENSION is applied. For the Upper Thoracic regions, the **MANEUVER is started with the head and shoulders hanging over the edge of the bed with the painful side up towards the ceiling** (See Figure 1). This constitutes the FLEXION IN TRACTION component.

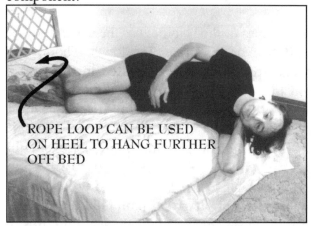

Figure 1 FLEXION IN TRACTION starting position by hanging Upper torso for right-sided high Thoracic disc pain

If the pain is in the posterior midline (which is uncommon for the Upper Thorax) then the MANEUVER is initiated in the face down posture.

When hanging the Upper Thorax over the edge of the bed, the weight of the head and shoulders are usually sufficient to cause you to slide off the bed when hanging. **So, I would say that you might as well just "get a rope" before you even start these MANEUVERS.** To avoid redundancy, I refer you to the ROPE-ASSISTED TRACTION Section in CHAPTER 4 for a general treatment on the use of a rope or strap to assist TRACTION. The use of a rope is also described in the CERVICAL (NECK) PAIN MANEUVERS Section with directions on the manner in which the rope is managed for Upper Thoracic pain by looping it around the foot or the knee. For lower Thoracic pain, the rope is looped around the chest and under the armpits as described in the LUMBAR DISC PAIN section or around the hands as described below.

How far the Upper Thorax hangs over the edge of the bed depends upon how low in the Thoracic spine the bad disc is located. If high in the Thorax, the elbows can hang over the edge and the hands can be used to support the neck and head. For more explicit directions on effecting a Low Cervical/High Thoracic lesion, combine this MANEUVER with the DYNAMIC POSITIONING described in the CERVICAL (NECK) PAIN MANEUVERS Section.

Start with the painful side up FLEXION IN TRACTION to recruit the peripheral fibro-cartilaginous ligaments and the posterior longitudinal ligament of the Cervical and Thoracic region. So long as the head and neck are supplying TRACTION to the affected disc, FLEXION IN TRACTION can be accomplished with the painful side up using the down-side forearm and elbow as a fulcrum. It may be necessary to actually put the downside hand or elbow on the floor if the problem disc unit is low in the Thorax. The same type of adjustments to achieve maximal flexion and tension on the ligaments can be made by moving the body towards the head or foot of the bed while keeping the head fixed and "teetering" off the foot of the bed with the hands and arms. By adjusting the position of the down-side arm relative to the edge of the mattress, the highest degree of tension can be generated by the weight of the head, neck, and shoulders being hung towards the floor. **FLEXION IN TRACTION is accomplished by simply letting the Upper body hang towards the floor with the painful side up.** The neck should be kept in a relatively straight configuration by using the hands because there is no reason to put FLEXION or EXTENSION pressures on Cervical discs not involved in the MANEUVER.

You must insure that the specific problem disc is in FLEXION by adjusting your position on the bed such that when the herniated disc is put in FLEXION, the character of the pain changes. When the appropriate disc unit is being stretched, the pain should not increase, but, in most cases, it decreases and you then know that you are at the correct level.

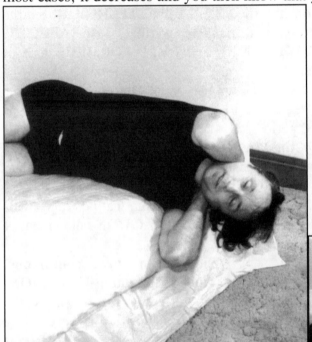

Additional TRACTION force can be supplied with the lever action of the down-side arm and elbow and the hands on the neck in a surrender type position (See Figure 2) as far down on the Thorax as possible using the medial surfaces of the forearms against the mastoid processes as described in the CERVICAL (NECK) PAIN MANEUVER Section of the book in THE HEAD-HANG. Those methods described earlier in the CERVICAL (NECK) PAIN MANEUVER

Figure 2 Hanging head, neck, and shoulders with arms in a "surrender" position for Upper Thoracic disc pain on right.

Section of the book can be applied here as well and reviewing the explicit manner in which they are applied can be done by referring to the HEAD-HANG Section of the book.

Gentle ACTIVE THERAPEUTIC CIRCUMDUCTIONS are helpful while the head is in TRACTION whether it is in FLEXION as it is now or, later, in EXTENSION. Only this time, you will be

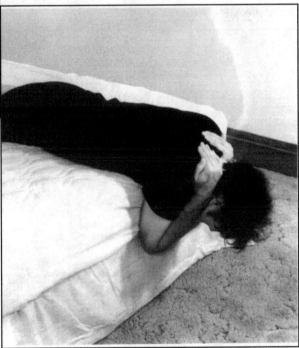

Figure 3 Face down position for Upper Thoracic disc

339

making a motion with your head, neck and Upper Thorax as if you were "drawing" ovals with your neck on the walls or the floor, respectively, when the Upper body is hanging over the edge of the bed or near the floor.

After sufficient FLEXION IN TRACTION is achieved at the site of the disc problem, you may begin gentle NARROW-ARC ROCKING. Rolling slightly from side to side while keeping the painful side mostly up while maintaining FLEXION IN TRACTION assists in centralizing disc material that has herniated to the far periphery of the disc.

RELAXATIONAL BREATHING is especially effective in the Thorax to relax those disc units. Many times when a Thoracic disc is involved, the simple act of breathing is painful. You will know that you are putting sufficient TRACTION on the problem disc unit because this aspect of the pain is usually relieved.

Here, too, is an excellent opportunity to practice the MOBILIZING TECHNIQUES if the disc material is difficult to centralize. If your disc is difficult to mobilize, THERAPEUTIC CIRCUMDUCTIONS, CHIROTATIONAL MOVEMENTS, and INCH-WORMING here, if desired, can be used to help centralize disc material.

At this point, DYNAMIC POSITIONING can be applied simply by remaining in this configuration or adopting one with a lesser degree of FLEXION and TRACTION that is comfortable enough to remain in for a prolonged period.

This FLEXION IN TRACTION stage of the MANEUVER is terminated by rolling to the face down position (See Figure 3) while maintaining as much TRACTION on the problem disc as possible. You may already be in the face down position if your disc pain is located centrally in the midline posterior. In that case, simply start your roll from that position. This constitutes the PASSIVE THERAPEUTIC CIRCUMDUCTION IN TRACTION component of the MANEUVER.

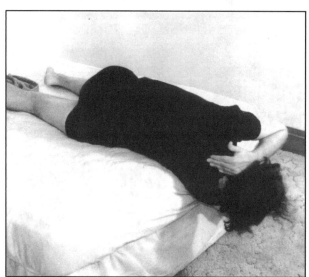

Figure 4 Roll towards painful side completed with painful side now in down-side position in EXTENSION IN TRACTION.

Then, in a slow, continuous, movement, while maintaining TRACTION, you continue with the roll towards the painful side to a position wherein the painful side is now the down-side (See Figure 4). This eventually puts the putative disc in EXTENSION IN TRACTION so long as you are sure to maintain TRACTION.

In this action, you must roll towards the side of pain until you are 180 degrees rotated from your original position while all the while maintaining TRACTION. At the end of the roll, **you want to have the painful site that was originally aimed towards the ceiling, eventually aimed towards the floor.** For example, if your right side was up during FLEXION IN TRACTION, the rolling should leave you with the right side down but still hanging in TRACTION when you finally

340

come to rest in EXTENSION.

In the case of a midline, posterior pain, you would eventually want to end the roll so that the anterior aspect of the body is in the up (supine) position.

In either case, **the affected disc should be caused to go from FLEXION IN TRACTION to EXTENSION IN TRACTION via a PASSIVE THERAPEUTIC CIRCUMDUCTION (rolling)**. By passive, I mean that the muscles at the disc unit being manipulated should not be activated. They should stay in the most relaxed and stretched-by-gravity condition. The roll can be accomplished by rolling like a log or be done in place by sequential adjustments in which you roll in place a little, adjust your torso to put the problem disc unit over the same spot that you were in before you rolled, and making sure your are in TRACTION, roll in place a little more, re-adjust, insure TRACTION, and so forth.

By adjusting your position relative to the edge of the surface upon which you are lying, the maximum amount of FLEXION at the onset and EXTENSION at the end of the roll should be kept at the problem disc level where the pain originates. For this reason, anticipating where you eventually want to end up in maximum EXTENSION IN TRACTION should dictate to what degree you are hanging over the edge of the bed or surface upon which you are rolling. Too, if you choose to roll like a log, you don't want to roll off the side of the bed before you complete your roll. So, in this instance, before you roll, position yourself on the bed so that you have a sufficient area on the bed to roll onto so you won't end up halfway through the roll without bed-space upon which you can come to rest.

Insuring that you have enough space to roll when you are actually rolling over like a log, you may find that the rope holding your foot causes you to roll in a "fan"-shape. The top of the "fan" being curved, changes the site upon which the FLEXION and EXTENSION forces are applied by the straight edge of the mattress.

By that I mean, all else being equal, a person starting their roll in the middle of the "fan" and rolling towards the edge will increase the degree of TRACTION because the disc unit is moving inferiorly relative to the edge of the mattress which restrains the upper body hanging over the edge. Similarly, if a person starts at the side of the proposed "fan" and rolls towards its center, TRACTION will be decreased. However, by using the arms in an improvisational manner, these rolls can be used in your favor to generate unique types of TRACTION when artfully coordinated with arm movements. Rolling-in-place eliminates this problem for those who cannot figure out how to use it to their advantage

The portrayals seen in the Figures of this book show a rolling-in-place, for the most part, because I have found that to be the easiest method to keep the disc at the same place relative to the edge of the mattress or on pillows and still be able to maintain TRACTION. Of course, this requires frequent stopping and relaxing to insure that you maintain maximum TRACTION before you proceed with the roll.

Once you have rolled to a painful-side-down EXTENSION IN TRACTION, you can use your legs to pull you back and forth on the edge of the bed to achieve the maximum degree of EXTENSION. It is important, during and after the rolling, to maintain TRACTION on the disc until the head, neck, and Thorax fall to the fully EXTENDED position. Then, the TRACTION supplied by gravity is usually sufficient.

To increase the degree of TRACTION, some RELAXATIONAL BREATHING can be used at this juncture, too. Some THERAPEUTIC CIRCUMDUCTIONS, CHIROTATIONAL MOVEMENTS, and INCH-WORMING here, if desired, can be used to help centralize disc material; however, try not to defeat the TRACTION when you successively contract the neck or Upper Thoracic musculature to effect any PASSIVE THERAPEUTIC CIRCUMDUCTIONS. On the other hand, a SEQUENTIAL ARCHING THERAPEUTIC CIRCUMDUCTION (see the so-named Section for details) uses muscular contraction to effect disc material movement. This stage of the MANEUVER is an excellent opportunity to use this MOBILIZING method if you have a difficult to manage disc. This effect is beneficial so long as you return to EXTENSION IN TRACTION before proceeding with the MANEUVER.

A rope loop, as described previously, should be attached to a foot to keep you on the bed. The farther you have to hang over the edge of the bed, the more you will need something to keep your body on the bed; but this can get complicated (especially when you attempt the CASCADE) because the feet aren't built to grasp and release ropes unless you are a chimpanzee.

You might experiment to figure out the best way to control and adjust the length of the rope. I think the easiest way is, first, to determine what the ideal length the rope should be. By positioning yourself and the rope on the bed before starting the MANEUVER; you can tie off the loop of rope into a fixed "lasso" large enough for your foot to easily slip into in but small enough to let your heel and forefoot still be caught by it when it tightens from your weight. For the most part, the rope length needs to be based upon at what point your problem disc lines up with the end of the mattress. The loop of rope should be able to be slipped off of your foot easily without the use of your hands because when you begin your CASCADE, later, you will need to have your legs free. An assistant such as your roommate, spouse, or any willing accomplice is necessarily valuable until you are comfortable with the effort. They can be directed to hold on to you, help with the rope to let you CASCADE, or even pull you back up on the bed as appropriate.

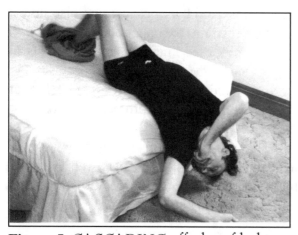

Figure 5 CASCADING off edge of bed in EXTENSION aimed towards Left-sided Thoracic pain.

Now, to complete this MANEUVER, you roll to a position in which the painful site is aimed at the floor and you are ready to CASCADE (See Figure 5). This can be done in two ways. The risky, head first, off the edge of the mattress method or the safer (but probably less effective) means by sliding your legs over the corner of the bed and going feet first.

You should be in EXTENSION, now, rather than FLEXION, **aiming your bent Thorax as much as possible towards the site of the pain.** This is more effective than flat on your back because usually in the Upper Thorax, the discs are laterally protruded due to the widening of the posterior longitudinal ligament that prevents directly posterior protrusions. The head-first progressive CASCADING of the head, then neck, then shoulders can proceed assisted with a balancing effect supplied by the down-side arm and hand by sort of launching off the elbow as an anchor to the fulcrum upon which the

Thoracic spine balances; or you can do it by just simply hanging. I have personally found that maintaining TRACTION while CASCADING IN EXTENSION is most effective right up to the moment that WEIGHT-BEARING IN EXTENSION occurs, but my Thoracic discs, when they go out, are extremely laterally-placed and this is about the only way I can be successful.

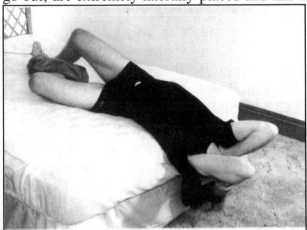

Figure 6 Maximum EXTENSION IN TRACTION preparing to dismount bed

The real difficulty comes when you have CASCADED as much as possible and your head is on the floor. By then, your veins may be bulging and your face getting edematous as, by now, you are literally hanging nearly upside down. This sensation is usually uncomfortable; and I think it sufficiently explains why those devices that lock one's feet in a boot, hooked onto a suspended "teeter-tottering-trapeze"-like gravity TRACTION device, never really became very popular or effective. By the time a person relaxed enough to effect a full TRACTION, they were ready to have a blood vessel explode in their brain. This is no joke,

because the blood vessels in this position can distend and, at the least, give a headache sensation if prolonged. Also, these devices only allow TRACTION without true, relaxed, EXTENSION; and the locking of the feet prevented any sort of side-directed MANEUVERING so all the lesions that had lateral components were not helped unless they were so minor that simply the sucking action of TRACTION was sufficient to effect a re-centralization.

So, at this juncture, you have a choice, either figure out some other way to get to your feet while accomplishing a inverted WEIGHT-BEARING EXTENSION, or continue to CASCADE

to the floor, landing on your extended head and neck (which succeeds in accomplishing an inverted WEIGHT-BEARING EXTENSION) and ever so carefully slide the rest of your body to the floor while bending towards the side of the pain. However, this can be scary, so I cannot recommend it to any but the most agile. It could even be considered dangerous because the weight of your body could be put on your neck and head in an uncontrolled fashion if one were to do it without assistance. One wrong move or loss of control and you easily could be made worse than when you started.

So, when you are ready to get up, it is probably safer and wiser for you to simply angle your neck and Upper Thoracic spine

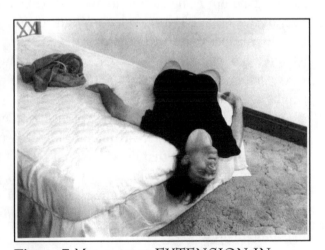

Figure 7 Maintaining EXTENSION IN TRACTION by dropping legs over side of bed in preparation for CASCADE

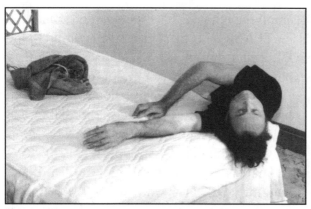

Figure 8 CASCADING in EXTENSION IN TRACTION towards Left for High Thoracic pain to Left

in EXTENSION, swing your legs over the edge of the bed (presuming you were CASCADING at the outset over the foot of the bed) and bring yourself to the upright position by using the weight of your legs as a counter weight to drag your Upper torso across the corner of the bed and wriggle to an upright position by CASCADING feet first until you are WEIGHT-BEARING IN EXTENSION on your knees (See Figures 6-9).

Alternatively, you could use your legs in an INCH-WORM fashion or have your assistant pull you back towards the head of the bed while your neck and Thorax remain in EXTENSION towards the site of the pain. Then, using the most efficient means your physical condition allows, get to your feet while MAINTAINING THE EXTENSION.

Also, the CASCADE effect can be had by a nearly identical action as is described in the dismount portion of the Section on LUMBAR (LOW-BACK) HIP-HANG; only, this time, you keep your head on the bed as long as possible while you get your feet under you. Then, so as to give yourself more room to MANEUVER your neck and Upper Thorax in EXTENSION directly over the site of pain, you lean your whole body far to the painful side and sort of collapse on the floor, landing on the non-painful side.

If you are very tall or your mattress is close to the ground, you can simply lock your neck and Upper Thorax in extension towards the painful side and simply stand up, being careful to avoid flexion at any level of the spine. The last part of your anatomy to leave the surface of the bed should be the back of your head on the painful side so that it is kept in the maximum amount of extension until it begins to bear weight again.

Regardless of what method you use, you must be careful not to persist if a pinching-type of pain ensues. This indicates that the disc is not ready to be seated; and you are crimping it. In that event, you must go back to the beginning FLEXION IN TRACTION and work with it more before attempting this component of the MANEUVER.

Once erect, you can use your hands and arms in concert with the bed if necessary to unweight that part of the body above the bad disc, then go through a PARTIAL WEIGHT-BEARING

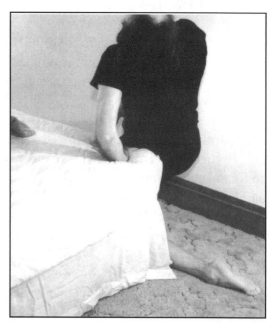

Figure 9 WEIGHT-BEARING IN EXTENSION towards area of pain for a more Left-sided Upper Thoracic pain.

344

CIRCUMDUCTION advancing to a FULL WEIGHT-BEARING CIRCUMDUCTION similar to that described in the HIP-HANG LUMBAR PAIN MANEUVER Section associated with Figures 16-18, wherein you use your hands pushing down on your hips to UNWEIGHT the upper torso while CIRCUMDUCTING in the appropriate EXTENDED direction (see THERAPEUTIC CIRCUMDUCTION Section) while progressively bearing weight.

To end the MANEUVER, bring your head to rest in the neutral position and go on with your usual activities, AVOIDING WEIGHT-BEARING FLEXION and MAINTAINING EXTENSION as much as possible.

LOWER/MIDDLE THORACIC SPINE MANEUVER

Thoracic pain originating in the Lower or Middle Thoracic spine is managed with MANEUVERS nearly identical to those employed for the Lumbar region. It would be unnecessarily redundant to reproduce all the details and directions to describe the movements and considerations that pertain to the lower Thoracic area when they are basically the same for the Upper Lumbar region. Of course, the exception is that the disc unit level that is put into TRACTION and where FLEXION, EXTENSION, and the change in pain character occurs should be in the Lower Thoracic region. However, simplistically lumping the MANEUVERS for these different regions together would have unnecessarily increased the complexity of both, distracted the reader, and led to confusion. So doing would have defeated the purpose of my intent to keep what is basically simple--basically simple.

Again, the most problematic consideration differentiating the MANEUVERS for the two regions is inducing enough TRACTION on the Thoracic region because when using a bed to perform the MANEUVERS, the legs usually hit the ground; and, therefore, gravity isn't able supply enough weight to sustain adequate TRACTION at times. This dilemma can be overcome by the use of pillows to raise the torso at the site of the pain so that it assumes a maximally bent configuration at a height sufficient to allow the legs to remain hanging.

The Thoracic MANEUVER, like the other MANEUVERS, can most easily be accomplished using a bed. A rope is similarly fixed to an area near the head of the bed and tied in an identical manner to that described in the ROPE-ASSISTED TRACTION and LUMBAR PAIN MANEUVERS Section of Chapter Five. The rope can be looped around the chest wall or wrapped around the wrists (See Figure 10). I prefer the chest method because, in actual practice, wrapping it around the wrists tends to cause ligature pressure on the wrists and discomfort; however, the reader is free to try either so long as the skin is protected with a soft barrier. There may be some advantage for certain persons to use the wrist method because it puts the arms and shoulders into TRACTION at the same time, which produces a slightly different dynamic than just the

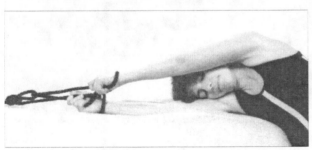

Figure 10 Using rope wrapped at wrists for Thoracic disc pain

shoulders being put in TRACTION by the rope under the armpits. Also, when the wrists are the securing point, the arms are drawn superiorly and parallel to the axis of the body, which makes rolling and circumducting easier. For particular, individual, disc problems, one method may be found to be more effective than the other. Either way seems to work, so the reader is free to try both.

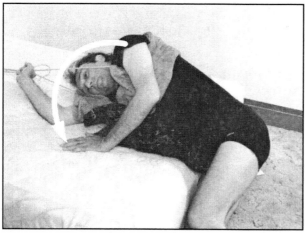

Figure 11 Initial position for Low Thoracic pain radiating to Left side

The LOWER THORACIC PAIN MANEUVER is started by lying down on the bed such that the painful site is aimed towards the ceiling with the legs and lower torso hanging over the end (See Figure 11). This constitutes the FLEXION IN TRACTION component. Pillows are placed directly under the site of pain so that maximum FLEXION can be achieved. You then rest in this position long enough for the ligaments, muscles, and fibro-cartilaginous disc components to come to full length. This position is varied by moving the body superiorly or inferiorly until the maximum stretching is felt at the painful disc level. The rope should be adjusted at this point so as to allow you to hang at this precise location without using the muscles of the arms because to do so would most likely activate the shoulder muscles. Any activation of the Thoracic or spinal musculature attached to the problem disc site will make TRACTION ineffective. This can be prevented by grasping the rope at the site where the rope of the large loop passes through the small, knotted, loop. In this way, you only need to use the muscles of your hand to keep your position. You will know that you are putting the ideal site in TRACTION when the character of the pain changes.

In the environment of Thoracic disc pain, a somewhat unique sensation is often encountered. While the pain is present and the disc material is displaced off-center, breathing deeply while erect and weight-bearing is quite often painful enough to cause one to be unable to take a full breath. It is as if you almost reach the end of a respiratory excursion and the pain stops you from taking a full breath. Patients often describe this pain as "taking their breath away." This sensation, if present prior to starting TRACTION, most probably will be relieved when the putative disc is placed in

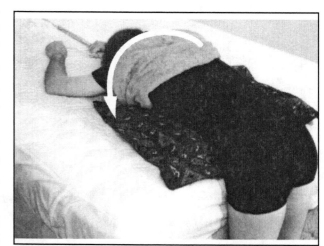

Figure 12 Arrow showing roll to face down position when pain is Left-sided (this is also initial position for Low Thoracic pain radiating to midline posterior).

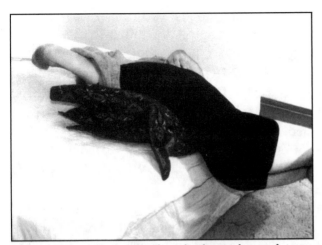

Figure 13 Rolled to Left-side down for Left-sided Low Thoracic lesion to end in EXTENSION IN TRACTION (for midline posterior pain roll is continued until flat on back)

TRACTION, indicating that the pressure on the peripheral ligamentous structures also has been relieved. If and when this effect occurs, you can be reasonably certain that you are stretching the correct disc.

As described above in the Lumbar disc MANEUVER section, combinations of "hula"-type ACTIVE THERAPEUTIC CIRCUMDUCTIONS, SHORT ARC ROCKING from side to side, INCH-WORMING, and RELAXATIONAL BREATHING to relax can be employed to maximize TRACTION and encourage disc material centralization. The reader here is encouraged to read/review the section on the equivalent bed-based MANEUVER for the Lumbar spine in the LOW BACK (LUMBAR) PAIN MANEUVERS Section of Chapter 5 since the activity is the same except for the site of the disc being more superior, in the Thoracic spine, rather than the Lumbar spine. All the associated motions and actions that are applicable to the Lumbar spine work similarly on the Lower Thoracic spine. Therefore, I need only summarize the salient features of the MANEUVER here.

Next, once the disc has been in FLEXION IN TRACTION long enough to allow for some centralization of the disc material to occur, you should roll onto the abdomen (See Figure 12) and continue rolling in the direction of the painful side. This constitutes the PASSIVE THERAPEUTIC CIRCUMDUCTION action. For instance, if the pain radiates to the left side, you will roll such that the left side is eventually in the down-side position. This action should be carried out while maintaining TRACTION on the affected disc, and you should end up with the problem disc in EXTENSION IN TRACTION with the painful side aimed towards the floor (See Figure 13).

The same MANEUVER can be done using the looped wrist method. If your particular disc frequently requires MANEUVERING or a daily regimen is found to be necessary, it is not absolutely necessary to loop the rope around your wrists or tie it. You can simply hold onto the rope so long as you do not tighten up the muscles attached to the spine. It may take some practice, but it is not difficult to learn to use only the arm musculature to grasp the rope while intentionally avoiding the activation or use of the spinal musculature. This method is depicted in Figure 14.

While positioned in EXTENSION IN TRACTION, any of the ancillary movements such as CHIROTATIONAL TWISTING, ACTIVE THERAPEUTIC CIRCUMDUCTION, INCH-WORMING, and RELAXATIONAL BREATHING can be employed to help centralize disc material. These MOBILIZATION methods, their proper execution, and their principles of action are described in their respective Sections of Chapter 4 and need not be re-described here.

At this point, while you are hanging in EXTENSION IN TRACTION one can feel free to

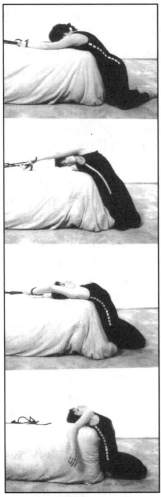

Figure 14 Wrist-rope MANEUVER for Thoracic pain in midline

test whether or not the disc has moved sufficiently centrally to complete the MANEUVER. This can be done by a passive rolling type of DIAGNOSTIC CIRCUMDUCTION while lying down. It is not necessary to remain in TRACTION to accomplish this, and one would probably be well-advised to INCH-WORM oneself up onto the bed while keeping the painful side down to do so. If it appears that there is no arrested movement during a DIAGNOSTIC CIRCUMDUCTION effort, then it is reasonable to complete the MANEUVER by CASCADING to a WEIGHT-BEARING EXTENSION stance.

To finish this MANEUVER, one again assumes the EXTENSION IN TRACTION position and simply slides off of the end of the bed with the Thoracic spine arched posteriorly in EXTENSION. As this is done, the successive discs are placed in maximum EXTENSION IN TRACTION as they slide over the "hump" that exists at the edge of the mattress. The most effective means of getting your legs directly under your torso is to position the toes and feet so that the superior part of the forefoot is tucked underneath the thigh like the traditional Japanese seated position. Your buttocks then rests upon your heels and the maximum amount of EXTENSION can be occasioned. If your bed is too low, you can collapse on to the side opposite the painful side.

Ideally, the EXTENSION should be directed towards the painful herniation site so as to capture it in a WEIGHT-BEARING EXTENSION. Due to the length of the torso relative to the height of the mattress off of the floor, it is sometimes necessary to allow your body to come away from the bed or by letting the feet slide out from under the buttocks, giving you a little more room to collapse to the floor. This motion serves to squeeze the disc material centrally in a "clam-biting" action so long as the displaced disc material is positioned sufficiently within the concavities of the vertebral body's adjacent surfaces. If not, WEIGHT-BEARING will again be painful and the onset of this pain coming signifies that more MANEUVERING will be necessary.

IF AT ANY TIME YOU FEEL EXTREME PAIN, SUDDEN NUMBNESS, or AN ELECTRIC-LIKE SHOCK GOING TO ANY PART OF YOUR BODY, STOP MOVING AND GET YOURSELF

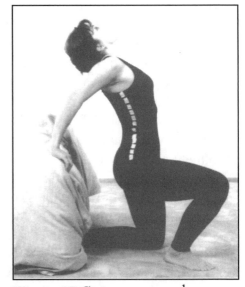

Figure 15 Coming to standing in WEIGHT-BEARING EXTENSION

348

BACK INTO A NEUTRAL POSITION ON THE BED AND REST FOR A FEW MINUTES. THEN, WHILE SUPPORTING YOUR THORAX IN A NEUTRAL, PAINLESS, CONFIGURATION, GET UP BY THE MOST CONVENIENT MEANS THAT AVOIDS PAIN; AND REFER TO THE CHAPTER ON DIAGNOSTIC METHODS. YOU MAY NEED AN NMRI or SURGERY TO SOLVE YOUR PARTICULAR PROBLEM, BECAUSE THESE SIGNS INDICATE THAT YOU MAY HAVE DISC MATERIAL IMPINGING UPON A NERVE ROOT.

You can come to a standing position by keeping the Thoracic spine in EXTENSION, getting your legs back under you, and rising to the erect upright stance as in Figure 15. You can use the bed to help support yourself while getting to the upright position. The face should necessarily be aimed towards the ceiling; otherwise, the Thoracic spine will not be in maximum EXTENSION. Of course, if the pain is to one side or the other, the EXTENSION should be directed and maintained towards the side that the pain is on, aimed directly over the peripheralized disc material.

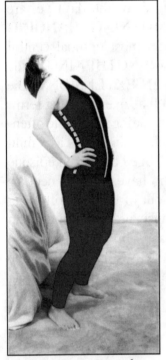

Figure 16 Seating disc material with partial UNWEIGHTING in EXTENSION

Once you are standing, you should put your hands on your hips and push inferiorly on them to UNWEIGHT the Thoracic spine. Then, by circumducting as best as you can at the affected disc, you can seat any disc material that was reluctant to centralize during the previous movements (See Figure 16). This MANEUVER is now completed.

THORACIC PILLOW-ROLL

The Thoracic spine is amenable to the use of pillows as is described in THE LUMBAR AND CERVICAL PILLOW-ROLL MANEUVER Sections as well as the STANDING EXTENSION TECHNIQUES for the Lumbar Spine previously described in the LUMBAR DISC PAIN MANEUVER Sections. For an Upper Thoracic disc problem, the CERVICAL MANEUVERS pertain and for a Lower Thoracic disc, THE LUMBAR MANEUVERS are effective. To repeat them here, by replacing the terms "Lumbar" with "Lower Thoracic" would unnecessarily increase the amount of paper in this already over-sized book and cause the purposeless sacrifice of too many trees.

One only needs to modify the technique so as to insure that the problem disc unit is being acted upon. This simply amounts to moving superiorly or inferiorly upon the pillow-mound until the change in the character of the pain indicates that you are activating the disc unit with the herniation.

The back of a couch can also be used as the platform for the pillows in order to especially increase the degree of FLEXION IN TRACTION for difficult to move disc material. This strategy is described at the end of the LUMBAR SEA LION MANEUVER Section of the book and portrayed in the COUCH-ASSISTED CERVICAL MANEUVER SECTION.

ROUTINE PREVENTIVE MAINTENANCE

Almost as important as terminating pain is the necessity for preventing it from recurring. **In order to prevent spinal pain at any level from returning, routine efforts often need to be made to maintain the disc material in a centralized position.** This consideration holds especially if the exacerbation of pain or the injury is recent. Now, the natural response to this information may be to be disappointed with the future prospect of every day having to perform some task to prevent pain; however, realistically, as time increases after an acute pain episode, the ROUTINE PREVENTIVE MAINTENANCE becomes less and less necessary and increasingly less complicated as your back improves. Eventually, it turns into a habit if you let it, then you don't even realize you are doing it.

These routine efforts can amount to something as simple as hanging the head or hips over the edge of the mattress before you get out of bed or carefully placing the problem spinal segment in a mild EXTENSION IN TRACTION then tightening the extensor muscles of the spine whenever you think about it (especially in the morning as your first act of the day) yet are designed to accomplish sophisticated goals. For instance, the MORNING HANGING EXTENSIONS serve to mechanically replace the disc material into its most optimal central position as the first action of every day. Also, the PREFERENTIAL STRENGTHENING of the muscles of extension selectively increases their tone so as to MAINTAIN EXTENSION at the putative disc sites both immediately after accomplishing the action as well as over the long term.

The theory necessitating this type of activity comes from an understanding that, quite often, the onset of back pain is not an event of sudden incidence. Frequently, the pain begins as a mild discomfort that predictably can mature within hours or days into a full-fledged back pain episode that makes you unable to work or puts you into bed. Often people who have suffered neck or spinal trauma find that they are at least functional until they try to get out of bed the following morning, whereupon they become disabled by pain. If one were to intervene in the initial and ongoing stages of this process before pain progresses too far, the pain reasonably can be expected to be arrested or largely prevented. What I am terming MORNING MAINTENANCE can be applied anytime of the day; however, the best opportunity comes in the morning before you get out of bed.

MORNING MAINTENANCE

Properly loading the spine as the first action you take in the morning is beneficial because it insures that the moment the back bears weight, the disc material is positioned more centrally and mechanically ideal. This opportunity to re-centralize gives the disc less probability of inducing pain by weight-bearing if the disc material has migrated to a decentralized configuration during the night. If a person wants to get out of bed and onto their feet, (s)he must bear weight on the spine. If one bears weight, especially in flexion, on a displaceable volume of mobile disc material, the fragments of disc material are moved more posteriorly and peripherally. Preventable pain is then unnecessarily created as the first event of the day when the pressure on the capsule stretches pain receptors.

Actual morning spinal MANEUVERS are particularly successful because they can prevent the onset of this pain, take advantage of relaxed muscles so that TRACTION is maximally effective, and ideally prepare the spine for the remainder of the day's forces. It takes advantage of the fact that most muscles are in a state of deep relaxation immediately upon waking. They are flaccid and easily placed into TRACTION so long as they have not been activated. So, to be maximally effective, it is important not to activate muscle groups and MANEUVERING must be done before any of those muscles are contracted for the first time of the day. However, **it takes conscious effort to avoid contracting the extensor muscles of the back until the TRACTION component of the MANEUVER is completed. This is done by judiciously avoiding the use of those muscles.**

One way this is insured is by stopping yourself from automatically "stretching" the moment you awake. Most people, without thinking, automatically arch and extend their spines immediately upon gaining consciousness from sleep. This is the yawning stretch that is usually accompanied by a "muscle builder" type flexion of the biceps and a side-to-side circumduction of the head, neck and shoulders. This is so universal and characteristic of land-dwelling vertebrates (animals with spines) that it has to have some evolutionary significance. I believe that it has been coded as a stimulus/response mechanism so as to protect the spine and re-set the discs centrally before they weight-bear. **I have observed cats, dogs, monkeys, and even infant humans do it; and I believe it is the natural, involuntary, equivalent to what *The O'Connor Technique (tm)* intentionally seeks to ultimately accomplish.** However, if the spine has been injured such that an EXTENSION MANEUVER, without prior FLEXION IN TRACTION, is accomplished, this instinctual behavior can serve to prematurely lock the spine into an extended position with the disc material still displaced, crimped, or trapped posteriorly. Once you contract the muscles, it makes them harder to relax in order to do a more effective MANEUVER. In fact, *The O'Connor Technique (tm)* is not in opposition to this evolutionary programming, on the contrary, it actually compliments it. A morning MANEUVER, if necessary, only delays the biologically programmed extension just long enough to FLEX IN TRACTION so as to make certain that when you finally do intentionally extend by contracting the muscles, the disc is in a position that will allow it to migrate anteriorly rather than posteriorly by a crimping action. For people with disc protrusions at the capsular margin that are capable of posterior crimping of the disc material in extension, a FLEXION IN TRACTION is necessary to prevent the pinching pain that comes with muscular extension or WEIGHT-BEARING IN EXTENSION. For those without badly damaged discs, a simple hanging in extension (EXTENSION IN TRACTION) will usually suffice.

It is helpful to temporarily disarm this natural morning stretching by pre-programming yourself to expect the stretching/yawn and consciously train yourself to remain motionless until the urge passes. Then, learning to use the other muscles of the legs and arms (rather than the spine) to move you into position for an EXTENSION IN TRACTION or a FLEXION IN TRACTION (depending upon your necessity), insures that you do not contract the spinal musculature so much that it cannot fully relax for the TRACTION that you will soon be putting on it. Doing this allows for maximum TRACTION because there are no contracted muscles to oppose this TRACTION. Sleep is probably the best relaxation vehicle, and it is better to rely upon it than drugs which achieve the same end yet carry the potential for dependence.

Most back pain suffers with conditions of significant duration already have learned by trial

351

and error their own most successful method of exiting the bed. Adopting a different more successful method should not be difficult for this subset of sufferers. What I suggest, is that **the back pain sufferer who wants to make** *The O'Connor Technique (tm)* **MANEUVERS requiring TRACTION have the highest probability of success, attempt to practice them immediately upon waking**. In this way, if they are successful, you are properly loaded for the day and you start fresh with centralized discs. Even if that goal is not immediately accomplished, then, you at least have the advantage of knowing that you have attempted them under circumstances giving you the highest probability of success.

Since all of the MANEUVERS end in a WEIGHT-BEARING EXTENSION (provided that no pinching pain intervenes), you end up in the same evolutionary advantageous position of extension with contraction of the erector spinae muscles, whose increased tone tends to prevent posterior displacement of disc material and the extensors of the back are locked so that, when weight-bearing occurs, any previous posterior displacement of disc material is more likely to move anteriorly as a result of this action.

All of the MANEUVERS that can be accomplished in bed or that were designed for the reclining position are applicable to the post sleep period. It is not necessary to limit their use to just routine maintenance after a night's sleep. They are excellent for the immediate, post-injury, period after sleeping under the influence of tranquilizers; however, one should sleep in a slight extension position such that you are prepared to enter into any one of the appropriate MANEUVERS which offer the best opportunity to centralize discs or those MANEUVERS that you have found most successful for your particular pain condition.

For the purpose of maintaining your discs in the pain-free state, it is not necessary to use a rope because what is being done in this instance is considered MAINTENANCE due to the presumption that the discs were configured normally during the pre-sleep period, and all that is necessary is that an insurance of maintaining that positioning is undertaken.

It is also not absolutely necessary to perform a FLEXION IN TRACTION movement every time. In fact, it is probably necessary to use a FLEXION IN TRACTION only when the disc is actually painful. **When it is non-painful (which is most of the time) and you want to keep it that way, simply using an EXTENSION IN TRACTION movement that effortlessly proceeds to a WEIGHT-BEARING EXTENSION while getting out of bed is probably sufficient.** This activity is not particularly inconvenient or complex.

For all levels of the spine, one only needs to place the problem disc in a relaxed hanging EXTENSION IN TRACTION before exiting the bed. For the Cervical and Upper Thoracic region, simply hanging the head over the edge of the bed accomplishes that end. For the Lower Thoracic and Lumbar region, hanging the hips over the edge of the bed is the easiest means of generating EXTENSION IN TRACTION. In each case, the final effort amounts to only keeping the affected disc in EXTENSION until WEIGHT-BEARING can be accomplished.

Most of the time, the means by which one can keep the disc unit in EXTENSION is by CASCADING out of bed feet first or by rolling on your side and simply placing the affected disc unit in a maximum EXTENSION by using your hands and/or legs to adjust your posture and coming to standing in the most advantageous manner that your bed situation allows.

If you choose to exit the bed feet first, CASCADING over the edge while keeping the affected disc relaxed in TRACTION and EXTENSION until it bears weight will automatically re-centralize minimally displaced discs. **Simply leaving the bed by first putting your legs on a waiting chair, doing a momentary hip hang, and then putting the feet on the ground and sliding off of the bed such that your head is the last body part to leave the surface is all that is necessary for the most common Lumbar lesions. In essence, there is nothing more complex about MORNING MAINTENANCE than getting out of bed in a different way than that which involves flexion.**

If you analyze how you usually leave your bed you will find that most of the time you start by raising your head up, then your thorax, then you come to sitting as you throw your legs over the edge. This constitutes a WEIGHT-BEARING FLEXION and should be avoided by back pain sufferers. **So, instead, you simply train yourself to take out a few seconds to put the problem disc in EXTENSION IN TRACTION then get out of bed by sliding over the edge such that the discs are sequentially placed in a small degree of CASCADING TRACTION AND EXTENSION as their first act of the day.**

Essentially, you are just accomplishing a dismount as described in the final component of the BED-BASED MANEUVERS in each region of the spine's MANEUVERS Section of the book as your first activity of every day. As your legs slide over the edge of the bed, the Lumbar spine is first put in EXTENSION IN TRACTION. The more you CASCADE over the edge, each successive disc is placed in the same EXTENSION IN TRACTION configuration. The weight of the body below the affected disc is supplying the TRACTION, and going over the edge of the mattress provides the EXTENSION. If you feel that a particular area needs a little extra help to seat the disc material, you can do some ACTIVE or PASSIVE THERAPEUTIC CIRCUMDUCTIONS or any of the other ancillary MOBILIZATION movements such as INCH-WORMING, SEQUENTIAL ARCHING EXTENSIONS, and CHIROTATIONAL TWISTING, amply described in the PRINCIPLES OF THE O'CONNOR TECHNIQUE Section. If your disc pain radiates to one side more than another, be sure to aim your extension towards that side so that you are putting the maximum EXTENSION directly over the herniation site as you begin the WEIGHT-BEARING.

This consideration may obviate that you select the ideal side of the bed to sleep on, depending upon your particular disc problem. For instance, if you have a disc that usually produces pain to the right, that means that the disc herniates to the right and you will find that it is much more convenient to exit the bed from the edge of your mattress to your right side when lying on your back. That way, all you have to do is hang your legs over the edge of the mattress closest to your body and slide out. This naturally involves the right side being bent preferentially into EXTENSION . Similarly, if your pain is in the midline, you may need to rotate yourself so that the axis of your spine is perpendicular to the edge of the mattress so that you extend directly to the posterior. This is probably more convenient than scooting to the end of the bed; however, if you have a bed partner, sometimes its difficult to rotate without waking them up when you bump into them.

If you give it some thought, it is really quite arbitrary how you exit a bed. **There is no reason not to leave your bed in this novel way.** All you need to do is remember to do it and avoid tightening or activating any muscles that act upon your problem disc until you are in EXTENSION. With a little concentration and practice, you can learn to use your arms and legs to position yourself and selectively avoid the use of any spinal muscles. Even if you do use some of them, you needn't tighten them or contract them strongly until you are in the extended and WEIGHT-BEARING position.

Eventually, you probably will find that you do not have to do this at all because your back will get progressively better and pain won't remind you that something is wrong. So, as you continue to improve, the need for articulate management will dissipate, leaving you with only one major taboo--AVOID WEIGHT-BEARING FLEXION.

Lumbar--Hip-Hanging Morning Extensions

For the Lumbar and Lower Thoracic Spine, probably the most gentle and least energetic means of encouraging prolapsed disc material to return to a central position is by the passive TRACTION MANEUVER of HIP-HANGING EXTENSIONS. The technique is prepared in advance by having a chair (or some equivalent structure) at the end or side of your bed such that one can relax comfortably with the Lumbar spine as nearly vertical as possible. Any way in which this can be accomplished is reasonable so long as the weight of the upper torso can be supported by the mattress and the hips can hang for at least a few moments.

This is, for the most part, simply a foreshortened modification of the BED-BASED LUMBAR PAIN MANEUVER OR "HIP-HANG" and can be used on a daily basis to "load" the Lumbar spine each morning upon arising (especially if back pain is a frequent early morning experience). It is arguably the most successful means of accomplishing a MANEUVER-EQUIVALENT without hardly trying.

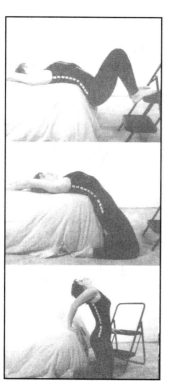

To initiate their leaving their beds, most people, without thinking, get up out of bed by doing a sit-up like activity before swinging their legs over the edge to standing. This is probably one of the most counter-productive movements I can recall. Think about what you are doing if you don't make an effort to manage your discs. If you have not made certain that you slept with a towel or pillow to keep your back in EXTENSION, you may have just spent as much as 6 to 8 hours completely relaxed, sunk into the bed with the back in a flexed posture, especially if your bed is soft. Then, before any tightening or toning of the posterior back musculature is accomplished, a mechanically unfavorable WEIGHT-BEARING FLEXION starts the day. This can only cause a nucleus pulposus or mobile disc material to be squeezed posteriorly. Any wonder many people complain that they can be in bed, just fine, then as soon as they get up. BAM! The back pain starts.

If you fall into this category, the HIP-HANG type of MORNING MAINTENANCE is the ideal solution. You start by positioning yourself in bed on your back so that your feet can glide off the end of the bed first. When your feet are off the edge of the bed, find the chair to place them on and allow the knees to bend and the

Figure 1 Morning Hip Hang EXTENSION

hips to flow off the edge of the bed (See Top Figure 1). When the area of the disc pain reaches the edge of the bed, stop and relax for a minute in the TRACTION which results from this position.

The muscles of the back should not be activated during this whole process; and they should still be in the relatively deep, relaxed, state that they had when the body was asleep. At this point, TRACTION will be most effective because there is no interference due to muscular contraction or spasm. Again, gently circumducting and rotating the hips in a hula dance/twisting, bump and grind fashion, sucking in and pushing out the stomach causes the spinal muscles to further relax and the disc material to be mobilized anteriorly. One can also see that the "clam" spoken of in the previous Sections on EXTENSION "eats" some disc material by rhythmic vertebral movements as you SEQUENTIALLY ARCH IN EXTENSION OR INCH-WORM. The back is then arched fully and completely backwards into a HYPEREXTENDED posture and the hands and arms are used to help the body to standing. As one stands, the disc begins to bear weight and, by definition, you go into a WEIGHT-BEARING HYPEREXTENSION.

This action re-sets all the lumbar discs into a central position; and, if you are willing to go through the minor inconvenience of this MANEUVER every morning, your back will start out properly loaded immediately upon rising. Of course, this can also be utilized for those periods when the back is going through a period of pain; however, during those periods it is probably better to use the full BED-BASED LUMBAR PAIN MANEUVER, including the preliminary FLEXION IN TRACTION component.

This MANEUVER doesn't need to be looked upon as a morning constitutional inconvenience. Rather, it can be accomplished by incorporating it into a means of putting on your socks and shoes or your pants and underwear, "killing two birds with one stone"--or, better: "filling one disc with two bones."

Putting on shoes or pants-wear in the mornings can be either a painful proposition that commits your day to misery or a complement to your back management. Think about what is happening when you "naturally" get up in the morning without any of *The O'Connor Technique (tm)* considerations. Your muscles are still maximally relaxed from a night's rest when you do a "sit-up" to rise out of bed. Then you usually sit on the edge of the bed and put that relaxed back in the most severe FLEXION it will probably experience all day, as you bring your feet and hands to the same level so they can touch your feet. You obligatorily flex the spine in order to put your socks on, tie your shoes or pull pants on. By so doing, the entire weight of the upper body (that portion above the site of pain) is pressing down on the affected Lumbar disc, causing it to migrate posteriorly in the first moments of the day's upright posture if it hasn't already had a good start by sleeping on a too-soft or too-hard bed. Then, when trying to pull on a tight shoe or pants, you increase the stress on the disc by the strength of your upper arm's pulling ability. Worse, is to try to do it while standing or jumping around, when the risk of losing your balance is added which could cause you to fall. These are forces the back should not be exposed to at anytime, let alone when all the muscles are just waking up.

To counteract this tendency, alternative dressing techniques can be designed into your morning behavior that incorporate principles of *The O'Connor Technique (tm)*. First, **elevating the feet to a position above the floor level by placement on the chair or box at the side or the foot of the bed can be used to make the flexion less severe or non-existent**. The elevated platform can be a fashionable end table, an antique trunk, or simply a chair. Make certain that whatever you choose, it is stable and will not slide out from under your feet.

Before going to sleep, you can place your clothing articles on the chair within easy reach of your hands. You can slide your legs over the edge, placing your feet on the chair. Continue to slide until your buttocks and Lumbar spine CASCADES over the edge of the bed while your feet remain on the chair. This action places the Lumbar spine in UNWEIGHTED EXTENSION without activating any muscle groups that would interfere with the TRACTION process which is simultaneously occurring and being assisted by the weight of the legs. The back is now especially able to be put in a maximum degree of EXTENSION IN TRACTION because there was not prior contraction activity of the back muscles.

Now, once the back is in this position, give it a few seconds to slowly equilibrate. It takes time for the ligamentous structures to come to full length, and they should not be forced. When waiting that few seconds, it is helpful to take in deep breaths and, as they are exhaled, an intentional effort is made to further relax the muscles of the back. Also, doing a mild "hula dance" circumductional movement gently with the hips alternating with relaxing again a few times can free up the disc space allowing the displaced fragments to re-centralize.

This is now the ideal time to put on your lower extremity garments. Putting one leg up and resting it across the other such that the lateral part of the ankle is positioned on the opposite knee. Brings the foot and hand together. The placement of the legs can be changed by moving the chair or repositioning the feet. The closer the legs are drawn to the body the more Lumbar flexion is induced. This is okay because the spine is UNWEIGHTED and in TRACTION. This FLEXION becomes advantageous because the posterior longitudinal ligaments are recruited to push the disc material more centrally into disc space opened by the TRACTION which is still being supplied by the hips.

You can also leave the feet on the chair, pull the chair very close to the bed, and reach them by simply flexing at the knees. Of course the thigh obstructs your view, but if you are old enough to have back pain, you probably have dressed enough times for it not to be necessary to see your feet to put on your socks. This positioning allows you to perform the lower extremity dressing functions without WEIGHT-BEARING FLEXION because you can remain on your back, on the bed, and relaxed. If flexion does occur, it is a NON-WEIGHT-BEARING FLEXION and lets the feet get close enough to the hands to let the clothing get on without pain. The shoes are put on in a likewise fashion and tied while the back is kept in hanging status. I would recommend that shoes without laces be worn because it lengthens the time of this process and loafer type shoes can be put on once you are standing.

The alternative, usual, means of dressing while standing or sitting on a chair "normally" does just the opposite because the back is, without fail, weighted and placed in flexion. Starting out the day with this activity actually puts pressure on the disc that can only increase its chances of further posterior migration and makes no sense.

After the garments are on and you are ready to stand, again, re-adjust the spine with the "hula"-type partially UNWEIGHTED CIRCUMDUCTION; and, then, allow the Lumbar spine to assume an extended position. Once it is in full EXTENSION, the feet are brought directly under the buttock by leaning backwards on the bed. You will find that in order to do this most effectively you can do it as described in the HIP-HANG LUMBAR PAIN MANEUVER Section;

alternatively , the toes can be bent (curled superiorly or dorsiflexed) but with the bottom of the toes flat on the floor as the heels are pointed upwards towards the buttocks. Either way, the Lumbar spine is then allowed to continue its CASCADE over the edge of the bed until it ends in a kneeling stance. At the same time this is happening, a steadily increasing ACTIVE EXTENSION should be attempted in the direction of the source of the back pain. If it is in the midline, then the muscles of the erector spinae system should be contracted equally. If the pain is to one side or the other, that side should be preferentially contracted so that when finally coming to rest with the buttocks resting on the heels the Lumbar spine is in full EXTENSION directed towards the site of the herniation.

Holding this EXTENSION, you then stand up as carefully as possible, using your hands to help bring you to the standing position without being caused to flex the Lumbar spine. The chair's back can be used to pull oneself to standing by pulling it towards the body, or the hands can be put behind the back and the arms used to push one's self to standing.

Alternatively, you can stand directly up from the point where the back is in full EXTENSION. However, the Lumbar spine must be locked in EXTENSION and standing up without going to your knees first seems to require that the Lumbar spine flex unless you have something very stable to grasp so as to pull one's self to full standing position.

With this MANEUVER, any subtle disc material migration that occurred during the night has a good chance of being reversed. If your day is started out with the discs centralized, the probability is increased markedly that they will stay that way and remain pain-free so long as no WEIGHT-BEARING FLEXION is allowed the remainder of the day.

Make certain that you never try to manipulate your feet or tie your shoes while sitting on the edge of the bed or standing while bending over in flexion to put on your socks. If you don't have the chair or time to go through the entire MANEUVER, it is usually sufficient to lay back on the bed with your hips hanging; and, tucking your knees to your chest, put on the socks while there is no weight applied to the Lumbar spine. If this is insufficient yet you find it inconvenient or unsuccessful going through an entire MANEUVER, try simply leaning back on the bed and pull your legs close to your abdomen with the knees flexed while moving your hips as though you were wagging your tail. Then simply relax your back muscles and let your spine go into EXTENSION IN TRACTION without activating any of the muscles. This can be done because you don't have to tighten the erector spinae muscles to let your feet go to the floor. Once they are on the ground, do a mild hanging "hula-dance"-type MANEUVER (THERAPEUTIC CIRCUMDUCTION IN TRACTION), letting the spine finish in EXTENSION; then, by selectively contracting the erector spinae muscles, lock it into exaggerated EXTENSION or HYPEREXTENSION aimed at the exact point where the discomfort originates.

Attention! If, at this point or any point in which you are putting a load on the disc, you feel a pinching sensation as though your vertebrae have something wedged between them, DO NOT PROCEED WITH THE ACTION . Either repeat the partial MANEUVER or do an entire BED-BASED MANEUVER until the pinching does not occur, or get up as best you can without increasing your level of discomfort. None of these MAINTENANCE MANEUVERS should result in greater pain than you are already experiencing. They may change the character of the pain or you may feel pulling or some other sensation; but an increased painful sensation means that you are not ready for the WEIGHT-BEARING IN EXTENSION part of the

MANEUVER.

The final stage of the MANEUVER is to get your feet under you and, keeping your back in HYPEREXTENSION aimed along a vertical axis of the site of the pain (which should be directly over the herniation), get to your feet without any flexion. This constitutes the WEIGHT-BEARING HYPEREXTENSION component of the MANEUVER.

Once up, put your hands on your hips, spread your legs apart till your feet are about shoulder width apart, lift the part of your body above the painful spinal segment by pushing down on your hips with your arms and swivelling your hips like you were painting horizontal lines back and forth on the wall with a paint brush held between your legs. The idea is to HYPEREXTEND the spine at the exact level of the involved disc and CIRCUMDUCT it through its posterior range of motion, as described earlier at the end of THE HIP-HANG MANEUVER. This action can centralize disc material that was partially moved by the previous actions. A disc on the verge of going in can be caused to be completely moved anteriorly at this point, if that hasn't been accomplished at any of the other stages of the total MANEUVER.

From here on out, for the rest of the day, make every effort to keep your back in EXTENSION and avoid FLEXION like the plague. You should walk away with the extensor musculature in tone. Oddly enough, this activity, especially depending upon the strength of the EXTENSIONS, strengthens the extensors through an isometric type exercise. Using the logic of the weight-lifter's arm getting so strong that he can no longer fully open at the elbow gives one reason to believe that the same thing done in EXTENSION at the back will keep the back from fully flexing. Thereby, on a daily basis you can AVOID FLEXION and accentuate EXTENSION to preferentially keep your back out of the degrees of flexion that predispose to posterior disc migration.

Cervical--Head-Hanging Morning Extensions

For the Upper Thoracic or Cervical Spine, a similar technique can be practiced. Of course, you would want to focus largely on CASCADING your neck off of the edge of the bed rather than your low back. For the Low Cervical and Upper Thoracic it is more valuable to initiate this MANEUVER with hanging your head over the edge of the side of the bed first with the painful side up in a FLEXION IN TRACTION effort so as to recruit the peripheral capsular ligaments into pushing disc material over the lips of the vertebral basins (that is the biconcave surfaces). Also, positioning your body somewhat close to the foot of the bed makes the ultimate dismount easier. The degree to which you would hang your head over the edge depends upon how low in the neck the pain is located. The lower in the neck the pain, the more you would hang it over the edge until you can feel the area of pain change its character.

Then, CIRCUMDUCTING the neck by rolling the body with the lower trunk and legs, while keeping the neck musculature inactivated, moves the disc material centrally enough to make the ensuing EXTENSION effective.

The EXTENSION component is most easily accomplished if you simply roll to the painful-site-down position and hang there for a few minutes, lock your neck into EXTENSION and get up by sliding your legs off of the end or side of the bed.

Alternatively, you can start by scooting your legs off of the end (foot) of the bed then let their weight pull the remainder of your face-up body off; and, since your head is hanging off the edge, it will necessarily have to be dragged up onto the bed or pivoted around until it can be CASCADED in into EXTENSION. It is almost impossible to effect this MANEUVER without going to the floor with your body or locking your neck into EXTENSION over the site of the pain and standing up in that position with your neck cocked fully to the side of the pain and slightly to the posterior. **However, if there is a pinching or wedge-like pain still felt when you go into EXTENSION as you CASCADED, the disc material is most likely still too far out peripherally to allow for WEIGHT-BEARING HYPEREXTENSION to move it centrally--so do not try to force it.** Either try again, do a full arm-assisted TRACTION MANEUVER as described in THE HEAD HANG section or wait until you have the time and opportunity to do a full arm-assisted TRACTION MANEUVER combined with some DYNAMIC POSITIONING.

Once in full EXTENSION over the site of the pain, the musculature of the neck's extensors can finally be activated and fully contracted. This action should trap the disc material and force it centrally as well as, if done repeatedly over time, preferentially strengthen those extensors to prevent future posterior displacement of the disc material.

Thoracic--Morning Extensions

For the Thoracic region, the wherewithal to self-design a combination of the movements, described above, that incorporate enough of both to effectively mobilize the vertebrae and discs at the region where the pain is located should be obvious by now. The process is so closely related to the MANEUVERS described under the Thoracic region that it only requires the reader to review the appropriate sections to gain full advantage of the principle and apply it to the getting-out-of-bed setting. For Upper Thoracic disc pain, refer to the HEAD-HANG section and for Lower Thoracic disc pain, refer to the HIP-HANG section. Simply positioning differently until your problem disc is the one undergoing the TRACTION, FLEXION, or EXTENSION is all the modification necessary to properly constitute a MANEUVER that functions at the Thoracic level.

CHAPTER SIX: ANCILLARY TOPICS

This chapter deals with numerous ancillary topics that have relevance for back pain sufferers yet have only a tangential relationship to the mechanical principles to which the bulk of this book is devoted. They are varied concepts of associative importance in the prevention and successful resolution of pain so as to "make bad backs better ;" however, they don't easily fit into any categorical grouping. The reader is encouraged to review them and read those sections that have pertinence to their individual concerns and needs.

ACUTE PAIN MANAGEMENT STRATEGY

If you have just injured or re-injured your back and the pain is intense, you can be said to be in "acute" pain. Trying to do MANEUVERS too close to the actual timing of a forceful injury usually is non-productive because often the pain makes every movement (even the therapeutic ones) untenable. After treating many patients immediately after a severe injury, I have learned that most of them are intolerant of any movement; so I have routinely advised rest in the acutely painful situation.

Immediately after the onset of severe, acute, pain, put the involved spinal segment into the position that puts slight comfortable unweighted TRACTION and mild EXTENSION on the disc in pain.

A simple rule of thumb would be to put the affected spinal segment in the most comfortable DYNAMIC POSITION IN EXTENSION with only a small, comfortable component of TRACTION. The degree of TRACTION should only be enough to adequately UNWEIGHT the affected segments. Figure 1 shows a

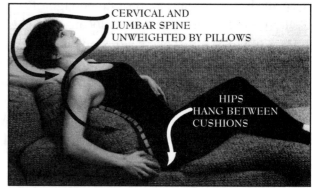

Figure 1 Ideal position for relieving acute Lumbar pain

generically stable position for most spinal pain especially the Cervical and Lumbar region. It is easily adopted by anyone who has a couch with cushions that can be moved. However, the same arrangement can be made on the floor or bed with enough pillows. Note that most of the weight is taken off of the spine by the slight reclining pose. All the natural lordotic (concave) curves of the spine are supported by selective positioning of pillows and cushions that put the spinal segment in an ideal DYNAMIC POSITION. The pillows provide support to maintain EXTENSION and unload the discs. Notice that the hips are between the separated seat cushions because this allows them to partially hang in slight TRACTION. Of course, this position can be modified to accommodate the exact site of pain.

Stay in this position as much as possible and make it your "bed rest" position for a

couple of days if necessary. Studies indicate that the bed rest period is ideally kept at around four days. I have found the position depicted in Figure 1 as the best Low Back Pain alleviating position for a number of reasons, one of which is that it allows you to eat, read, watch TV, etc. without the necessity of much movement, especially WEIGHT-BEARING FLEXION. Should it be necessary to get up, by not being in a recline, you are already half-way there when you need to accomplish an activity of daily living. Taking yourself to a bed is okay so long as pillows are correctly used to create a mild DYNAMIC POSITIONING in EXTENSION IN TRACTION; but, since you will have to eat and being in bed is usually boring after awhile, with this position, you can sleep if necessary but remain in a position allowing some level of function. Also, the knees, you will note, are supported in a semi-flexed position. This takes a stretching pressure off of the sacral region that can aggravate Lumbar pain.

When the pain is so intense that you need to be immobilized, **pain medicines are not only justified but usually are a necessity**. A simple guideline for using medicines during back pain episodes that are brought on by trauma or lifting wrong or "over doing it," is to take only enough to **control the pain**. If you are familiar with the MANEUVERS to get out of pain, you can **immediately attempt the MANEUVERS that you have found successful. Then, if the pain is not immediately and dramatically alleviated, using acetaminophen or/and narcotic pain killers during the first few days, while also taking an anti-inflammatory medicine to get control of inflammation as soon as possible, is a good way to reduce the predictable severity.**

If the episode is severe, the events of pain frequent or prolonged, you can expect inflammation to play a role. Don't wait until it gets well-established before acting against it with the anti-inflammatory medicines like Ibuprofen, Naproxen, Aspirin, etc. For severe, sudden onset pain, it is not unreasonable to take relatively powerful narcotics so long as they are decreased in dosing at the earliest possible opportunity. There is no reason to suffer just because you fear that you might get addicted. You have to get these drugs from doctors anyway, so just mention that getting addicted is a concern of yours and request that he make certain you don't over-use them. Doctors in general are now reluctant to prescribe powerful and effective pain relievers because the Drug Enforcement Agency has so intruded upon the practice of medicine that they fear losing their license to prescribe if they happen to fall outside of some secret computer surveillance calculation. Also, some people tend to abuse these medicines. One way of approaching this is to make it clear to your doctor that you only need them for a short time and you have no intention of requesting repeated refills.

Once you have the pain under control and are relaxed, **direct your focus to, or actually feel, your back muscles that are found on either side of the midline spinous processes (the line of bony bumps that run down the middle of your back), if the muscles are hard, enlarged by a constant contraction, and unable to relax or jerk and spasm with the slightest movement, consider taking a muscle relaxant.** By all means, if you do, do not attempt to function normally, bend over, work, or exercise while under their influence.

Since you should be at "bed rest" until the severe pain subsides, do everything possible to stay immobile. I do not recommend lying in bed, flat on your back or even (as some advocate) in a fetal position with a pillow between your legs. You are free to try these positions, but they usually allow the Cervical and Lumbar spine to remain relatively flexed. Depending upon which side you choose, you could be lying such that the affected disc is put in postero-lateral flexion away from the side of the herniation, which will result in greater protrusion pressure and consequently more pain if the fissure is laterally oriented.

A couch is a better place that can allow you to use pillows to position yourself so that the affected segments can be put in the ideal degree of TRACTION and EXTENSION and kept that way. Realistically, the back pain sufferer is managed easier if kept in the living room and remains an actively involved family member rather than shut away in the bedroom. In essence, it is no small coincidence that this position is the one adopted by astronauts, since the gravitational forces during lift-off have to be evenly distributed. Back pain makes gravity your enemy. Since this position allows you to read easily, I would recommend getting out this book and reviewing its principles while you are immobilized.

If you are in severe pain, getting up to go to the bathroom should be your only activity; but, depending on your situation, you may have to take care of children, live alone and have to feed yourself, or perform real world *et cetera*. In that event, dismount from your position of most comfort slowly and carefully, making an attempt to begin bearing weight in mild EXTENSION only so long as a pinching sensation doesn't occur. If pinching occurs, then that indicates that the disc is still protruding; and, you should make attempts to do the appropriate MANEUVERS to get it "in" as soon as possible. One of these MANEUVERS should be to dismount the couch with a HIP-HANGING EXTENSION IN TRACTION. The transition from this position to an EXTENSION IN TRACTION is simplified since the manner in which you recline minimizes the need to activate muscles and reduces their opportunity to go into or stay in spasm. Spasm, as you may recall, prevents MANEUVERS from working because it closes the space between vertebral bones; and anything you can do to prevent it is advantageous.

If the spasm is too significant, don't attempt the MANEUVERS until the analgesics and the muscle relaxants have had time to work and your back "quiets down." Attempting these MANEUVERS too soon in the presence of spasm is usually unproductive. Be patient, the spasm usually doesn't persist all that long, even if you don't use muscle relaxants. In my own experience, after an acute injury or a bad exacerbation, the first day of the pain is usually the worst; and, regardless of what you do, it decreases after that because the mind becomes accustomed to the pain, the nerve fibers get exhausted from being activated so frequently, and it doesn't seem so novel to the brain after about the first 24-48 hours.

After the spasm is controlled and the acute pain is somewhat tolerable, you may assume that it is safe and prudent to carefully perform the DIAGNOSTIC CIRCUMDUCTION and MANEUVERS in an attempt to centralize the disc material. Of course, this is assuming also that you failed in the opportunity to prevent pain immediately by applying the previously described principles or did not perform a MANEUVER soon enough to get the disc material centralized prior to its extreme peripheralization. One of the major points of this book is to raise the readers' intellect to the point where these events rarely or never happen; however, I'm enough of a realist to write this chapter for that possibly inevitable occasion and for those who are suffering their first episode.

The sooner you accomplish a MANEUVER to put the disc material back in place, the sooner you will begin to substantially reduce the pain. If the MANEUVERS are unsuccessful in achieving a restoration of full range of motion, it can be because spasm or pain is too great to properly accomplish them. Too, fear plays a role at this point. Since you have just felt the worst pain you possibly can conceive of outside of an amputation or a gunshot wound, you are most likely very reluctant to perform **any** movement that may reproduce that pain. All I can do at that point is ask you to trust in *The O'Connor Technique (tm)* as the most highly probable method of resolving the pain and slowly proceed with the most appropriate MANEUVER. If you follow the instructions and adhere to the precautions, you are highly unlikely to come to any further harm or increased pain overall.

The MANEUVERS can be stopped when you have achieved a return to a full range of motion. However, all of the pain may not necessarily have terminated. Don't forget, in most herniation or protrusion injuries, there was sufficient force to break cartilaginous and ligamentous tissues. That is certainly enough force to tear adjacent structures and do damage to other innervated tissues like muscle, ligament, and bone. So, don't expect the pain of that trauma to immediately dissipate simply because the disc material has re-centralized. In my own experience, a couple weeks is not unusual to expect these damaged structures to heal to the point that they are largely pain free. That is why the use of Non-Steroidal Anti-Inflammatory medicines should probably be used continuously for at least this amount of time.

Once the pain has subsided and you are convinced the disc material has re-centralized, it is time to start gradually strengthening the extensor musculature while all the while maintaining the maximum amount of comfortable EXTENSION. This activity must necessarily wait until full range of motion is consistently maintained because, if you cannot fully extend without a crimping-like pain, the disc material has not yet centralized. If it is not centralized, EXTENSION and strengthening of the extensors will be too painful to tolerate and not in your best interests.

SUPPORT DEVICES AND APPURTENANCES

Some back pain experts recommend against spinal braces, corsets, or supports; however, I think their concerns are misplaced. A national survey revealed that less than one percent of orthopedists responded that they never used them. A number of my patients wouldn't be without them, either. Not because they are so weakened that they can't be without them, but because they are nice to have around when performing activities that might stress the back or, when their back has been bothering them, to achieve an increased degree of stability.

The usual argument against back braces alludes to the possibility that the back muscles will weaken if brace use is prolonged. No standard, commercially available, Lumbar support that I'm familiar with will restrict or limit movement to the extent that muscles atrophy to a substantial degree. Regardless of its shape or type, it cannot be so tight as to make you unable to comfortably breathe. If you can breathe, it is not so tight as to prevent the reasonable degree of movement necessary to prevent the back or abdominal muscles from significantly weakening. Atrophy only occurs when muscles are prevented from moving such as in a cast. Back supports don't prevent movement inasmuch as they restrict movement at the furthest reaches of the range of motion. When you try to bend too far forward while in the brace, its abdominal tightening reminds you that you shouldn't be making that movement.

Too, I find when my back is acting up, **simply sleeping with a rigid Lumbar support or brace in place can provide the ideal amount of Lumbar support necessary to most times put**

the disc back in effortlessly while I sleep and keep it "in" when I am caused to sleep in a strange bed or while camping out. I usually take it with me on vacations because I routinely find myself over-doing it; and, the result is a ruined vacation if I get into pain. So, I wear it for protection sometimes and for therapy other times. I, like most patients, have found that following the principles of *The O'Connor Technique (tm)* leads to having to wear the brace less and less. I am to the point that I only use it about every six months and only then for a night or two at the most.

LUMBAR SUPPORTS

For persons who are in acute low back pain or find their Lumbar spine frequently "going out," I recommend the temporary use of back supports or braces. My personal favorite is a flexible, elastic corset-type device with a *CONTOUR FORM* moldable plastic insert (See Figure 2). I have found it to be very comfortable and effective, with no risk of inducing atrophy. The plastic is heated and placed into a pocket in the girdle while it is being worn and, as it cools, it forms to the desired Lumbar curvature to induce a mild degree of EXTENSION. This is very effective for at least two reasons: It interferes with WEIGHT-BEARING FLEXION; and, when seated or reclining, it provides wide-spread Lumbar support. It can be combined with a weight-lifter's belt to add strength or simply put on under your clothes with a regular belt that also holds up your pants when worn over it.

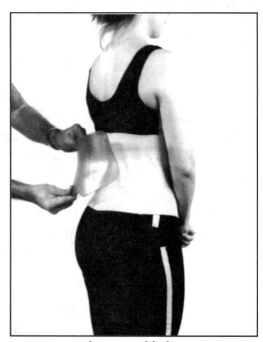

Figure 2 Plastic molded insert corset-type device

CRUTCHES

Try to avoid bearing weight on a herniated Thoracic or Lumbar disc until you are reasonably certain that the disc material will only move anteriorly when you do. One means of doing this is to use crutches during ambulation attempts. **Crutches allow you to take the weight off of the affected disc and still walk around.** You should coordinate your crutch use so that, whenever your weight is on your legs, your back is in slight extension if you can manage it. If crutches are not available, simply a long, strong staff, higher than your own height, can be put to the same purpose, just like in Biblical times.

Crutches are an excellent means of getting through the immediate post-traumatic period in order to walk around. Even though bed rest is frequently given as a prescription for the time period following an acute injury, it is sometimes realistically impossible to manage. Life would be grand if everyone with an acute back injury were able to lie in bed and have someone take care of them for the several days necessary. Back in the days when the medical system truly took care of "people" and "patients" rather than "consumer units," one could be expected to be admitted to a hospital for adequate nursing care. However, since the administrators took over the system, a doctor would be criticized and hounded by the utilization-review nurse for having the fiscal irresponsibility of taking care of the needs of a human being. So, one is forced to remain at home to ambulate without assistance to the toilet, table, and automobile, to traverse to and from the doctor's office, the diagnostics facility, and place of employment. When in unremitting pain, even standing up can be a feat of Herculean endurance. So, crutches come in handy.

If you can't afford a new pair of crutches, any Goodwill or Salvation Army usually has a barrel full of them. They function by allowing the body to prevent WEIGHT-BEARING. The weight is taken off of the hips, and placed under the armpits. With the weight removed from the damaged disc, the pressure of the herniated disc material impinging upon the peripheral ligaments and nerves is reduced. They also assist in getting up and down by providing a support structure for the arms and hands to use to UNWEIGHT the affected disc.

When using crutches to walk, you will be constantly weighting and un-weighting. The more time you spend in an unweighted state, the less pain you will experience. Recall, the force of WEIGHT-BEARING contributes to the pressures acting on a herniated disc. The crutches can be managed to keep the affected disc unweighted most of the time. As you hang your upper torso from the crutches, you capitalize upon the TRACTION created when the crutches are bearing the weight of the body. Eventually, you must ambulate, and WEIGHT-BEARING is unavoidable. So, in the process of WEIGHT-BEARING, a concerted effort should be made to place the affected disc in EXTENSION so that a WEIGHT-BEARING IN EXTENSION can function. How this can function to re-centralize disc material can be appreciated by reviewing the STANDING TRACTION/EXTENSION MANEUVER for Lumbar pain in Chapter 5 and treating your crutches as the platform for repeated MANEUVER equivalents as you use the crutches to ambulate. Then, while accomplishing the necessary task of walking, you can centralize the displaced disc material. If not, at least your actions can keep the disc unit in the ideal environment for central migration of disc material; and, when the damaged disc is ready to centralize, it can.

CERVICAL SUPPORTS

Commercially available Cervical braces function reasonably to maintain the neck in an UNWEIGHTED condition for daily upright activities. Routinely, one sees people walking around with various types of neck braces. They actually do help relieve pain quite often or all those people wouldn't be putting up with the embarrassment and inconvenience of the brace. I see little advantage in people wearing the soft collars since they don't have sufficient structural support to unload the head off of the neck; but the hard collars with padding can provide genuine support that is often the only source of relief in the acutely painful situation. However, sleeping with either is probably not in one's best interest. They are uncomfortable and supply no support to the natural lordotic curvature to MAINTAIN EXTENSION. Rather, I would sleep with the Cervical supports described and portrayed in this book's section on CERVICAL DYNAMIC POSITIONING and shown in that Section's Figure 1.

Note, in Figure 1, there are two supports. The one wrapped around the neck is for Higher and Middle Cervical discs. The other is aligned perpendicular to the spine and placed more inferiorly directly under the site of pain. This type of support (even if it is only a folded towel) would be used for Low Cervical or High Thoracic discs. The standard, commercially-available, soft collars are too thin to provide proper EXTENSION MAINTENANCE during sleep and the hard collars are too uncomfortable in which to sleep. It is not unreasonable in the presence of a Low Cervical or High Thoracic disc problem to use both types of support at the same time. The neck roll keeps the Cervical lordosis maintained while the more inferiorly placed support keeps the affected disc in slight EXTENSION IN TRACTION.

The cheapest, simplest and most effective means for supporting the Cervical spine is a common "terry cloth" towel rolled to the comfortably ideal size, put around the neck like a collar, and secured in the front either with a light string or a large safety pin. Unfortunately, it is bulky and difficult to wear during the daytime upright activity period; so, a standard, commercially-available soft or "Philadelphia" collar is sometimes the only available support, although inadequate.

DEPRESSION

Provided that you have done everything right, you should be out of pain and back to functioning by following *The O'Connor Technique (tm)*; however, the realist in me must raise its ugly head. During the painful episode in which back pain pervades your consciousness and regardless of whether you get better or not, coming to terms with this new state of affairs can result in a prolonged grieving response. **This longing for what cannot be is sometimes referred to as depression.**

With persistent back pain, anyone can get depressed. After all, one can be unequivocally confronted by the loss of cherished or even routine activities. Once this is recognized and accepted into the psyche as a permanent, or probably permanent, reality--it is a natural, human response to grieve the loss of a significant component of your former self.

If you are in pain, you relate to people differently, and they relate to you differently. You usually, out of necessity, become more dependant upon other people; and, in some ways, that can be self-defined as degrading, especially if you have been a strong and independent personality up until then. Prolonged pain often changes people's personalities, they become less tolerant, more argumentative, impatient, and "cranky." Stay like that long enough, and you begin viewing the world in a different light.

There is a profound amount of uncertainty involved in pain of this level and duration. You can never be certain if you will ever get out of it. The prospect of living the rest of your whole life feeling as you do during an acutely painful episode, is anxiety producing and, consequently, after a prolonged period, depressing. How deeply and how long the depression lasts varies from person to person; but I'm pretty convinced it is universal in the presence of a genuine, chronically painful, disc condition. Many people would argue otherwise; however, I would counter that they just haven't experienced ample agony to develop a competent perspective.

I have had the opportunity to observe numerous patients who were young, fit, active, and suddenly forced to live the life of a "cripple" (their choice of words, not mine). No, they don't mean "alter-abled" or "physically challenged," They mean "crippled." They have shared with me their fears and profound disappointment at having been dealt this sudden insult to their bodies, psyche, and life-style. In that context, **it is not an admission of further imperfection to resort to the use of an anti-depressant**. The drugs exist, they are effective and do not, in the majority of cases, have to be looked upon as a life-long support therapy. Neither are they addictive; after the pain resolves, they usually can be stopped.

When you find yourself crying, frequently sighing, having feelings of worthlessness, thoughts of death or disease can't be shaken from your usual thought patterns, you're getting tired of living, constantly in a foul mood, even the things you can do that used to be fun no longer are, you aren't enjoying the company of people, or your eating or sleeping patterns become bizarre and unusual, you have a good chance of being depressed. In most cases, this passes without pharmaceutical assistance; however, if it is prolonged and you sustain a grief reaction for too long, you get into a state of chemical imbalance of the neuro-transmitters in your brain that may prevent you from recovering by your own will power, even if your back gets better. Depression is a strange bird, sometimes you don't even recognize it because you are too depressed to see it. That's probably an excellent time to try an anti-depressant. There's no shame in it, anymore than there is "shame" in your back becoming "bad." It is a sometimes unavoidable consequence of the major loss and constant pain accompanying the disability of disc disease. There is no reason not to treat it the same way you would the pain--you do what is necessary to make it better, even if it means taking a medicine for your "mind".

I would not recommend a "self-medicating" alternative with alcohol or prolonged use of narcotics, as people so often do. It's a better idea to turn to the same primary care physician who manages your back pain for antidepressants because they are available only by prescription and he/she would be the one most likely to be knowledgeable of your situation to prescribe them without the attendant stigma of going to a psychiatrist.

I have arrived at a simplified means of determining which of the two major classes of depression medicines should be tried first that serves my patients rather well. If you have trouble getting to or staying asleep, first try a low dose of an anti-depressant that has the side effect of sleepiness. This includes drugs like Amitriptyline, Maprotiline, Trazodone, etc. They are effective, safe when used as directed, not addictive, and widely used.

If you seem to be tired all the time, you can't seem to stay awake (and it is not due to the narcotic analgesics or other medicines such as anti-histamines or other drugs taken for other reasons), or getting-going in the morning is a Sisyphian task (that's the Greek mythological character who was sentenced by the Gods to an infinity of rolling a great boulder up a hill in Hades only to have it roll back down before reaching the top), first try a low dose of the new Serotonin Re-uptake Inhibitors, like Prozac, Paxil, Zoloft, etc. One of the advantages of these medicines is that they seem to control diet. You eat less while on them. That can be important because with boredom and depression people often tend to eat more. This, combined with the back pain enforced inactivity, can cause people tend to gain weight, which ultimately increases their back pain problems.

Monitor your behavior and reactions over the next few weeks to months. Count your sighs per hour and if they don't markedly decrease or you still find yourself crying when you see Lassie pulling the child from the fire or watching emotional dramas, consider the need for an increased dose. Your doctor should advise you on that score.

PAIN MEDICINES

Pain medicines can simplistically be divided into two main categories on the basis of their mechanism for decreasing pain. Those that largely function by simply interfering with pain sensations in the brain and those that stop inflammation. Neither of them will solve the pain problem if the cause is mechanical. If the disc material is physically de-centralized and inducing pain by impacting upon nerves and ligaments as described earlier in Chapter Two, a person might take any and all of them that can be put into a body; and, when they wear off, the pain will still be there. More often than not, **the pain will remain regardless of the amount you take until the mechanical source is alleviated, only you will be too "doped-up" to care**.

The medicines that interfere with the pain sensations when they reach the brain are usually referred to as **opiates or narcotics** and include Codeine, Vicodin, Talwin, Darvon, Demerol, Morphine, etc.. They are best used during the acute episode when the sharp, disabling, pain makes even bed rest agonizing. They **should only be used for a short period because they require increasing doses to maintain the same level of pain control and often result in a dependence upon the medicine--if not outright addiction.** It is unfortunate that many physicians in today's *UNHOLY DRUG WAR* feel intimidated into believing that they cannot prescribe these medicines as frequently as necessary because of fear that the Federal Drug Enforcement Agency's computers will single them out for reprisal. This is not some perception I alone have, this thought comes to me through a conversation with one of the most competent, intelligent, and ethical physicians I have ever met. He is an anesthesiologist who recently went into the field of pain management and voiced this fear to me. It is not an unreasoned fear if one considers the federal government's response to California voters' *Compassionate Use of Marijuana Law*. They told physicians that they would revoke the DEA license of any doctor who so much as discussed the use of marijuana with patients. The *DRUG WAR* seems to have given them the power to ignore the Constitutional Right of Free Speech. The DEA also seems to feel it can ignore the results of democracy if it doesn't suit its purposes since it also threatened to revoke any Oregon physician's license if he were to prescribe a drug of the type that can be used for assisted suicide. Such is the state of affairs when a government declares war on its people.

The fact of the matter is that some patients, as a consequence of the arguments put forth in Chapter One regarding the inadequacy of our society's management of back pain, are genuinely in recurrent pain so often that they require substantial amounts of narcotic medicines for repeated periods of time. However, if they end up addicted, the doctor gets blamed, sued, or has his license revoked regardless of whether he was treating legitimate pain or not.

The fact of the matter is that for many patients, narcotics are the only source of relief; and, unfortunately, when no other option is forthcoming, they desire refills. Statistics say that 70% of back injuries recover in 2-3 weeks and 90% resolve within six weeks. If 90% of adult Americans will experience the problem at some point in their lives[1], then 30% of those adult Americans will be in pain greater than 2-3 weeks, 10% will still be in pain after 6 weeks (and probably will always be in pain). If you are one of those sufferers, you will be the one asking for refills after six weeks. This is sometimes interpreted as "drug-seeking behavior" and narcotics are refused or, the physician, fearing lawsuits or Drug Enforcement Agency intimidation, severely limits their prescriptions. Since most of the time (in the absence of *The O'Connor Technique*) the mechanical source of the pain is not adequately addressed and removed, millions of patients are caused to experience pain for prolonged periods of time. They, then, do engage in "drug-seeking behavior" to limit their discomfort or mask the pain enough so that they can continue with their work or daily activities. Its a sad state of affairs, but the warning stands, do not depend upon narcotics for long term pain relief.

These medicines should only be used occasionally, for severe pain events, and in doses only high enough to make the pain manageable. One should not take narcotic pain medicines so that physical labor can be accomplished. If it hurts bad enough to necessitate pain medicines, the mechanical problem must not have been solved and has to be surmounted before putting any more stress on the disc system. The risk for functional damage is too great. Of course, I say this only in the context of the new understanding engendered and hopefully communicated by this book. In the past, prior to *The O'Connor Technique (tm)* such a pronouncement would have been unrealistic due to an absence of alternatives. Now, there is an alternative because the mechanical problem can be rapidly solved, in most cases. If you are certain that your disc is "in," then a narcotic can be taken for a very short time to cover any residual pain in order that one may continue to function. Incidentally, I have not had to resort to narcotics for ten years.

Many people believe that they cannot take these medicines because they get sick to their stomachs while on them. They assume that this is an "allergy" and avoid the medicines even when in severe pain. Most of the time, this is simply a side effect of the narcotic. Almost all narcotics slow the involuntary muscular actions (peristalsis) of the stomach and intestines so that food does not move through as well. If food is left in the stomach too long, one can experience nausea; and the stomach can be expected to vomit its contents. This should be predicted anytime one prepares to use these medicines and take them only with a tiny amount of easily digested food or limit yourself to small to moderate volumes of liquids while they are acting. Also, don't plan on using your mind while under their influence because they can interfere with judgement, response times, and ability to think or concentrate.

The other major type of pain relievers are the anti-inflammatory medicines such as aspirin, ibuprofen (Advil, Nuprin, Motrin), and the other Non-Steroidal Anti-Inflamatory Drugs (NSAIDS). These are very effective because most back pain is felt to have an inflammatory component[2]. There are many of them on the market and different people respond differently to the various types. Most doctors usually try their favorite brand and, unless that fails to achieve results, stick with it. A person should try a number of them by asking their doctor for samples of different classes of NSAIDS (oops, I forgot, the government's incursion into the practice of medicine has been so heavy-handed that the sampling of these medicines has largely stopped) then rely on the one that provides the most relief with the least side effects.

These medicines should always be taken with food and be aware that they can have significant side effects, especially on the stomach, intestines, and kidneys. About 10-15% of people have to stop the medicines because they get stomach aches or diarrhea. They often cause the stomach to become inflamed. If this happens, take antacids like TUMS, Maalox or Mylanta.

If that doesn't work, discuss the problem with your doctor and he may want to use one of the agents that reduce stomach acid such as Pepsid, Tagamet, or similar agents.

Most importantly, use these medicines for pain of an inflammatory nature. Inflammatory pain usually is a persistently aching pain that is continuous and steady with a sensation of warmth as though the area had been burned. When a disc puts continuous pressure on a ligament or two joint surfaces rub together in an abnormal way, cellular damage is occasioned. This results in white blood cells migrating to the area to clean up the damaged tissue. They release chemical mediators that induce pain. The NSAIDS block the production of these body chemicals.

Again, until the disc material is repositioned and the pressure taken off the adjacent structures, the pain will persist regardless of how many of these medicines you take. However, they are excellent as a means to reduce pain and should be used frequently to manage pain whenever they work effectively because, the longer one lets an inflammation persist, the more damage to the joint occurs. The longer the inflammation goes unopposed, the harder it is to manage.

Give these medicines a sufficient time to work before giving up on them. Don't expect them to ablate all the pain immediately, some do and some don't. It is important to see which ones give the most relief and continue them, if possible, for an appropriate trial. That, in many cases, requires at least three consecutive weeks of use before it can be said that they are ineffective. If you recognize relief while taking them, even if it is not complete, that particular compound probably is working for you as much as can be expected, and that brand should be the one you rely upon most. Also, for conditions that are accompanied by long periods of inflammatory pain, it is a good idea to plan on going on the medicines for a prolonged period of time to keep the inflammatory process suppressed. If you stop these medicines too soon, the inflammation may return and you might constantly be playing "catch-up." Plan on continuing the medicines for a couple days after the pain has resolved until the biological chain of events that produced the pain have been given sufficient time to quiet down and stay that way before stopping the medicines.

Understand too, that these medicines act by stopping the production of pain chemicals. The earlier that they are employed, the less chemicals are produced that will attract more white blood cells and increase inflammatory pain. These medicines are not accepted to be addicting so there is little danger of becoming dependant upon them; however, rather than letting the joints be slowly destroyed by the chemical reactions of inflammation, it is theoretically better, in the absence of side effects, to use these medicines for sufficient periods until, when they are stopped, the inflammatory pain does not return.

Be aware, though, there is another drawback to these medicines and that involves the long-term use causing kidney disease (analgesic nephropathy), making them a two-edged sword. If your lower legs or feet swell (watch for indentions made by your socks) while on them, one has to make a decision between risking the damage caused by prolonged arthritis or the damage to the kidneys from prolonged use. If these drugs are required frequently, the compromise I feel most comfortable with is to take the medicines during periods of pain in the dose necessary to control the pain then, as soon as possible, try to reduce the dose to the lowest effective dose that provides enough relief to make your activities tolerable. Also, you can alternate between these drugs and others like acetaminophen.

If you only get occasional flare-ups or when the back is sore from "over-doing it," after the pain is suppressed for a sufficiently long period (a week is not unusual), you can experiment by stopping them and seeing if the pain returns or increases. If it does, then you have not used them long enough; so go back on them for about an other week and try again until the inflammatory pain stays away after you have discontinued the medicine. Usually, when the back is sore, even after successfully re-centralizing disc material with the MANEUVERS, there is often a residual aching pain that seems to remain even though you can CIRCUMDUCT through the spine's full range of motion in EXTENSION without any inhibition of movement. This implies that the mechanical component is not acting to produce the pain and, by default, the pain is probably inflammatory in nature and best addressed with NSAIDS.

Also, if you predict that your work or unavoidable physical activity will result in pain afterwards or you know that the same level or duration of activity you have planned has resulted in an aching back in the past, take some of these medicines **before** you engage those activities and continue the medicine until you are sure you have controlled the pain.

For a good example, let's say you have to move your household and you are forced to lift, stoop, and carry weight. You know yourself and your back well enough to assume it is unlikely that you will not be able to escape back pain. Despite knowing how to be careful to avoid the WEIGHT-BEARING FLEXION or squatting yet, by experience, you nevertheless usually end up putting your disc "out" and so can expect several days of aching afterwards. Take a dose of the medicine prior to the activity so that it will be in your system for the time that you will be doing the activity. Then, depending upon how much of that activity results in solely inflammatory pain or soreness, let that determine how long you will stay on the medicine. Usually it will be shorter.

Last but not least, don't forget acetaminophen or Tylenol. It is somewhat in a class by itself because no one really knows how it stops pain, but it works. It can be taken safely with NSAIDS or Narcotics and has few side effects except for prolonged use of high doses can cause kidney or liver damage, especially in those with pre-existing liver disease.

MUSCLE RELAXANTS

Muscle relaxants have a definite role in the management of back pain; but this role is limited to those times when there is actual spasm of the back muscles that will not be relieved by heat, massage, and gentle TRACTION.

In my opinion, they are too often inappropriately prescribed and frequently misused. Some are frankly dangerous when taken to excess, especially Flexeril. Many times the back pain is so severe that the patient, after being told the problem is muscular in origin, will take more than the recommended dose to totally eradicate the pain. This can lead to irregular heart rhythms that persist for prolonged periods of time, long after the drug's muscle relaxant properties have been exhausted.

The back muscles spasm as a protective mechanism best referred to as "physiological splinting." When damage occurs to the vertebral column, the muscles undergo spasm, presumably to protect the integrity of the central nervous system. This makes evolutionary sense for every creature from the most primitive segmented worm to modern homo sapiens. Spasm prevents further movement-induced injury and enforces rest. However, in deference to this mechanism's intent, most people with acute back pain and spasm seek and acquire muscle relaxants then attempt to continue with activity. Therein lies the fault. **Once the spasm mechanism that prevents movement is disarmed, the vertebral column is left without protection and the traumatic damage can be magnified by movements that result in posterior migration of the disc.** This can cause a stable injury to advance into further neurological damage that would otherwise have been preventable if muscle relaxants were not misused.

Ideally, muscle relaxants should only be used when one can relax in a position that affords the greatest probability of the disc migrating forward or anteriorly. They should never be used when there is a probability or expectation that WEIGHT-BEARING FLEXION will result in the disc moving posteriorly or backwards. The ideal position in which to rest while the back is in spasm is described earlier as sort of modified seated HIP-HANG utilizing mild EXTENSION IN TRACTION.

Also, muscle relaxants can be used to release the spasm when it prevents the back muscles from relaxing sufficiently to allow TRACTION to be effective on the problem disc unit. When attempts are made to re-position the disc material back into its correct, anatomical position, centrally, in the intervertebral space, muscle spasm can prevent the TRACTION necessary to give the disc material a place to re-locate. If every time TRACTION is attempted the spasm pulls the vertebrae closer together, there is no place into which the misplaced disc material can migrate; and the pressure it is placing on the outer bands of the annulus fibrosus will persist. As long as the pressure remains, the pain will persist. **The muscle relaxants can, in this scenario, intentionally and effectively disarm the spasm mechanism to allow for the disc to be re-positioned with the proper movements so long as while under their influence NO WEIGHT BEARING FLEXION is allowed.**

TRAVELING WITH A BAD BACK

Anyone with a history of spinal pain can probably recall at least one vacation that was ruined due to back or neck pain. A lot of people "on vacation" actually do more physical exertion than at any time during the year. Usually, it also involves activities that they are not accustomed to and consists of a lot of stooping, bending, lifting and prolonged sitting while in transit. There is a tendency to travel more while on vacation, and this implies carrying heavy luggage or remaining in awkward positions for long periods. Many people with bad backs actually avoid traveling because of this phenomenon and tend to consign themselves to routine behaviors that are safe and less likely to result in back pain. This is unfortunate because people with bad backs who do not know the basic principles that cause the pain, how to relieve it, and prevent it, must simply gravitate to those activities that they have learned through experience don't result in pain. This can lead to a very confining lifestyle.

By systematically exploring the most common movements and activities most encountered during traveling, a person can be better equipped to avoid pain and have an enjoyable vacation.

First, avoid lifting luggage. Get someone to help you. Most of the time another person is available to get your luggage into the car. Two people can lift the heavy bags, and you can make several trips at your leisure. Don't hang things around your neck unless you are certain that it stays very close to the center of gravity. Leaning forward with a heavy camera bag strapped around your neck can instantly jerk your neck into flexion and put a disc off center.

If you are required to lift, make sure that your back is in the locked and loaded EXTENSION position (refer to the PRINCIPLES Chapter on AVOIDING WEIGHT-BEARING FLEXION). One of the most dangerous efforts a traveler can make is to lean over a trunk and jerk out a heavy suitcase (See Figure 3). Here, your back is at an extreme mechanical disadvantage; you are horsing up an amount of weight that you rarely lift on a regular basis and are markedly unprepared to do properly.

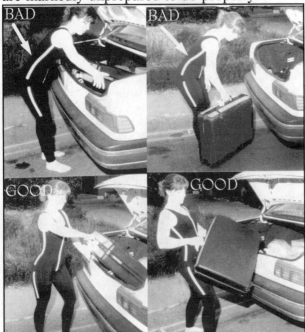

Figure 3 Bad (Flexed) and Good (Extended) ways to remove luggage from trunk

Easy to say, just don't do it, but how can you vacation if you can't lift baggage? Do it in stages, with your arms. Lean over the trunk, place your non-dominant arm locked in EXTENSION on a stable platform (such as the edge of the trunk or another object in the trunk) and lift the object to be moved to the edge of the trunk with just the strength of the dominant arm while keeping the back in EXTENSION by looking upwards.

In fact, while resting your upper body on your arm, step backwards with your feet until your back goes into a swayed position. That way, you have very little probability of accidentally going into WEIGHT-BEARING FLEXION. When you are ready to stand erect again, be certain to shift one of your hips towards the weighted arm, slightly bend your knees to get under the arm to keep any weight off of the Lumbar spine, and keep it in EXTENSION when bringing yourself to the erect, upright position. This way you prevent your Lumbar spine from feeling the weight of the upper body until you are in a full upright stance.

Once the suitcase is on the edge of the trunk, it only needs to be lowered to the ground. Don't forget, similar forces involved in lifting an object are felt on the spine when lowering the object to the ground so keep your back in EXTENSION.

When lifting anything out of a container like a car's trunk, you don't have to pick it up and carry it in one move. Break the moves down into a series of small lifts. Lift one corner and turn the object on its edge. Balance it on a corner and swing it so that when it falls, it will fall onto the edge of the trunk. As it balances, pulling it lets it fall out of the trunk. As it falls, slow the fall with your hand, your legs, or your body, and let it slide onto the ground. Or, you can pull the suitcase to your upper thigh, and then rest its weight on your leg, letting it slide down your leg. That way, you do not use your spine to bear the weight of the object.

The inverse of this concept can be applied when your luggage is on an airport carousel.

Ordinarily, it is necessary to lean over the moving conveyor and jerk the luggage over a retaining barrier. Usually, there is an effort to do this rapidly so that you won't collide with other people or luggage. **Avoid this impulse, allow the movement of the conveyor or other luggage to push the baggage by simply guiding one edge over the retainer wall.** The point is to only lift a part of the suitcase so that you are never caused to lift the weight of the whole.

Whenever you find it unavoidable to manage weights that are knee level, lift objects such that their weight can be supported by an elbow resting on a knee (as in Figure 4). In that manner, the weight is communicated to the tibia of the leg and not felt by the spine.

Many times while traveling, boredom or exhaustion leads to the attempt to sleep in the seated position. Usually, little effort is made to protect the spine from flexion. Heads nod forward and are jerked up spontaneously when discomfort triggers a protective response. The consequence of repeating this activity is that the discs are progressively displaced posteriorly so that by the end of so much as a little nap, the traveler is committed to potentially weeks of neck pain.

The same forces at work on the Lumbar spine are acting to displace the discs when in an attempt to sleep one reclines in a airline or automobile seat. Usually a person loosens the seat belt and slides down in the seat until the Lumbar spine and the Cervical spine are put into relaxed, WEIGHT-BEARING FLEXION. Whether in an

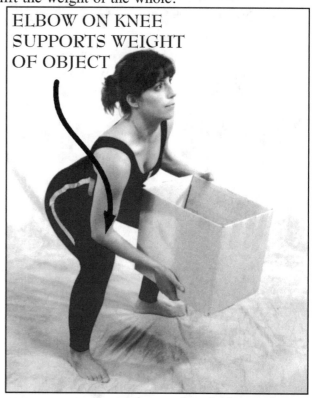

ELBOW ON KNEE SUPPORTS WEIGHT OF OBJECT

Figure 4 Managing the weight of a box at knee level while maintaining Lumbar EXTENSION and causing leg to carry weight.

automobile, a bus station, or an airplane, attempts to sleep in this disadvantageous circumstance can result in a painful vacation without any obvious cause or trauma. You just wake up with pain for no apparent reason.

The solution to these problems when traveling by air is to start by acquiring a couple pillows and a blanket as soon as you board before they are all taken by others. The pillows are used to support the Lumbar spine and the blanket can be rolled into a support for the neck by wrapping it around the neck like a bow-tie and simply tying a large knot in it. By keeping your seat-belt fastened, you can eliminate the natural slumping into flexion. You will be surprised at how much more effective this is than buying those funny little pillows that they sell in catalogues and in airports.

Another tragedy in progress comes when the plane has landed, after slouching in your seat for hours, you jump up so as to be the first person to stand hunched over for another critical ten minutes, long enough to put any number of discs "out" that were not already protruded from

374

hours of WEIGHT-BEARING FLEXION in relaxation. Avoid this by performing an UNWEIGHTING with your arms on the elbow supports, CIRCUMDUCTING IN TRACTION (Hanging "Hula-" type); and, in essence, perform a modified SEATED LUMBAR EXTENSION MANEUVER (see the so-named Section in Chapter Five for directions); however, you can't be expected to go to your knees. Simply rising up in EXTENSION and waiting until you can stand up straight before rising from your seat should suffice.

Sleeping with a large pillow to which you are unaccustomed or on a too soft or too hard a bed, can result in a back pain episode capable of ruining your vacation. By now, it should be apparent to the reader why simply sleeping in a strange place can result in back pain. First, every motel or hotel I've ever been in seems to have huge foam rubber pillows that cock your head into a position almost perpendicular to the plane of the sleeping body. I suspect their intent is to have a large, well-formed, firm, pillow that makes the bed look as though it is new and inviting so you will rent the room. In reality, it is one of the worst enemies of the traveler's neck. My suggestion here is to use something else for a pillow (a folded fluffy towel to support your Lumbar concavity), sleep without a pillow, or bring your own in your suitcase. The best pillow is a feather-type pillow with about a half to a third of the filling that the pillow would ordinarily take if it were full. This allows for the easy shaping of the pillow and tucking of it into the neck spaces to afford the optimal individualized support without causing the neck to go into WEIGHT-BEARING FLEXION.

PREGNANCY AND DELIVERY

Countless women who go through a pregnancy and subsequent delivery relate that their back problems began with these events. **Studies indicate that up to one-third of women in labor have severe, continuous low back pain,** typically described as exceeding that of the contraction pain.[3] **In one study 67% of women reported the presence of pain at delivery, 37% had some back pain at the follow-up examination, and 7% still reported significant back pain at 18 months.**[4] This is not surprising since, usually, the equivalent of a thirty pound increase in weight has been added to their bodies with relatively little time for physical accommodation. Much of this weight is centered at the abdomen which pushes the Lumbar spine into EXTENSION simply while lying supine, not to mention the additional weight that the water retention and fat contribute during WEIGHT-BEARING FLEXION. Too, their ability to sleep in the prone position is denied by a basketball size abdominal mass, thus eliminating an unconscious source of EXTENSION MAINTENANCE during sleep time. Then, to add the final coup-de-grace at delivery, **they are encouraged to lie on a flat, hard surface, without Lumbar support, forcibly flex forward, and brutally load their Lumbar discs by the weight of their body in combination with contracting their abdominal musculature while well-meaning but back-protection-ignorant assistants grab them around the neck and force them into unnaturally violent WEIGHT-BEARING FLEXION while pushing on their abdomens.** All of this activity places the worst of all possible stresses on the Lumbar disc system at a time when some poorly understood hormone-like substances designed to soften cartilaginous tissue is coursing through the body so that the symphysis pubis (the disk-like material composing the junction of the anterior aspects of the pubic bones) can separate to widen the pelvic canal to give the baby's head more room. This same substance acting on the discs might very well be increasing their propensity for damage. The combination of all these conditions cannot do anything other than pre-dispose these women to disc herniation or prolapse.

If these forces aren't bad enough, shortly after the baby is born, the woman enters a period in her life when she will be doing more bending over and lifting than she has probably accomplished in her life when compared with her non-child-bearing years. This may be the reason why **one study of asymptomatic women found disc degeneration on magnetic resonance imaging already present in over one third of women aged 21-40,** the prevalence of one or more degenerate discs increasing linearly with age.[5] Since a good percentage of these women do not have back pain, some researchers argue that the presence of disc degeneration is a "natural phenomenon" that cannot be the source of back pain. I interpret this as faulty logic. Just because a certain percentage of people with NMRI findings of disc disease do not complain of back pain doesn't mean that they do not have disc problems. They may have accommodated to the pain, they may have physiologies that heal more adroitly, the disc material may not be in a position to put actual prolapsing pressure on the capsule, or by unconscious means they may have changed their movement patterns to not utilize the damaged disc units.

Certainly such findings cannot be used to argue that the presence of disc disease on an NMRI is meaningless in the context of pain diagnosis; yet that is a common philosophy and interpretation made by current back pain clinicians and repeated *ad nauseam* over and over when denying people disability claims.

Any woman undergoing a pregnancy should understand that her back is made vulnerable to disc disease by pregnancy, labor and delivery, as well as the post-partum care of the child; and she should make efforts to protect it. First, applying most of the techniques described in this book that relate to preventing back pain by lifting correctly with the disc units in EXTENSION, performing hip hangs to properly load the back every morning, and **AVOIDING WEIGHT-BEARING FLEXION** will help to reduce the probability that the back will be damaged by pregnancy.

Avoiding heavy work can also be assumed to be able to prevent subsequent back problems since, in the same above referenced study, heavy work during the prenatal period and before pregnancy was correlated with pain. A valid conclusion drawn from this study's findings is that women engaged in heavy or monotonous work should be extra diligent to avoid back pain inducing movements, especially prolonged WEIGHT-BEARING FLEXION. Any bending forward with the additional weight of the pregnancy can be damaging. **If a pregnant woman finds herself with pain during a WEIGHT-BEARING FLEXION event, she should immediately stop the movement, unweight the portion of the back where the pain exists and go into EXTENSION by the most immediate means. Do not attempt to straighten up before UNWEIGHTING the painful segment.** Unlike other situations in which only objects are lifted, the additional weight of pregnancy being lifted cannot be dropped because it is attached to the abdomen. **Instead, I recommend that if pain occurs while lifting, no effort should be made to straighten up; but, rather, any weight being lifted should be abandoned and an attempt should be made to immediately find something to grab onto or support the upper body to take the weight off of the affected segment.** If no support object can be reached, carefully lowering yourself to the floor on hands and knees to make the painful segment immediately NON-WEIGHT-BEARING is the best response. Then, letting the affected segment slowly move into an EXTENSION IN TRACTION posture before resuming WEIGHT-BEARING is essential. How you accomplish that is up to you, but a HIP-HANGING OR STANDING EXTENSION on the nearest piece of furniture is probably the best response. During these protective movements, the spine should be guarded so as to insure that no motion is allowed which increases the pain.

The arms must be used to support the body whenever possible. Basically, the pregnant woman should treat her back like a sixty year old's. Elderly people often use their arms to "walk" the upper body's weight to the fully upright position. They use convenient, chairs, tables or any other stable object to help support their weight whenever possible. They don't usually do that because they are tired, they do it because it takes weight off of the Lumbar discs. I've become so adept at observing this phenomenon, I can often identify people with Lumbar disc disease instantly by just watching how they rise from a seated or reclining position. Believe it or not, a person naturally and unconsciously makes those postural concessions because it eliminates pain; or, rather, they learn that if they do not do it, pain results. Unconsciously or consciously they are rewarded for that behavior by some relief of pain.

So, the advantage this book's pregnant (or nonpregnant for that matter) readers have is that they needn't go through that painful learning curve or conditioning process. Going into the pregnancy you can prepare for the probability of pain, predict it, and prevent it. If you don't believe that the disc damage will result from *your pregnancy* because you feel lucky or superior, you can foolishly wait until it does come and then act on it by applying the PRINCIPLES of this book--better late than never. My advice is to **practice the techniques of this book before the pain *makes* you do it.** However, most people have to be convinced that extra effort is necessary before they will accomplish it. I suspect that is human nature. So, rather than preemptively preventing pain, the majority will wait till it starts. Therefore, at the first onset of Lumbar pain, the pregnant woman should stop any WEIGHT-BEARING FLEXION instantly and carefully lower herself to the floor until on her hands and knees rather than continuing to perform the painful flexion activity. Then, carefully, in the absence of flexion, get to a couch, bed, or large pillow so a HIP-HANG can be done to take the load off of the Lumbar disc as soon as possible.

It is very difficult for a pregnant woman to perform FLEXION IN TRACTION so it is essential that the disc material is prevented from moving too far peripherally before intervention is attempted. If the disc material gets too peripherally positioned, one cannot rely upon the FLEXION IN TRACTION to get it back in because there is a baby in the way. That's why I'm placing such an emphasis on prevention. The disc disease should not be allowed to progress to the point where FLEXION IN TRACTION becomes necessary.

An important consideration here is that most women have not lived with back pain for years and do not have the experience to recognize pain-provoking movements before they are executed or know when to alter the dynamics of the particular movement when it becomes painful. Take for instance the pregnant woman who experiences pain when bending forward to pick up an object from the floor. Usually, the almost natural response is to put the free arm on the hip near the pain and straighten up. It may be a means of taking some weight off of the Lumbar spine, but it is inefficient. That action, although providing a mild UNWEIGHTING, still requires the erector spinae muscles to contract which puts added pressure on the flexed disk until it reaches the neutral position or EXTENSION, increasing the probability of further pain and damage.

The next most important consideration is for the pregnant woman or her partner to judiciously monitor the labor and delivery process to protect the Lumbar spine. Monitoring the activity during labor to **insure WEIGHT-BEARING FLEXION at the Lumbar region is avoided** is essential. Using a delivery chair that has good Lumbar support or arranging pillows and the bed during labor and delivery so that the Lumbar spine is not allowed into forced WEIGHT-BEARING FLEXION at any time can prevent the forces being applied that result in disc herniation damage. If a woman is fortunate enough to attend birthing classes or has a partner who will help attend the delivery, one of his/her responsibilities should be to make sure pillows are available and that no one forces the delivering woman into spinal WEIGHT-BEARING FLEXION unless absolutely necessary to push out the baby. I seriously doubt if there is any situation in which WEIGHT-BEARING FLEXION is absolutely necessary since there are certainly less traumatic options available to the prepared and knowledgeable pregnant woman and her care-givers. Considering these issues well in advance and discussing them with the obstetrician or delivery room staff can be reasonably assumed to be in one's best interests especially if a "bad back" is already present or back pain accompanied the previous delivery.

Ideally, finding an obstetrician who employs a birthing chair or an equivalently positionable delivery room table that allows gravity to aid in the delivery of the infant serves most to protect the spine from WEIGHT-BEARING FLEXION and the forces predisposing to disc prolapse. In a reclining chair, the woman's back is allowed to remain in a partially upright, largely vertical posture, with the weight of the upper body supported and usually in a small amount of EXTENSION. In this position, "bearing down" can be accomplished without the contraction of the abdominal musculature in flexion. Contracting the abdominal musculature is the most important participatory activity a woman can accomplish during labor to help push the baby out. "Bearing-down" does not require WEIGHT-BEARING FLEXION, nor does it require assisted flexion by one or more burley nurses. A polite request asking them to avoid forcing the back into flexion prior to the excitement of delivery and reminding them to try to keep the back in EXTENSION when they position themselves to "help you push" is in the best long-term interests of the delivering woman with or without prior back injury.

If laboring in a standard hospital bed, raising the head of the bed to a near maximum, moving one's upper body high up on the raised portion, putting a pillow in the Lumbar region for support, and bringing the legs into a squatting posture with the heels on the cheeks of the buttocks such that they separate the pelvis is as close as one can comfortably come to the "natural" manner in which Asian women have delivered babies for centuries. Some primitive cultures suspend a rope from the ceiling to facilitate squatting while delivering, intuitively understanding the proscription against WEIGHT-BEARING. Unless one can convince the labor and delivery staff to allow a "trapeze bar" to be set up, putting the head of the bed up usually has to suffice (the trapeze bar would usually interfere with the obstetrician working at the foot of the bed). Alternatively using the side rails in the fully up position and your arms locked in EXTENSION so as to take weight off of the pelvis can allow safe abdominal pressure to be generated without the risk to the spine.

With appropriate care and diligence, I am convinced that most back pain associated with pregnancy, labor and delivery could be prevented if WEIGHT-BEARING FLEXION

is prevented. I predict that studies eventually will confirm this. But it will only come after enough women who have had deliveries which allow them to compare the pain they experienced without employing the considerations inherent in *The O'Connor Technique (tm)* with those deliveries in which the PRINCIPLES are applied and practiced. I trust that the "word will get out" about the superiority of this practice and women, as knowledgeable consumers, will insist that the labor and delivery room environment be modified to accommodate their back pain considerations over the previously painful and poorly justifiable alternatives.

After the delivery, caring for an infant and toddler begins another stage that I have seen numerous times give new mothers permanent back problems. They are constantly caused to bend over for bottles, babies, and extra house work. Usually this extra "back-breaking" effort is initiated following a "back-breaking" delivery that sets them up for future damage and disc disease. If the same PRINCIPLES outlined in this book are applied during those endeavors, the joy of children needn't become a torment.

First, predict that you will be doing a lot of lifting when the baby comes and make certain that you keep your hamstrings (those muscles at the posterior thigh that attach to the lower leg below the knee) long and flexible by stretching them daily before the baby arrives. Ideally, this exercise regimen should begin early in pregnancy and be maintained until well after the baby learns to walk and doesn't need to be picked up so often. This is done with the back in an extended posture while the torso is allowed to bend forward at the hips. Gradually increasing the degree of flexion at the hips (not at the Lumbar spine) is done by progressively increasing the numbers and extent of the hamstrings stretches. Of course, this may be done without the need for dedicating special time or buying a membership to a private fitness emporium. Simply incorporating these movements into your daily regimen is sufficient. When you need to bend over to pick something up off of the floor, you position your back into EXTENSION, lock it that way then bend at the hips to get to the floor with your hands. When you are first doing this, you will find it easier if you spread your legs apart to bring your hips lower to the ground and reduce the distance you have to bend to get your hands on the ground. After awhile, you can bring your feet closer together gradually as a means of progressively increasing the stretching of the hamstrings. Spreading the legs widely apart when bending over to pick up objects prior to labor and delivery will also help to place widening stresses on the symphysis pubis, the cartilaginous area in the front of the pelvis that allows for the natural widening of the hips that comes from hormonal influences during the later stages of pregnancy. Daily adopting a wide-based stance and purposefully flexing only at the hips whenever going down to pick up objects can get one into the habit of picking up things in this fashion and can prepare you for the day when you will automatically adopt this posture when attempting to pick up the baby.

If this is not satisfactory for any number of reasons, making sure that you bend at the knees, pull the baby or the object as close to the body as possible, insure that the Lumbar spine is in EXTENSION, the Thoracic spine is straight, and the head is looking up whenever lifting will also accomplish the same goal of protecting the Lumbar spine (See Chapter Four's, Section on Lifting Heavy Objects for more articulate directions). And, of course, understanding and applying the PRINCIPLES of *The O'Connor Technique (tm)* in your daily activities goes without saying whether it is before, during, or after delivery.

The PRINCIPLES of MAINTAINING EXTENSION and AVOIDING WEIGHT-

BEARING FLEXION pertain as much for the pregnant state as the pre-and post-pregnant state. Never bend over a crib, car seat, play pen, tub, or bassinet when the Lumbar or Thoracic spine is flexed. Putting down the crib rails and rolling the baby to your trunk or resting the upper trunk on the object being leaned over then using one arm to hold up the upper body while the other lifts and brings the baby towards you until you can safely lift it with the arms, while MAINTAINING EXTENSION of the spine, will prevent you from turning into a chronic back pain sufferer like so many other young mothers I have witnessed. Also, don't let a young baby hang onto your head or neck while it is flexed. Be very careful about diaper bags, the appurtenances of child-rearing (portable cribs, car seats, etc.) especially if they have straps because the tendency is to load them over the neck or shoulders and bend over. This puts the Upper Thoracic and Cervical spine at high risk of injury. Make several trips, get someone to help, or do without some of those luxuries if carrying them induces back pain. Relying upon a stroller is probably much more safe with regards to back pain prevention than carrying the baby around for long distances. Suffice it to say, a little thought applied to protecting your back will pay off in the long run so pay attention to the carrying and lifting details of baby care.

Getting out of bed several times a night to manage the newborn can also aggravate back pain. Usually, one immediately commits WEIGHT-BEARING FLEXION to get up, then again when leaning over the baby's bed to adjust the bottle, hold the bottle, or pick up the baby. The back musculature is usually completely relaxed and very vulnerable to injury. What's worse is that these are repetitive actions almost as bad as sit-up and toe-touch exercises.

It is not necessary to re-capitulate the entire book as it pertains to pregnant women; however, the weight-gain of pregnancy is probably worth discussing. In my practice, I have seen innumerable very attractive young women not only ruin their figures but set in motion the conditions that will eventually ruin their backs by gaining too much weight during pregnancy. I feel that any woman and especially those with histories of back pain should judiciously avoid gaining too much weight during pregnancy. **The pregnant woman should learn from her doctor how much weight is safe to gain during pregnancy and rigorously stick to a measured dietary and exertion strategy that prevents excessive weight gain.** If this is not done, regardless of all the other detrimental effects of obesity, you can count upon back pain as a result. By simply managing your excess eating and increasing your energy output during pregnancy, you can avoid the pitfall of obesity on the journey of life. It is so hard to convince people that back pain is a result of obesity because they argue that they were "heavy" for most of their lives and didn't have back pain. The point they seem to miss is that the disc system cannot tolerate those extra load-bearing stresses forever. Eventually the discs break down under the stress.

This needn't happen if a woman understands that pregnancy, and the related, genetically-driven, appetite-enhancement it brings, puts her at risk for obesity and its many complications. Simply managing this problem adequately during the short duration of pregnancy can prevent years of agony from coming to pass. **Trust me on this one, those extra cookies cost dearly, and you will pay for them in back pain for the rest of your life.** Especially those that gained and retained an excessive amount of weight during the pregnancy.

SPORTS

It would be idealistically sufficient and efficient to simply state: **Adhere to the PRINCIPLES of *The O'Connor Technique (tm)* while performing sports as well as avoid any sport that subjects you to the risk of uncontrolled forces that can lead to a traumatic WEIGHT-BEARING FLEXION injury of the spine; and you probably won't develop disc disease from sports**. Realistically, however, I am compelled to specifically address several sports with some insights that may not easily come to the reader until it is too late to prevent disc problems. So, I have identified the following sports because they particularly influence and impact upon back pain in general.

Understand at the outset that athletes who injure their backs often fall into a unique category. Depending on the sport, especially those sports like gymnastics, tennis, football, diving, weight-lifting, etc. in which HYPEREXTENSION injuries are routine, athletes can predispose their backs to another statistically much less common form of back injury. This injury, spondylolysis, can come as a result of HYPEREXTENSION forces and cause a break in the bony bridge, the *pars interarticularis*, between the vertebral body and the posterior anatomical components of the vertebral bone. This bridge is often fractured or naturally separated in athletes; but, when compared with the general population, it is an uncommon problem. When broken, this allows one vertebral body, usually L5-S1, to slide forward on the other. **This is spondylolisthesis, and the PRINCIPLES of *The O'Connor Technique (tm)* cannot be relied upon to pertain in the presence of this problem. This is one reason why an athlete who injures the back should get an X-Ray examination of the spine to insure that this lesion is not present before applying the techniques or following the recommendations of this book.**

Despite the minimal risk of presuming a disc problem exists when spondylolysis or spondylolisthesis is the real cause, it should be recognized that, by far and away, more athletes suffer disc herniations from WEIGHT-BEARING FLEXION injuries than they do from HYPEREXTENSION injuries. A reasonable recommendation coming from that understanding would be that **if your injury was sustained when you were bent backwards, a spondylitic or articular problem can be suspected. In that case, trying *The O'Connor Technique (tm)* would be worthwhile to insure that any component of existing disc disease is addressed; but, if unsuccessful, one needn't persist. By all means, if pain is increased, don't continue any of the MANEUVERS until properly evaluated by an orthopedist skilled in back problems.**

One concept that I feel needs to be advanced here is specifically directed at a person who has sustained a significant back injury and is considering investing a great deal of effort and energy into a physical endeavor such as a sports career. **If the injury and its accompanying pain are sufficiently severe to alter one's ability to move painlessly for a time after the injury, I would counsel those individuals to presume the injury is disc-related and not persist in any athletic pursuit that would put the injured disc at risk for further injury, even if, at the time, no pain exists.**

Also, I would caution any adult parent with back pain, preparing a son or daughter for life, to make the presumption that their child is at high risk for the same fate. Not only should the parents consider adopting the PRINCIPLES and following the instructions of *The O'Connor Technique (tm)*, but they should be clearly communicated to the children at an early age and taken into consideration when deciding if a career or major goal in life should be sports, as opposed to some less traumatic pursuit. If not for acting on the belief that the genetic probability exists for a ligamentous weakness to be an inheritable defect, then it should be for the general "common sense" of the matter. **Once the disc system is significantly traumatized, the risk of persisting in an endeavor that subjects it to further, predictable, injury is foolish.** Young, injured, athletes should at least be given this risk/benefit discussion so that if they elect to continue a sports activity they can learn to incorporate the PRINCIPLES of this book into their behavioral choices. For instance, if grandpa has a "bad back" and dad has a "bad back," the son with a back injury that makes him unable to play or work for a few days should abandon the consideration of making a career out of physical labor or sports. Even if the youth only takes away from the lesson the two easily understood and applied edicts to AVOID WEIGHT-BEARING FLEXION and MAINTAIN EXTENSION, they will have acquired valuable preventive measures that pertain to just about any sport.

These recommendations, I presume, might be met with criticism by "sports medicine physicians" for such pronouncements' alleged audacity in the absence of "scientific proof;" but I, nevertheless, will stand by them because discogenic back pain is such a prevalent plague in our society that its prevention demands Draconian edicts. After a genuine disc herniation injury, no amount of strengthening, "work-hardening," or physical therapy will repair the damaged cartilaginous components of the disc's annulus fibrosus. What may have been the initiating injury that resulted in perhaps a few days of significant pain, resolving in a short time, that otherwise could have been lived with, can be transformed instantly into perpetually crippling pain by continuing a sport that predisposes one to the same traumatic forces.

I have listened to too many patients relate histories of back injuries that seemingly resolved only to return later with renewed fury and increased degree as a result of relatively paltry stresses later in life to not make this recommendation. In light of the far greater stresses placed on the disc system by sports and having the personal experience of sustaining three of the most significant injuries in my own experience at the hands of unnecessary sporting actions, I cannot, when counseling athletes in my sphere of influence, in clear conscience, make any other recommendation. Of course, everyone must make such decisions for themselves based upon the risk/benefit ratio of what is entailed by not playing those sports, yet I can't think of any reason a person with disc disease should persist in a sports-directed career path, or for that matter, a career involving physical labor. **If it is indeed a herniation, (and if *The O'Connor Technique (tm)* is successful in relieving the pain, that is reason enough to make that assumption), they will never reach their goal anyway because the probabilities are that eventually their backs will fail before they reach the height of any such career involving WEIGHT-BEARING FLEXION.** Too many competitors without disc disease will have eclipsed their performance before the benefits of a sporting career can be realized. So, it makes little sense to risk the possibility of not being able to perform any major physical activity for the remainder of their lives in lieu of the transient glory of winning a meaningless high school football game in an attempt to foster a fantasy that they will someday play professional football.

In a similar context, I really cannot remain silent about the multitudes of young athletes intimidated and enticed to continue sports despite injuries that should have otherwise caused them to "retire." Someone has to call a halt to this carnage by instructing the young, disc-injured, would-be-professional, athlete in the reality that their chances of going professional are slim in the first place and reduced even more in the presence of significant disc trauma so as to place such aspirations into the realm of fantasy, and their further pursuit only a promise for a later life of pain.

Any sport (or martial art like Karate, Ju-Jitsu, etc.) in which it is routine to fall with a flexed spine should be considered dangerous for anyone and especially those with a family history of back pain or a prior history of significant back pain. If one has no prior injury to the back and wishes to engage in these sports, exercises that strengthen the paraspinous musculature should be done to fortify the spine and the PRINCIPLES of *The O'Connor Technique (tm)* should be understood before an injury occurs. A muscularly stronger back has less chance of injury especially if the strengthening includes preferentially building up the extensors. Realistically, I doubt that most people engaging these sports will follow this advice; however, it discharges my responsibility to the reader by that recommendation's making. To be honest, it has been my experience that most people don't practice preventive measures that require significant expenditures of energy or time. I understand this; but to the extent that perhaps trainers and coaches reading this take it to heart, they might keep their athletes winning longer decreasing their chances of injury.

One thing that young athletes especially lack is the wisdom to understand that the damage they do to their bodies (especially cartilaginous structures) usually will plague them the rest of their lives. It is up to those adults who have experienced this phenomenon to take charge and not allow injured athletes to persist in any sport that would serve to complicate or compromise the injured individual's future well-being. I find repugnant coaches and trainers whose selfishness places their need to win above the youth's future interests. Usually they assuage their consciences by reassuring themselves that they are letting the athlete decide if they are too injured to play while neglecting the intense psychological pressure they have previously put on the youth to perform to their coach's expectations. The "guilt trips" that are laid on kids when they "let down the team" lead these injured children to perform feats that commit themselves to futures of disability and pain. **I look upon this phenomenon as a subtle, poorly recognized, inadequately addressed, but prevalent form of child abuse in our society, exceeding in damage much lesser forms of abuse that are severely punished when identified by the authorities.**

This phenomenon is rarely recognized or paid anything other than lip service; but it is typified by the 1996 Olympic decision made by the little female gymnast who was encouraged by her coach to not default after it was obvious to the world that she had sustained an injury to her ankle. Her "heroic" decision was so insignificant in the grand scheme of things that I can't recall her name. She nevertheless did perform in pain and most probably turned a significant sprain into a quantifiable ankle ligament rupture. My knowledge of her specific injury is limited, of course, but I can prove that one ligamentous injury to the ankle usually is followed by repeated injuries due to the damaged ligaments' inherent instability and inability to ever completely heal. This gymnast, now, faces the unnecessarily higher probability of ankle arthritis when she reaches her fourth decade. Some orthopedists would contend that the arthritis is inevitable. If she is unable to run or walk without pain in her 50's and her kidneys are ruined due to taking years of pain relievers, her coach will most likely not be around to pay her medical bills or pat her on the back in the year 2030; and all she will have is her dusty gold medal to offer solace. Of course, she will, for time immemorial, provide an excellent "bad example" of the "agony of victory."

I seriously doubt that this behavior will be addressed by our society in the near future because it is routinely argued that the injured athlete is the "only" person who can tell how much pain they are in; and, if they can tolerate the pain, they should be allowed to be the best judge. Quite frankly, this is a disdainfully pragmatic attitude placing a decision of monumental magnitude upon a person incapable of understanding the consequences of their "choice." The argument that they have competent judgement skills does not withstand moral scrutiny in a child abuse or neglect situation involving a minor regardless of the presence or absence of consent; so it shouldn't be tolerated in athletes under the age of consent. Our legal system does not defer to a child's discretion by asking: "Do you choose to live in a home where you are routinely injured?" And it shouldn't ask: "Do you want to play with a coach who talks you into breaking your own bones." Of course, this won't be the first hypocrisy identified in our society; so the duty is left to the parents of these children to be alert to this behavior and intervene to prevent future pain and disability when applicable.

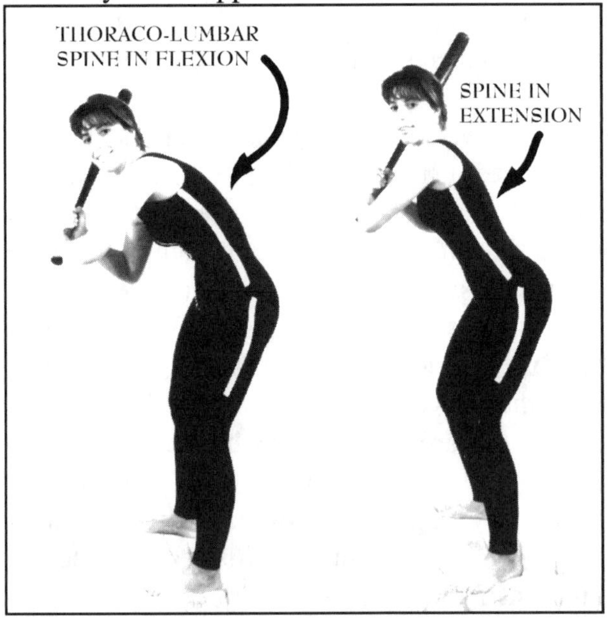

Figure 5 Batting position options: Left incorrect and Right correct

I cannot stress how important it is to act defensively with regard to the spine. The following dissertations on sports categories can give the reader (young or old) some specific insights into how to act to protect the spine and avoid injury.

BASEBALL

Baseball could best be described as a moderate risk sport; but the risk is largely dependent upon the position of the Lumbar spine during the batting activity. The batter has three postures in which to allow the back to rest while waiting to hit the ball-- neutral, extension or flexion. Neutral and extension are far more preferable to the dreaded WEIGHT-BEARING FLEXION. In a flexed swing, suddenly, a great deal of force is applied to the disc while twisting. In a neutral position, it isn't so bad, but in EXTENSION the disc is actually protected. I would recommend that anyone with Lumbar disc pain or a history of same, re-learn their batting stance to make sure it is in mild EXTENSION before the swing.

Not long ago, I recall reading in the newspaper of a famous baseball star who was unable to play due to a back pain problem. I decided to watch the news to see if they showed his batting stance. Sure enough, he leaned way over towards the plate with nearly his entire Thoracic and Lumbar spine in WEIGHT-BEARING FLEXION. It was easy for me to see how his back pain could be prevented and probably remedied. I sent him a letter, but he never responded.

The lesson here is that the same PRINCIPLES applying to everyday life apply to sports.

384

Any time you expose your back to WEIGHT-BEARING FLEXION, you risk damaging the disc. The stances adopted in Figure 5 demonstrate the subtle but important difference between a protected back in a batting stance and one which is a set up for disc pain. Note how the Cervical, Thoracic, and Lumbar spine are flexed on the Left (incorrect) and in slight EXTENSION on the Right (correct).

The weight should be centered over the vertebral bodies and the Cervical, Lumbar, and Thoracic spine placed in slight, comfortable EXTENSION. Any bending should be done at the hips. This way, when the force of initiating the swing is felt and the centrifugal force of the bat is felt on the arms at the end of the swing, the spine is in a much more mechanically advantageous position to sustain it. The ease with which the stance can be changed with such little effort is inversely proportional to the damage prevented. There is so little inconvenience involved in protecting the spine from WEIGHT-BEARING FLEXION as well as MAINTAINING EXTENSION and so much benefit to be gained that the effort can be looked upon as negligibly simple. The sooner it is practiced, the better.

FOOTBALL

Football should be considered a dangerous sport for the back. Oddly enough, it is practically considered a "rite of passage" for most male high school students who eventually will engage in occupations requiring physical labor. Therefore, it is probably the worst sport they could choose from the standpoint of their future comfort. I wish it were possible for me to quantify how many backs have been ruined by high-school football. Perhaps the terms quarter-, half-, and full back should be looked upon as the degree of disability remaining after their respective careers are terminated by being tackled and landing on a flexed spine.

Again, an individual incident comes to mind to typify this reality. Joe Montana, quarterback for the San Francisco Forty-Niners, received a disc injury requiring surgery. He reportedly "recovered" enough to return to football--which was amazing; but, to my observation, he was never able to reproduce equivalent performances. If he doesn't already know it, he can look forward to back pain for the rest of his life. Whatever level of pain he has, it was only increased by persisting in his career after such an injury. I'm not certain that the money he received during his playing career is adequate compensation for the years of pain he will inevitably experience. However, that isn't newsworthy, and it is unlikely that anyone will ever learn the true extent of his pain, because to publicly elaborate it might discourage similar performances in the future by sensible athletes as well as cast an uncomplimentary light on our society's values.

I see no realistic means of protecting the spine from football injury. I seriously doubt that any level of exercise will prepare the back for the stresses engendered in the predictable trauma sustained. I leave it to the readers' discretion if they choose to play this brutal sport. Personally, I believe the wise individual will avoid it, the wise parent who comprehends the realities of back pain will discourage it, and anyone who has back pain significant enough to have been motivated to read this book should consider it contraindicated. It makes no sense to damage your body in such a manner.

Watching young men permanently injured due to the prevalent attitude in sports that it is acceptable to try to hit another player in such a manner to hurt him enough to knock him out of the game is unacceptable in a civilized society. I think that this practice could be stopped simply by permanently banning from the game any player who injures another player in the commission of a foul. Since violence is what fills the stadiums and the teams owners' pockets, I seriously doubt any efforts will be made legislatively in that regard.

GOLF

I could probably write a book about golfing as it relates to back pain. Maybe, I will eventually; however, some principle points should be made, herein, due to the high probability of alleviating a lot of golfers pain since it is my belief that this sport is one of the major unrecognized sources of back injury in people who can least afford it. I think the current interpretation of the frequent news reports of professional golfers not able to play tournaments due to back pain looks upon these athletes as having back problems that coincidentally catch up to them in their golfing professions. Or that they sustain an injury in some other manner that effects their golf "game." Golfing is not really a game, from the perspective of a vertebrologist. It is a dynamic, high energy, violent sport. When one looks upon a elderly group of septuagenarians walking around the course, they tend to believe that it could not constitute much of a vigorous activity. However, I have "played" golf enough times to get sore and appreciate the stresses put upon muscles, ligaments, and especially discs. I had to consciously protect my back to insure that the pain I experienced in my extremities, as a novice never making those movements before, did not extend to my spine. I was successful and my hopes are that the protective insights I have made will be communicated to the golfing reader whether a professional or a retired dilettante.

The golf swing constitutes a rather powerful set of forces that, if misdirected, has the capacity to damage discs. The position adopted by many golfers during the swing can very frequently be a **WEIGHT-BEARING FLEXION of one or more disc units. These extraordinarily rapid forces combined with the WEIGHT-BEARING FLEXION can easily be seen to be sufficient to herniate a disc**. The golf club might seem to be too small a weight to substantially effect spinal mechanics; however, one must consider that the kinetic energy of the club constitutes enough force to propel the ball well over 100 yards. If one tried the same feat by using one's arm, it would be impossible because that much force cannot be generated by the strength of anyone's arm. But, surely, the strength of one arm is sufficient to herniate a disc, especially if one considers that lifting a garbage can is capable of the same consequence and a person's arm is clearly capable of accomplishing that effort. One can then conclude that when the club strikes the ball it has enough centrifugal force pulling it away from the body to be equivalent to a substantial weight. Consider, too, that this force is not only repeatedly but rapidly applied; and, by virtue of that, after a certain point when the golfer is committed to the full swing, nothing one can do will change the forces and their directions in mid-swing. There is too much force, too rapidly applied, for anyone to be able to reasonably retract it once a certain point has been reached.

In light of and in spite of these admittedly inexact physical comparisons, the means of preventing injury cannot come during the swing when you have already committed yourself to damaging forces resulting from a mechanically disadvantageous movement. Therefore, **in order to prevent damage, it is essential to design, practice, and program your posture and swing, in advance of the generation of these forces, to prevent WEIGHT-BEARING FLEXION at any area of the spine you do not wish to expose to disc trauma**. Depending upon the particular golfer's stance, either the Cervical, Thoracic, and/or Lumbar vertebrae are placed at risk. The individual area at highest risk depends largely upon what section is put in the most WEIGHT-BEARING FLEXION during the most forceful component of the swing. This may involve some compromises for the golfer who has back pain or one who wants to prevent it. That is, if a good golfer has previously trained with a particular stance and now realizes that it is detrimental to his back (yet to alter his stance will necessarily sacrifice accuracy)--some compromise may need to be made. Time may be required to gradually make the transition. A risk may have to be taken to accept a poorer stance from a back pain perspective if more "harm" will come by his golf game suffering. Pretty much, I would argue that the back is most important; however, we live in the real world where compromises must often be made and risks are willing to be taken for the perceived benefit. So, I leave it to the discretion of the golfer. For all I know, all golfers properly swinging should already have their backs remain in a neutral position; yet I doubt that to be the case since I so often hear of professional golfers hurting their backs and having quit the circuit. If they were protecting their backs already with the ideal golfing technique I think this would be less frequent a phenomenon.

   The goal of every golfer should be to maximally adhere to the PRINCIPLES of *The O'Connor Technique (tm)* **while at the same time aspiring to adopt the classically successful golf swinging techniques.** This can be accomplished by a number of means. First, selecting a **longer club length** than one might otherwise choose without the consideration of spinal WEIGHT-BEARING FLEXION in mind. The longer club length helps keep the Lumbar and Thoracic spine out of flexion during the forceful component of the swing. Some other back pain books might try to convince you that it is the swing itself that generates torsion forces to damage the discs; however, I disagree. **The torsion can have some participation in the injury, but it is the WEIGHT-BEARING FLEXION that is the larger culprit and only complicated by the torsion.** The same considerations given for lifting heavy weights should be applied during the swing. The entire spine should be placed in the neutral or slightly extended configuration. If this cannot be accomplished and still maintain a reasonably accurate result, then at the very least, any area of the spine that is uncomfortable after golfing should be considered an especially vulnerable area and accordingly protected by being placed in EXTENSION even if this causes some other area to allow something closer to flexion.

   Above all, if a person has a back problem already, that area of the spine should not be afforded the luxury of compromise. **The particular problematic disc level must, at the very least, be kept in EXTENSION.** Now, this doesn't mean that a golfer of 20-40 years should suddenly go out and swing with his back bent backwards. Let's be real. Gradually, an effort should be made to protect the painful disc by, as judiciously and slowly as effectively possible, making an alteration to insure that no rapidly violent moves are made on a disc system that has accommodated over the years to an entirely different set of forces and movements.

   Another issue is the closeness to the ball. If one treats the point of impact with the ball as the effective "weight" that is being lifted, the closer that "weight" is brought to the center of gravity, the lower amount of force will be felt at the flexed spine. This may seem hard to accomplish because centimeters are in question, but **the closer one gets ones feet to the ball, the better**. The farther from the body, the more the body has to flex to reach it with the club.

Also, **consider how you look at the ball**. There are two ways of taking a person's gaze from the horizon to the ball. One can keep the neck rigid and bow at the Lumbar spine until the eyes meet the ball, one can bend at the thorax, neck or any region in between. More effectively and safely, one can choose to bend the neck at a point higher than the attachment of the shoulder muscles by simply tucking the chin close to the neck. This way, the forces felt on the arms are not acting upon the area at the base of the neck because it is not allowed to go into FLEXION. This would eliminate the FLEXION component and the WEIGHT-BEARING component of danger to discs susceptible to harm.

Getting the Lumbar spine into EXTENSION may not be so easy, but it probably is the most important consideration. This can be facilitated by **widening the stance** and **using the hip joints to sustain the most flexion**. This stance allows the Lumbar spine to remain in EXTENSION, yet the hip region of the body can still engage in flexion if necessary to maintain an effective and successful swing. Understandably, this can result in a stance that feels and appears awkward and may fall outside of the stance that is accepted by others as classically appropriate and ideal. Everyone is motivated by different concerns and modifications from the traditional are sometimes necessary to effect beneficial outcomes. I doubt that anyone would fail themselves by making their priority the elimination of pain and the retention of a successful golf swing regardless of how their posture may appear to other golfers who have little understanding or concern about the safety of the spine.

Too, **carrying a golf bag around, lifting it frequently, and bending over constantly to place tees or pick up balls contribute to repetitive WEIGHT-BEARING FLEXION**, the majority of which can be prevented or modified by adhering to the PRINCIPLES of *The O'Connor Technique (tm)*. Simply using the club as a cane to reduce the weight on the discs can eliminate a substantial portion of the load placed on the disc and reduce the weight-bearing component of WEIGHT-BEARING FLEXION. If you watch golfers carefully, you will notice that some do this spontaneously and many probably have come to use their clubs as supports because it reduces pain.

Also, when the wise golfer goes down to pick up a ball or place a tee, he will lift a leg when flexing at the hip rather than flexing at the Lumbar spine. When he rises back up, he only needs to let the leg drop and make the Lumbar spine rigid which allows the weight of the leg to act as a counter balance to lift the upper body. The club, in this stance, is used to stabilize the upper body and help it keep its balance.

Finally, golf carts were not designed for back pain sufferers. The roof is usually not high enough for a tall person not to have to bend over repeatedly getting in and out, and the distance from the seat to the floor is so short as to almost require the knees to be higher than the level of the waist. This automatically places the Lumbar spine in repetitive WEIGHT-BEARING FLEXION as the little cart goes jostling over the irregularities in the course. Needless to say this is an ideal condition for posterior migration of disc material and should be understood. An accommodation to this reality can be accomplished by employing a modification of the DRIVING AND VEHICULAR EXIT MANEUVER described in the so-named Section of this book.

WINTER SPORTS

Throughout the entire skiing, snow-boarding, or skating process, the Cervical and Lumbar spine, especially, should be kept in EXTENSION as much as reasonably possible. This consideration should include the action of falling. This may seem difficult because falls are usually seen to be "accidents" and therefore uncontrollable. Not so! With these types of sports, one can expect to fall a lot. Falling in WEIGHT-BEARING FLEXION on the buttocks is the worst of all possible injuries from a back pain perspective.

When falling cannot be avoided, at least **how you fall can be modified**. An effort should be made to fall forward or to the side if at all possible. In most cases of low speed falls, a person can choose to fall in such a way as to use the rigidly flexed arms to absorb most of the fall's energy. **One should not commit one's self to these activities to the extent of relinquishing the control necessary to be able to modify a fall.** If you find yourself moving so fast as to not be able to control the fall, then you should slow down.

Consider while skiing that one of the worst positions is the squat-like "tuck" that downhill racers assume with both of their legs close together. This maximizes the WEIGHT-BEARING FLEXION and opening of the posterior intervertebral spaces during the bumps and extraordinary G-forces placed on the spine during the UNWEIGHTING and re-weighting activities that cannot be avoided during skiing. This position should be avoided by the routine skier and left to the conditioned experts who most probably will have back pain later in life and wonder why.

When sledding or tobogganing the position in which you sit can determine the danger to the disc. Lying prone or with your legs directly under you while sitting upright keeping your back in EXTENSION on your heels is as safe as can be, considering the overall risk of the sport anyway. Sitting upright with the legs out stretched in front of you is dangerous and if you have a back problem will probably be too painful to tolerate unless you lean posteriorly, support your upper torso with your hands, and keep your Lumbar spine in EXTENSION.

TENNIS

Tennis can be more safely played if you use your legs more than your back. By that, a person should try to run faster and closer to the ball rather than allowing a reaching with the back in WEIGHT-BEARING FLEXION. This is especially pertinent for very low flying balls outside of the normal reach of the arms which cause the player to flex to bring the racket to the ball. A person with back pain can successfully play tennis if he programs himself not to commit WEIGHT-BEARING FLEXION. Either you let those low-flying balls go or find a way by increasing your speed or bending the knees to reach those them without flexing the spine, especially at the Lumbar region.

A means to that end is to adopt a stance while waiting for the ball that maintains an extended spine because flexing while launching forward puts unnecessary stresses on the spine. An equivalent agility can be developed by flexing more with the hips. This may be more difficult to remember, but that is what training is all about. The athlete with back pain has to train himself differently than someone with a genetically stronger or previously uninjured spine.

WRESTLING

Wrestling can only be considered a dangerous sport for the spine. Attempts to lift the opponent with the back in WEIGHT-BEARING FLEXION can be expected to damage a disc if done enough times. Also, it is not uncommon for a person to fall in FLEXION or have their neck forcefully flexed while attempting to push forward. All the damaging forces are compounded and probably any given level of damage is magnified by the twisting and unexpected pressures of a fight with another human.

Having been a former high school wrestler, I can speak from experience. I distinctly recall events of back pain routinely causing me to convince a fellow wrestler during warm-up to line up with me, back to back, locking elbows, and lift me off the floor while I was relaxed in EXTENSION by his bending anteriorly to carry my weight. This was done to "loosen up" the back and it was usually accompanied by wriggling and bouncing. The way I view this retrospectively, is that the wrestling activity had been displacing the central components of the discs; and we were unwittingly performing an EXTENSION IN TRACTION MANEUVER to re-centralize the discs material. This is sufficient to convince me that wrestling was probably a contributor to my early disc damage and can just as easily damage other young backs

Wrestling also gave me my first dose of how coaches subtly intimidate players into performing in the presence of injuries. During several matches, my knee dislocated to the extent that the match had to be stopped while the coach re-located my dislocated knee joint by carefully extending the knee. I made a decision that to wrestle in the final tournament would be foolishly placing my knee at risk for future, potentially worse, injury. I'll never forget the disappointed disgust on the face of my coach who convinced me that I was "letting down" my team. From then on, he would not establish eye contact with me and let me know that I was *persona non grata* in his realm. He intentionally made me feel bad; however, I still had enough sense to not wrestle again. My knee still bothers me to this day. It caused a permanent instability in the joint that still becomes painful if I put stress on the same ligament. It never quite healed, and neither did my respect for the coach.

1.   Deyo RA. Rethinking strategies for acute low back pain. *Emerg Med* 1995;27(11):38-56.

2.   Anon, Quoting Dr. Henry J. Bienert at the annual meeting of the Florida Academy of Family Physicians, Most Low Back Pain Is Said to Have an Inflammatory Component, *Family Practice News*, October 1-14, 1991;21;19:p 3,61.

3.   Melzack R, Second European Congress on Back Pain, reported in *Family Practice News*, August 15-31, 1988; 18(16):50

4.   Ostgaard HC, Andersson GBJ, Postpartum low back pain. *Spine*, Jan 1992;17:53-55.

5.   Powell, MC, et al., *Lancet*, (1986)2:1366.5.

CHAPTER SEVEN: OPTIONAL THERAPIES

The purpose of this book is not to obsessively evaluate the merits of all the available therapies with exhaustive statistics and intricate details; however, it would not be complete unless I gave some direction to those who's back pain is not alleviated by *The O'Connor Technique (tm)* and are forced to seek other relief from disc herniation pain. I am not so arrogant as to believe that my method will solve everyone's pain; so, for those situations, I believe I have a duty to give some of my perspectives so that at least some pitfalls can be avoided.

TENS (TRANSCUTANEOUS ELECTRICAL NERVE STIMULATION)

This methodology relies upon a small pulsating current of electricity to basically confuse the nerve impulses going up the spinal cord to the brain. It is possibly functioning on the same level as acupuncture, the effect of which is poorly understood and explained; however, in some people it works. What probably is happening is that a small amount of stimulation is carried in the fast fibers that carry information to the brain related to the position of the body, touch, and vibration. These fibers' connections have a hierarchy of order in which they pass on to the brain as if there were a "gate" that only lets one nerve impulse at a time pass through. This is called the gating theory of pain proposed by Melzack and Wall. It explains why when a person slams their knee into an object, it helps to rub it when one would logically assume that further stimulation of damaged tissue would increase the pain. The rubbing stimulates sensory nerve impulses which seem to beat the pain impulses to the "gate;" and the pain is reduced when the pain impulses do not travel up the spinal cord to the brain. I have found that, initially, it can help the pain; but, after awhile, the nervous system accommodates to the electrical impulses and the pain breaks through. Therefore, they may help in an acute situation for a short time, but do not look to these devices for anything approaching long-term relief in the presence of a disc herniation.

ICE AND HEAT

The Gateing Theory of Pain also probably explains why ice and heat both seem to reduce pain. They are often called "therapies," but I never use them because they only work during the time period that they are physically being applied. The minute the heat or cold leaves, the pain returns. I tend to like my method of going to the source of pain and eliminating it rather than masking it. For the most part, if you have an actual disc problem, it would be impossible to expect the temperature change at the skin level to have any effect on structures deeper in the disc realm of the spine.

This does not deny that when a piece of ice is rubbed on your back that the disc pain won't go away temporarily, because it does. Sometimes, if the pain is extremely severe, this is not an unreasonable alternative so long as you are willing to sustain the ice touching your skin, getting you wet, and you accept the fact that when you stop rubbing with ice the pain will return.

However, if you have been out of pain for the minutes to hours that the ice or heat was applied, at least you did get some relief during the most severe component of the episode, which in some cases, can be a great relief.

ACUPUNCTURE

Not one to immediately dispel the possibility that acupuncture helps pain, I feel that it is highly unlikely that sticking a little needle in a distant part of the body will have any effect upon the physical nature of herniated disc pain. I would be inconsistent if I supported any other view. I suspect that some people can get temporary relief from the pain in that fashion; but, as for remedying the origin of that pain--I can see no possible way in which it could function in that regard. Therefore, I cannot make any recommendation to resort to routine treatments unless there is no other means of ending the pain and you get dramatic relief with the first therapeutic trial. If it works, my suspicion would be that the patient didn't have discogenic pain in the first place.

TRIGGER POINT INJECTIONS

These rank very close to acupuncture in my view as a therapy. If someone thinks they can permanently affect pain caused by a mechanical impingement upon nerves by injecting an anesthetic at some distant point, they are only masking the pain if it helps at all. My suspicion is that when it is used for focal inflammatory conditions of the back but not the spine, it can be successful; however, this relies upon the misdiagnosis of tendinitis or fasciitis (inflammation of fascia, tendons or other ligaments, etc.) with disc disease. If it does work in the presence of disc pain, it is probably only deadening any input from the nerves that provide input for referred pain or capitalizing upon the above described "gating theory." If the nerve supplying the same area as the fibers that travel from the disc region are anesthetized, nothing will be felt from that area to be confused with pain. But admittedly, I can't give any reason for why it would even help in discogenic pain, that's why I don't use it, and never have, in my practice.

EPIDURAL STEROID/ANESTHETIC INJECTIONS

I rank this therapy within the realm of last resorts and believe it is treating only the symptoms, not the source. Of course, if you want to take the risk of someone putting a needle into your spine only millimeters away from the nerves that work your legs or arms, you are welcome to use your discretion. Early in the injury, the steroids will certainly reduce the inflammatory component, and the anesthetic (novocaine like drugs) will immediately eliminate the pain. However, the effect is reported to be not long-lived; and I fear that the steroids well-established propensity to weaken ligamentous tissues makes it a less optimal therapy. I can see little point in permanently weakening a containment structure for the short term, transient, gain of pain relief. If the mechanical source of the pain is not eliminated, the result is probably equivalent to acupuncture or TENS--No cure, just a time-limited treatment. Be certain that, if you do resort to this therapy, you choose a physician highly skilled in this technique and the proposed benefits vs risks be clearly explained.

There is another important consideration inherent in the decision to subject yourself to this therapeutic modality. Cortico-steriods are rather powerful drugs in that they cause tissues injected with them to shrink and weaken (atrophy). When a body tissue is inflamed, to shrink it is sometimes helpful because it causes the inflammatory process to be reduced as well. Injections for tendonitis or bone spurs are very effective in producing long-lasting benefit because they are injected into tissues that can tolerate the potential atrophy. In the case of a bone spur, the atrophy is intentional. However, the use of these drugs in the presence of a herniation can easily be seen to cause the intervertebral or capsular ligaments to be weakened. Doing so, I believe, is potentially counter-productive in the long term because those are the precise ligaments that you are relying upon to retain, move, and re-centralize the off-center disc material. If these ligaments are weakened, they might not be strong enough to perform the functions for which they were designed.

Usually, by the time patients seriously consider this modality, they are desperate for pain relief. I would caution against making any desperate decisions without some certainty of true, long-term, benefit as well as the absence of permanent harm. I would insure that any genuine presentation of the risks, benefits, indications, and contraindications divulges the actual long-term success rates and quantifies the number of people who went on to have surgery, anyway. Ideally, anyone faced with this dilemma should try *The O'Connor Technique (tm),* first, and be certain that they cannot benefit by it before potentially atrophying the inflamed ligaments. They are most likely inflamed because of a constant abnormal physical pressure and traumatic stretching due to a bulging or off-center piece of disc material. If they are treated with cortico-steroids, they can be expected to not perform to their capacity and fail. This could result in a nerve-damaging disc protrusion that otherwise would not have occurred–thereby potentially committing the patient to an inevitable open discectomy or fusion surgery. There lies grave importance in this decision because the new percutaneous discectomy and internal fusion procedures might not be attempted in the presence of a disc protrusion or extrusion that came as the result of an un-naturally weakened intervertebral ligament, since these procedures theoretically rely upon an intact disc capsule to be successful.

CHEMONUCLEOLYSIS

This is a technique in which a protein digesting enzyme (chymopapain) is injected into the central disc space and allowed to actually digest the disc material. It is reserved for patients with a documented herniated disc that have failed at conservative therapy. It fell out of favor a number of years ago, and probably for good reason, since more than 50% of patients experience increased back pain and muscle spasm after the injection and **nearly 80 percent have incapacitating back pain for up to three months after treatment**.[1] However, 70-80% of patients have a resolution of radicular pain within six weeks of injection.[2] Although considered a legitimate therapy, I am a little leery of someone injecting an enzyme capable of indiscriminately dissolving human tissue anywhere close to my spinal nervous system. If it is injected into the wrong place, it can digest the wrong structure. Once the enzyme solution is injected, it cannot be taken back. It is very difficult to insure that there is no breach in the disc capsule that would allow the solution to enter the spinal canal or contact nerve tissue. In that event, a digestion of the nerve roots or other elements could occur. The person doing the procedure has to be skillful and accurate every time. Allergies to the enzyme have also been known to result in anaphylactic (severe allergic) reactions.

An additional thought is that, over the long term, even a poorly functional disc is better than no disc. Without the disc, the vertebral bones would rub together or shift due to the lack of support inherent in the concentric structure. In the case of a posteriorly damaged disc, one still has the anterior component to provide some shock-absorbtion. There is little ability once the chemical is injected to differentiate good disc material from bad disc material. Everything is digested the same. For this reason, I really cannot recommend the therapy. In fact, I am not knowledgeable of a physician who performs this in my area; and I have practiced medicine for 15 years without making a single referral for this modality. Moreover, I have never attended upon a patient who has had the procedure. Therefore, I would say be very careful if this option is considered and become fully-informed prior to your decision.

SURGERY

Everyone with severe back pain is confronted by the inevitable concern--Will I need surgery? Too often, the decision is not well-thought out, made in desperation, or undertaken with unreasonable expectations. It is encouraging to note that only 5-10% of patients with radicular pain end up with surgery. Surgery should be **strongly considered** in the presence of demonstrable neurological compromise (that is if you have lost strength or absence of sensation in an extremity) that remains for more than a couple of days immediately after injury. This loss should be consistent and documentable by objective means such as NMRI and EMG (Electo-MyeloGraphy: a diagnostic technique wherein electrical impulses are measured from the spinal cord to the muscles to determine if the nerve is damaged.) It should be **considered** if intolerable symptoms have not been significantly alleviated after six weeks of failed non-surgical alternatives. The length of time elapsed without relief is probably the best indicator that the pain will not resolve without surgery.

Removal of the herniated disc material or "diskectomy" is warranted when the annulus fibrosus shows unmistakable signs of a prolapsed or extruded disc material. All of the surgical approaches to disc disease have one defining characteristic in common. They involve the removal of the offending nucleus pulposus or disc material from what ever abnormal anatomical space it finds itself, including the intervertebral space, the foramina (space where the spinal nerve root courses on its way out of the spinal canal), or the spinal canal.

When deciding whether to undergo a procedure in which someone is going to enter deep into the structural part of your body and remove some material wherein an error or bad luck can leave you a paraplegic, make every effort to determine the advisability of the technique and the qualifications of the physician. Don't go uninformed into one of the most important decisions of your life. Don't let your HMO intimidate you into accepting only the procedure they decided to pay for and don't fear doing research outside of your community to find the best institution in which to have the most appropriate procedure done by the most competent surgeon you can afford.

Of tantamount importance, if an immediate and persistent loss of function in an extremity occurs with a spinal injury or a progressive loss of neurological function occurs, surgery should be strongly considered to prevent permanent damage from compression of a nerve root. The presence of a foot drop (weakness such that you cannot lift the weight of your foot at the ankle) or a definite loss of sensation (that is, if you can stick a pin in the affected area and not feel it) constitutes a **medical emergency**. Weakness should not be defined as just a "giving out" with pain, and tingling feelings like the area is "asleep" (a paresthesia) are usually not signs of nerve damage that necessarily require surgical intervention. A significant weakness constitutes a profound failure of strength that doesn't allow normal movement, usually resulting in an inability to walk on your heels or toes or hold yourself up on the painful leg with a bent knee.

Surgery is said to not be indicated and should not be performed for a disc herniation without symptoms even if it appears to be compressing a nerve root on an imaging study. Surgery is also said to be not worth the pain, risk, and assumed benefit in syndromes of back pain without accompanying radicular pain (pain shooting down the extremity) or simply changes in sensation. If there is no loss of neurological function, surgery exposes the patient to the dangers of surgery without any predictable benefit. However, I have seen patients with such bad discs, that so continuously de-centralize and are so unstable that their only hope for a reasonably normal life would be to undergo surgical fusion of the offending disc unit. I even accept the reality that I may someday be forced to make this surgical decision for my own back.

If you are uncertain whether you need surgery or not, don't fear alienating your medical providers by asking sufficient questions to insure that you are making a fully informed decision. If they take any offense at your attempt to truly understand the risks, benefits, and alternatives, reconsider your decision to put your trust in that individual. They should never be too busy to adequately explain the merits and rationale for their particular approach to your problem. If you get the same anxious feeling as if when someone selling you aluminum siding is becoming visibly irritated when you attempt to actually read the fine print of the contract, hold off on your decision until you feel better about it.

Think about it, even if the success rate of percutaneous diskectomy is only fifty percent, it is only the equivalent of a large needle going into your back. The recovery from that is relatively minuscule compared to a spinal fusion or laminectomy in which the skin, muscle and sinew are splayed open, cut, torn, stretched and dried out by bright lights and every blood vessel that makes the fatal mistake of bleeding is electrically burned by a small smoking probe. Then, in the laminectomy, portions of the spinal bones are chipped away so that access can be gained to the posterior aspect of the disc. In the case of a spinal fusion, portions of the hip bone are harvested and used to build a plate of bone to make the formerly mobile spine, immobile.

Deciding to have anything like that done should only come after an attempt is made to exhaust all other opportunities for remedy and to acquire all the information possible to make an informed decision. A decision should be based upon the degree of symptoms compared to the alteration of lifestyle necessary without it as well as after it is done. There are people who have had the surgery and are glad they did because they were effectively healed. There are others who were surgically treated appropriately; but nevertheless got worse as well as those who got no appreciable benefit.

In my opinion, if it is determined on the basis of an imaging study (either CAT, NMRI, and/or Myelogram) that shows a compressed nerve in combination with an EMG (Electro-Myography = a test involving the use of tiny needles to measure electrical impulses reaching the muscles) that proves nerve damage, and the methods described in this book fail to help, then surgery is the only alternative to losing the neurological function of the extremity. Having a paralyzed leg or arm is no small matter and surgery is probably the only chance one has of preventing that complication. Usually, now-a-days, most surgeons won't proceed without satisfying those criteria; however, I still occasionally interview patients who have gone to surgery without actual documentable nerve damage, but this is rare lately in this litigious environment.

An important consideration that is sometimes over-looked in deciding to perform surgery is whether or not the nerve is permanently damaged to some degree when the disc is not actually compressing it. I don't feel that this situation is well treated or understood in the "black-and-white" world in which modern medicine sometimes paints itself. There are, you may be surprized to learn, grey areas of medicine still out there. **I have seen several cases in which, immediately following the injury, there is definite nerve impairment that later resolves because a disc fragment at the instant of the injury transiently compresses the spinal nerve root then recoils back into a position closer to the center of the vertebral disc.** This instantaneous collision with the nerve root can produce permanent nerve damage yet not be seen to be actively compressing the nerve on an imaging study. In this case, surgery probably cannot be expected to restore nerve function lost as a result of that happening. The nerve is permanently damaged, yet there is no continual compression by a piece of disc material. Even though the person may experience repetitive pain, the surgery probably isn't going to be that productive in the long run and, following the back pain management techniques delineated in this book is probably a superior plan.

There is good reason to believe that if one can keep the disc material centralized and prevent it from further impacting upon the nerve root, the body's healing process will fill in and scar down the area where the peripheral ligamentous structures were damaged and the granulomatous material that the body uses to fill in damaged spaces will additionally help prevent the disc from migrating to a position wherein it impacts upon the nerves.

In this event, operative diskectomy that does not remove the entire nucleus pulposus (as opposed to percutaneous needle diskectomy) would have been of no real, long-term benefit because, if anything, the process of taking out the disc material would only have made a larger opening in the ligamentous capsule of the disc unit which, over time and with continued flexion forces, would allow additional degenerating disc material to migrate out through the pathway created by a combination of the injury and the surgery.

However, if the imaging study shows continued compression that can't be helped by the techniques in this book and, the patient has neurological damage, there may be no genuine advantage to waiting. In this case, the nerve damage can be reduced or prevented by physically removing the putative piece of disc material. Here, the decision is not whether surgery is indicated, it is a matter of what type of surgery is best. I would favor percutaneous diskectomy; but if the disc material is so close to the nerve that the diskectomy needle might damage the nerve more in the process of trying to remove it, an open procedure might be the only alternative that makes sense.

There are several gradations of diskectomy which are arranged here in order of least to maximum trauma.

PERCUTANEOUS DISKECTOMY

Of all the available therapies for degenerative disc disease the most promising and least traumatic involves the use of a large needle-like device that enters the disc space and removes the painful disc material in a piecemeal fashion with a cutting device on the tip (or a laser which vaporizes the offending disc material) allowing it to be vacuumed out. This is called percutaneous diskectomy. One current and hopefully temporary drawback with this method is that there are too few competently trained and expertly experienced physicians who are capable of meeting the demand for the procedure. Consequently, a lot of patients who would be best served by this method approach the neurosurgeon contracted by their HMO and are convinced that an open procedure is necessary. Not being totally aware of the alternatives, they can be easily convinced that the open procedure is the only alternative because the HMO would otherwise have to pay a special neurosurgeon with whom they do not have an existing reduced fee contract.

Understandably a surgeon that has become competent and familiar with laminectomies and fusions is unlikely to abandon these procedures in favor of an alternative until forced by the marketplace. On the other hand, the "consumer" in pain has little opportunity or ability to truly evaluate the merits of a medical procedure and is only interested in relieving it. Pain and disability tend to make people dependent and trusting. That is not to say that one should decline to place trust in physicians, but if this alternative is not offered, then I would suggest that you ask if the procedure is "contraindicated" in your particular case. That will put the surgeon on notice that you know what you are talking about and, if his decision is legitimate, he will give a reasonable answer. If not, find out "*why not*?" with further exploration before going under the scalpel.

Some of the reasons why a percutaneous discectomy may not be appropriate are those cases wherein the disc material has pushed completely through the annulus fibrosus's capsule and/or the posterior longitudinal ligament and entered the spinal canal. In that case, it would be too dangerous to put a microtome into potential contact with the spinal cord or nerve roots. As long as the displaced disc material is shown (by imaging study such as NMRI, CT, Discogram, or Myelogram) to be definitely within the capsule and well away from the spinal nerve elements, this technique can be used, provided (of course) that *The O'Connor Technique (tm)* has failed

Although I clearly can't match my surgical credentials with those of the neurosurgeons and this book constitutes the only forum in which my opinion on how surgical procedures should be performed can, currently, be voiced, I would argue that the most lateral and anterior approach would serve patients best. Any procedure that compromises the integrity of the disc capsule should be performed such that it minimizes the future probability of disc material ultimately migrating through the surgically weakened capsule. During surgical manipulation, a pathway should not be created in the disc's capsule to allow pieces of disc material to travel outside of the disc space when future WEIGHT-BEARING FLEXION resumes.

In percutaneous diskectomy, disk material is removed through essentially a large bore needle. There is a reasonable probability that the nerve root decompression could be incomplete, more nucleus pulposus material could herniate in the future through the hole made, infection could occur, or facet joint damage could result. The success rate is highly dependent upon the expertise of the physician and by 1991 it was as high as 70% and as low as 50%.[3] In patients with classical herniated disc findings, its success rate is 85%.[4] It is described as an extremely safe technique, with over 20,000 of these procedures having been accomplished without a major nerve or vessel complication.[5] Advances in optics which allow for direct visualization of the intervertebral anatomy have recently improved upon these success rates.

The most recent advance employing a LASER to vaporize the disc material holds some greater promise once its use becomes more widespread. In this method, the same approach is used as in the microtome-facilitated diskectomy, but a laser removes the material by vaporization and suctioning. Even if all the herniated disc material cannot be removed, by removing a substantial portion of the disc, this method can create a larger cavity into which the most peripherally (furthest from the center) protruding nucleus pulposus can re-centralize and thus relieve pressure on the affected nerve root. It remains to be seen whether removing non-herniating disc material does not prematurely predispose the disc to degeneration and ultimately requiring a fusion later in life due to instability of the disc unit.

Not everyone is suited for this method, only about 15-20% of patients requiring back surgery qualify, and it is ideally suited for individuals who have a largely intact disk with only a small protrusion. Candidates for this procedure should meet the same criteria for standard diskectomy: 1) a positive imaging study evidencing Lumbar disc herniation, consistent with clinical findings, such as no significant pain relief following 6 months of conservative treatment, 2) significant unilateral leg pain greater than back pain, 3) demonstrated specific paresthetic complaints, 4) demonstrated indications from a physical examination, and 5) demonstration of neurologic findings indicating a herniated disc.[6]

It is contraindicated for those with broken off pieces of discs, previously operated on discs, failed chemonucleosis, spinal stenosis, or the elderly with chronic degenerative, bulging discs.

A recent advance in this method incorporates a fusion of the vertebral bones from within by injecting a slurry of bone into a disc space that has been largely evacuated of its contents while leaving the intervertebral capsular ligaments intact. The bony slurry later solidifies and transforms two vertebrae into a single solid structure. This "internal fusion" may prove to be an excellent procedure for those whose discs have severely degenerated and have become unstable due to spondlylolisthesis wherein one vertebral bone slides relative to an adjacent one.

MICRODISKECTOMY

Often, adequate decompression of the spinal cord or nerve root can be achieved by microdiskectomy. In this procedure, a hemilaminotomy (partial removal of the disc) is done through a tiny skin incision, and herniated disk material is removed with the aid of an operating microscope.

Microdiskectomy is basically the same procedure as a laminotomy, but an operating microscope with special small tools are used. With this method, the soft tissue damage and trauma of surgically approaching the herniated disc is significantly reduced, which also reduces the post-operative morbidity. It usually only requires one or two days in the hospital. The drawback of both this method and the laminectomy is that in order to remove the protruding disc material, the protective posterior ligamentous portion of the annulus fibrosus (the capsule) and posterior longitudinal ligaments usually must be surgically cut. In that case, there is a weakness created that can allow for future degenerated disc material to re-enter the spinal canal space through the surgically cut ligaments. For that reason, I would advocate these procedures only for those instances when the disc material has actually already herniated through the posterior ligamentous capsule, which can be determined when a discogram reveals the dye escaping through the torn capsule. If it hasn't, then a logically better approach might be to attempt a percutaneous diskectomy because that will better maintain the integrity of the capsule. It that fails, then an open approach might prove necessary, later; but, the trial with the percutaneous route stands a much greater probability of never requiring open surgery especially **if the PRINCIPLES in this book are adhered to post-surgically because *The O'Connor Technique (tm)* reduces the pressure and consequently the probability that disc material will put enough pressure on the posterior ligamentous structures to result in a herniation.**

LAMINECTOMY

One of the alternatives to diskectomy include laminectomy (or more properly termed a laminotomy) in which a portion of the vertebral bone directly posterior to the site of herniation called the lamina is removed. This allows direct visualization of the herniated disc material and facilitates its removal with grasping instruments. Sometimes this may be the best alternative, as in situations described above, wherein the herniated or sequestered disc material is too close to the spinal nerves to risk going in with a "blind" needle.

FUSION

The more disc material that is removed or the more surgery that is done increases the instability of the spine, often necessitating fusion surgery.

Fusion is the procedure whereby bone from other parts of the body (such as the pelvic bone) is harvested, and the spinal column has its discs cut out so that bone is touching bone. The posterior elements of the vertebral bones as well as the centers of the spinal vertebrae adjacent to the disc are cut into, then the bone grafts are placed between the vertebrae so that they grow together into a solid mass. This is probably the most traumatic surgical option. In an attempt to limit the severity of surgery, fusion is usually not done on the first surgical procedure (unless there is an existing spondylolisthesis or other anatomical exception); but remains as an option if diskectomy fails or repeated diskectomy results in instability.

This is the most drastic of therapeutic options for disc disease. **Considering the pain, the damage to associated ligaments, muscle trauma, prolonged discomfort of recovery, and potential for complications, it is not an option to be looked forward to as the next alternative. Fusion should not be considered a reasonable resort if you approach the other non-open surgical alternatives with a lackadaisical attitude that assumes you can ignore *The O'Connor Technique (tm)* principles of back protection and continue to abuse your discs by assuming**

that you can always have the fusion done, if worse comes to worse.

I would advise you not to rely on fusion as the final solution when "all" else fails and, by a careless spinal protection attitude, insure that all else does fail. Recent retrospective analysis of published series of back pain surgeries, with and without fusion, showed that **fusion offered no statistically improved benefit to the clinical outcome.**[7] In other words, just as many people were no better after this surgery as those who went through all the agony of having their back sliced open, their muscles torn, and bone chiseled with a hammer.

It is no small feat to direct a needle into a space deep within the body. Nor is it easy to perform an operation deep within the spine. I ask the reader not to interpret my assertions as failing to respect the skills of spinal or neuro-surgeons in general. **I have the utmost respect and frank awe of their skills and dedication to their patients.** The neurosurgeons I have had occasion to know work so hard and get unfairly sued so often, that I often wonder what could compel a person to subject themselves to such abuse. Sure, the money is good; but, in reality, they are probably underpaid when you take into consideration the sacrifices they undergo by choosing that career (This probably could apply to any physician, and does to most that I have had occasion to work with). I'm glad someone does it. My back would not have tolerated that laborious a career. Imagine bending over for hours upon hours without a break, night after night, day after day.

Those doctors deserve the utmost respect by their colleagues and the public in general; however, their decisions should not go without scrutiny, because they are human, too, and not all of them make decisions solely based upon what is best for the patient. Often, their needs and training impact upon their decision process. For instance, if a surgeon is up in his years, doesn't feel the need to acquire the skill of percutaneous diskectomy, and prefers to stick with the procedure he feels most comfortable with, he may be inclined to convince a patient to go with an open operative procedure when a percutaneous solution would have been better.

Given this scenario, it would require of him the largess to refer the patient to another neurosurgeon. If it just so happens that he hasn't been too "busy" (which in medical parlance means making money), he may be reluctant to offer that as an alternative. This is a consideration which the wise patient should be aware of, yet not assume to be the case unless definitive evidence exists to demonstrate it. If you suspect yourself being put in such a situation, it would behoove you to obtain a second opinion or a third opinion from a different neurosurgeon who does both procedures. It is unnecessary to be confrontational or accusatory, but in the same vein, do not assume a totally submissive role.

My intent is not to alienate neurosurgeons by this choice of words; however, if they are honest with their patients and themselves--they have nothing to be offended by because they are not of whom I make reference. Yet, they know, as well as I do, that there are some surgeons out there (the decided minority) that are motivated by something less than altruism.

Nevertheless, if, after you have devoted a legitimate and conscientious effort to rehabilitating and protecting your back, studied and practiced *The O'Connor Technique (tm)* on a daily basis, and you unfortunately are caused to resort to surgery, then you cannot be seen to have sold yourself short. Be aware, too, that often a surgeon's decision to operate or not depends upon the pressure put on the surgeon to operate. Patients who unrealistically believe that surgery is the answer, can influence a physician to decide in favor of surgery simply due to the patient's plaintive encouragement.

If you accidentally fall in flexion and your condition worsens, of course, no one can blame you; however, putting yourself in a position that would cause you to be in flexion when you fall can be seen as a failed opportunity to prevent future pain and problems. **If you are constantly conscious about the mechanisms of injury, you will judiciously avoid situations in which you put yourself at risk of a flexed fall that could result in a disc herniation.** If you fall while playing football, its not exactly an "accident" because, if you have a bad back, you shouldn't be engaging in a sport that has such a high probability of flexion falls.

An equivalent situation would be if one were to leave home without one's glasses and drive to the store. Not being able to read a one-way sign causes one to get into an "accident." Well, sure, it was an auto "accident," but by putting oneself knowledgeably into that circumstance, the person actually can be seen to have caused the "accident". Same with the bad back, if you carry packages up wet steps knowing that if you lose your balance you will be unable to grab the hand rail to prevent a backwards fall in flexion, you have just set yourself up for a prolonged period of pain. Sure, the fall was an "accident" in that you didn't plan it to happen, but you have pushed the probabilities that if something untoward did happen, the worse possible consequence for you would occur. It is better to think about these considerations in advance, and make several trips up and down the stairs so that you have a free hand to catch yourself in case you fall backwards. It may sound like an imposition, but if you ever have to experience the grinding agony of a surgical fusion procedure, looking back on whether you would have desired to sustain that inconvenience if you knew you could prevent it, I'm willing to bet you would choose the less traumatic option.

Finally, if you undergo a surgical procedure, you are at just as much risk of damaging the same disc unit as you were before surgery if you don't intentionally change the mechanical forces on your back. A diskectomy usually only removes the herniated volume or a portion thereof. There probably is loose disc material remaining, that with the same forces applied, will probably eventually migrate along the path the other material took on its exiting of the central area. This residual material has a good chance of returning you to the same pain you were in before the surgery. I believe that the above described mechanisms are the major cause of surgeries that do well in the immediate post operative period but, later, end up as long-term failures.

One concept that must be understood following surgery, a fusion or, for that matter, the prolonged wearing of a back brace to stabilize a painful segment of the spine, is that the damaging flexion forces that originally caused the affected discs to deteriorate will be communicated to the adjacent disc if you continue to commit the same flexion mistakes. If you persist in WEIGHT-BEARING FLEXION, put stresses on the disc level that had to be surgically or mechanically corrected, and you do not alter your motion behavior, you can expect the same herniations to happen again at either the repaired level (if it is not fused) or the level above or below the fusion. If for no other reason, knowledge of the operant mechanical forces and the protective measures elaborated in *The O'Connor Technique (tm)* is of value for any stage of disc disease or repair because it manages the problem on a minute-to-minute basis to prevent further damage from occurring. It is this ongoing damage that contributes to the surgical failure rates and, I believe, is largely preventable.

The point to remember is that, even **if you have to resort to surgery, the basic mechanical problems are still lifelong and still have a profound effect up the surgically treated unit and other adjacent discs. Surgery does not alleviate that reality**. Surgery may temporarily end the pain, but it has a good chance of returning unless you actively work to prevent it. *The O'Connor Technique (tm)* is, in part, designed to eliminate that event or at least forestall the eventuality if it should exist as your ultimate predictable destiny.

1.   Spencer DL, Lumbar intervertebral disc surgery In: Bridwell KH, De Wald RI, eds. The Textbook of spinal surgery. Vol 2. Philadelphia, Lippincott, 1991:675-93.

2.   Vlok, GJ, Hendrix MR, The lumbar disc: evaluating the causes of pain. *Orthopedics*, 1991;14:419-25.

3.   Spencer DL, Lumbar intervertebral disc surgery In: Bridwell KH, De Wald RI, eds. The Textbook of Spinal Surgery. Vol 2. Philadelphia, Lippincott, 1991:675-93.

4.   Kambin P, Gellman H. Percutaneous lateral discectomy of the lumbar spine; a preliminary report. *Clin Orthop.* 1983;174:127-129.

5.   Mooney V, Percutaneous discectomy. *Spine, State of the Art Reviews.* 1989;3:103-112.

6.   Overmyer R, Herniated disk: New laser therapy is more efficient and rapid than standard technique, *Modern Medicine*, June 1990;58:32-34.

7.   Turner JA, Ersek MN, Herron L, et al., Patient outcomes after lumbar spinal fusions. *The Journal of the American Medical Association*, 1992;268:907-11.